Early Detection and Intervention in Audiology

An African Perspective

Early Detection and Intervention in Audiology

An African Perspective

Edited by **Katijah Khoza-Shangase and Amisha Kanji**

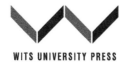

WITS UNIVERSITY PRESS

Published in South Africa by:
Wits University Press
1 Jan Smuts Avenue
Johannesburg 2001
www.witspress.co.za

Compilation © Editors 2021
Chapters © Individual contributors 2021
Published edition © Wits University Press 2021
Images and figures © Copyright holders

First published 2021

http://dx.doi.org.10.18772/22021026567

978-1-77614-656-7 (Paperback)
978-1-77614-661-1 (Hardback)
978-1-77614-657-4 (Web PDF)
978-1-77614-658-1 (EPUB)
978-1-77614-660-4 (Open Access PDF)

Project manager: Catherine Damerell
Copy editor: Lee Smith
Proofreader: Tessa Botha
Indexer: Sanet le Roux
Cover design: Hothouse
Typeset in 9 point Stone Serif Std

Contents

List of illustrations   vii
Abbreviations and acronyms   viii
Acknowledgements   x

Section One: Early Detection of Hearing Impairment

1   A Paradigm Shift in Early Hearing Detection and Intervention in South Africa   3
Amisha Kanji and Katijah Khoza-Shangase

2   Exploring Early Detection of Hearing Impairment in Sub-Saharan Africa   15
Amisha Kanji

3   Approaches to Early Detection of Hearing Impairment in Low and Middle-Income Countries   33
Amisha Kanji

4   Implementing Early Hearing Detection in the South African Health Care Context   42
Luisa Petrocchi-Bartal, Katijah Khoza-Shangase and Amisha Kanji

5   Confronting Realities to Early Hearing Detection in South Africa   66
Katijah Khoza-Shangase

6   Contextualisation of Risk Factors for Hearing Impairment   89
Jane Fitzgibbons, Rachael Beswick and Carlie J. Driscoll

Section Two: Early Intervention for Hearing Impairment

7   Approaches to Early Intervention for Hearing Impairment   117
Amisha Kanji and Aisha Casoojee

8   Models of Care in Early Intervention for Children with Hearing Impairment   137
Amisha Kanji

9   Continuity of Care at School for the Hearing-Impaired Child   155
Katijah Khoza-Shangase

Section Three: Complexities of Early Hearing Detection and Intervention

10 Sensory Impairments in Early Hearing Detection and Intervention   177
Nomfundo F. Moroe

11 Family-Centred Early Hearing Detection and Intervention   196
Ntsako Precious Maluleke, Rudo Chiwutsi and Katijah Khoza-Shangase

12 HIV/AIDS and the Burden of Disease in Early Hearing Detection and Intervention   219
Katijah Khoza-Shangase

13 Ethical Considerations and Tele-Audiology in Early Hearing Detection and Intervention   243
Alida Naudé and Juan Bornman

14 Best Practice in South Africa for Early Hearing Detection and Intervention   264
Katijah Khoza-Shangase and Amisha Kanji

Contributors   279

Index   283

List of illustrations

Tables

Table 2.1   Summary of findings from studies related to early hearing detection in South Africa   25

Table 3.1   Factors to consider when weighing up the approach to NHS   38

Table 4.1   Audiology services at all levels of health care in South Africa   46

Table 4.2   Practicability and efficiency of NHS in various South African health care contexts   50

Table 4.3   Assets facilitating the efficiency of hearing screening at PHC immunisation clinics   56

Table 4.4   Barriers influencing the practicability of hearing screening at PHC immunisation clinics   56

Table 5.1   SLH professionals registered with the HPCSA in January 2020 by province   70

Table 12.1   Overview of otological and audiological manifestations in paediatric HIV/AIDS   225

Figures

Figure 5.1   SLH professionals registered with the HPCSA nationally, January 2020   70

Figure 8.1   The influence of factors and their interaction on children with hearing impairment   148

Figure 12.1   Audiological presentation in the general HIV/AIDS paediatric population   233

Figure 13.1   General and specific ethical guidelines and rules for tele-audiology   248

Figure 13.2   Checklist for ethical decision-making in tele-audiology service delivery   252

Figure 13.3   Example of informed consent documentation related to telemedicine practice   256

Figure 14.1   Quadruple influence on risk   272

Abbreviations and acronyms

AAA	American Academy of Audiology
AABR	Automated Auditory Brainstem Response
ABR	Auditory Brainstem Response
ANSD	Auditory Neuropathy Spectrum Disorder
ART	Antiretroviral Treatment
ARV	Antiretroviral
ASD	Autism Spectrum Disorder
ASHA	American Speech-Language-Hearing Association
ASSR	Auditory Steady State Response
AVT	Auditory Verbal Therapy
BMI	Body Mass Index
cCMV	Congenital Cytomegalovirus
CHC	Community Health Care Centre/Clinic
CHW	Community Health Worker
CMV	Cytomegalovirus
CRPD	Convention on the Rights of Persons with Disabilities
CSTL	Care and Support for Teaching and Learning
DBE	Department of Basic Education
dBHL	Decibels Hearing Level
DCST	District-Based Clinical Specialist Team
DoH	Department of Health
DPOAE	Distortion Product Otoacoustic Emission
DPSA	Department of Public Service and Administration
EAR	Effectiveness of Auditory Rehabilitation
ECD	Early Childhood Development
ECI	Early Childhood Intervention
EHDI	Early Hearing Detection and Intervention
EI	Early Intervention
ENT	Ear, Nose and Throat
FCEI	Family-Centred Early Intervention
FDC	Fixed-Dose Combination
HAART	Highly Active Antiretroviral Therapy
HEU	HIV-exposed uninfected
HI HOPES	Home intervention: Hearing and language opportunities parent education services
HIV/AIDS	Human Immunodeficiency Virus/Acquired Immune Deficiency Syndrome
HPCSA	Health Professions Council of South Africa
HSV	Herpes Simplex Virus
HTA	Health Technology Assessment
HUU	HIV-unexposed and uninfected

ICT	Information and Communication Technologies
ILO	International Labour Organization
JCIH	Joint Committee on Infant Hearing
LAMI	Low and Middle Income
LOCHI	Longitudinal Outcomes of Children with Hearing Impairment
LSL	Listening and Spoken Language
LSLSA	Listening and Spoken Language South Africa
MDG	Millennium Development Goal
MOU	Midwife Obstetric Unit
NCD	Non-Communicable Disease
NHI	National Health Insurance
NHS	Newborn Hearing Screening
NICU	Neonatal Intensive Care Unit
NID	National Institute for the Deaf
NIH	National Institutes of Health
OAE	Otoacoustic Emissions
PCHL	Permanent Childhood Hearing Loss
PHC	Primary Health Care
PHIV	Perinatally HIV-Infected
PREM	Patient-Reported Experience Measure
PROM	Patient-Reported Outcome Measure
SAAA	South African Association of Audiology
SASL	South African Sign Language
SASLHA	South African Speech-Language-Hearing Association
SDG	Sustainable Development Goal
SLH	Speech-Language and Hearing
SWOT	Strengths, Weaknesses, Opportunities, and Threats
TB	Tuberculosis
TEOAE	Transient Evoked Otoacoustic Emission
TNHS	Targeted Newborn Hearing Screening
TOWS	Threats, Opportunities, Weaknesses, and Strengths
UHC	Universal Health Coverage
UNAIDS	United Nations Programme on HIV/AIDS
UNHS	Universal Newborn Hearing Screening
UNICEF	United Nations International Children's Emergency Fund
VLBW	Very Low Birth Weight
WHO	World Health Organization

Acknowledgements

We would like to acknowledge the chapter authors for their significant contributions to this book. We wish to also acknowledge our precious families for their unending and unconditional support during the journey of putting this book together. We are also greatly indebted to the following scholars and academics who generously agreed to serve as reviewers for chapters, contributing significantly to the quality assurance of this valuable output: Dr S. Moodley (Centre for Deafness Studies, University of the Witwatersrand [Wits]); L. Petrocchi-Bartal (Wits); Dr J. Fitzgibbons (Healthy Hearing, Queensland Health); Dr R. Beswick (Healthy Hearing, Queensland Health); Prof. C. Driscoll (The University of Queensland, School of Health and Rehabilitation Sciences); A. Casoojee (Wits); Dr N. Moroe (Wits); N. P. Maluleke (Sefako Makgatho Health Sciences University); R. Chiwutsi (Wits); Dr A. Naude (University of Pretoria); Prof. J. Bornman (University of Pretoria); N. B. Khan (University of KwaZulu-Natal); S. N. Adams (Wits); K. Masuku (Wits); Dr K. Coutts (Wits); T. Cloete (University of Cape Town); Dr S. Besharati (Wits); Dr L. Joseph (University of KwaZulu-Natal).

This publication was made possible through a grant received from the National Institute for the Humanities and Social Sciences (NIHSS).

Section One

Early Detection
of Hearing Impairment

1 A Paradigm Shift in Early Hearing Detection and Intervention in South Africa

Amisha Kanji and Katijah Khoza-Shangase

Early hearing detection and intervention (EHDI) has been extensively researched internationally, with a significant focus on the efficacy of implementing early identification through universal newborn hearing screening (UNHS) programmes (Kanji, 2016). However, most of this research has been conducted in high-income countries, and is not easily generalisable to low and middle-income (LAMI) contexts such as Africa, which differ in terms of populations, resources (human, equipment), health priorities, the burden of disease, as well as the neonatal protocols adopted. These differences require African countries to carefully consider context in EHDI programme implementation in order to ensure best practice that is contextually relevant and responsive. We thus call for a paradigm shift in EHDI initiatives within the African context. This chapter offers an introduction to such initiatives in South Africa, detailing the rationale for their value and relevance in this context. We outline approaches to EHDI, factors that influence its implementation, the positioning of these factors in the various levels of service delivery in the South African health care context, as well as continuity of care of the hearing impaired within the educational setting. Also addressed are the complexities surrounding EHDI implementation in South Africa, including EHDI in the context of other sensory impairments, in the context of the family, in the context of HIV/AIDS and in the context of tele-audiology. The goal is to recommend a paradigm shift for best/next practice for children at risk of, or with confirmed hearing impairment.

EHDI encompasses the earliest possible identification, diagnosis and provision of intervention for newborns and infants with hearing impairment in order to enable them to develop to their maximum potential and communicate effectively. This approach supports their individual needs as well as their later involvement in society and the country's economy (Health Professions Council of South Africa [HPCSA], 2007). The implementation of EHDI has been clearly associated with positive developmental outcomes, including communication (Fulcher, Purcell, Baker, & Munro, 2012; Kennedy et al., 2006; Sininger, Grimes, & Christensen, 2010). These outcomes have been specifically recorded in high-income countries where EHDI programmes, particularly early identification programmes, are well established.

EHDI arguably falls within the broader focus area of early childhood intervention (ECI), particularly as ECI programmes encompass a range of specialised services extending from service planning, rehabilitation and family-centred support to special education. Previous definitions of early intervention (EI) define ECI as the early identification and management of children from birth to three years of age (Rossetti, 2001). However, this definition has evolved, with the Consultative Group on Early Childhood Care and Development (2012) specifying early childhood as the period from prenatal development to eight years of age. The South African National Integrated Early Childhood Development Policy refers to the provision of early childhood development (ECD) services, and defines this period from conception until the year before children enter formal schooling. In the case of children with developmental difficulties and disabilities, this period is defined as the year before the calendar year they turn seven, as this is the age of enrolment in compulsory schooling or special education (Republic of South Africa, 2015). To position this book within the African context, the definition we adopt falls within the ECI programmatic outlook, and stretches to the elementary, basic education age.

EHDI remains a significant need for Africa, given the global prevalence and incidence of childhood hearing impairment. Recent estimates indicate that globally, 34 million (7 percent) of the 466 million individuals with disabling hearing impairment are children, of whom 7.5 million are below five years of age (Neumann, Chadha, Tavartkiladze, Bu, & White, 2019). Within these global estimates, prevalence rates have been reported to be higher in LAMI countries, specifically in South Asia, sub-Saharan Africa and the Asia Pacific regions. LAMI countries comprise 80 percent of the world's population, and are home to two-thirds of individuals with hearing impairment (Tucci, Merson, & Wilson, 2010). These prevalence and incidence rates are further exacerbated by the health care realities in LAMI countries, such as the burden of disease and poor social determinants of health, which place individuals at greater risk for hearing impairment.

The health care systems, as well as linguistic, cultural and socio-economic diversity in the sub-Saharan African context, present a unique setting for knowledge generation in terms of research, as well as academic and clinical teaching and practice in this field. Published evidence has acknowledged the impracticalities of attempting to implement developed world models for EHDI in LAMI countries such as South Africa (Moodley & Störbeck, 2015; Swanepoel, Delport, & Swart, 2004; Swanepoel, Hugo, & Louw, 2005). While research findings from high-income countries may be of value, it is vital to acknowledge that outcome-based recommendations from these studies may be costly and more difficult to implement in practice in LAMI countries. This is due to a number of reasons, including contextual differences, disease definition and response, as well as a different focus on disease prevalence. The sole reliance on evidence from international contexts may result in the specific, local needs of LAMI countries being neglected (Chetwood, Ladep, & Taylor-Robinson, 2015), leading to inappropriate and inefficient interventions and impacting negatively on the health outcomes of these populations. This highlights the need for a paradigm shift in EHDI in (South) Africa to a more contextually relevant and responsive approach driven by research that is sensitive to context while being internationally comparable.

Various initiatives are in place to address the gap in transferring theory into practice in the area of EHDI. The South African government's heightened focus on increasing access to health care through the re-engineered primary health care (PHC) model, and the efforts to achieve universal health coverage through National Health Insurance (NHI) as well as ECD programmes, make this an opportune time for establishing and documenting evidence-based research for clinicians, researchers and students. The existing body of literature in the field is almost entirely from the global North. This book therefore aims to provide evidence-based and contextually responsive information on EHDI from the global South, covering both detection and intervention aspects of hearing impairment. The information provided extends beyond the strictly defined age period of seven years. EHDI implications and possibilities are explored in the educational setting as part of the continuity of care for hearing-impaired children.

The book has deliberately adopted an African rather than a South African perspective, for several reasons. Firstly, the contextual realities under which health care delivery occurs are similar across the African continent. These include:

- resource constraints
- reliance on international aid and guidelines for some health care initiatives
- inadequate human resources across sub-Saharan African health systems, resulting in the use of task shifting in attempts to increase access (Maphumulo & Bhengu, 2019)
- negative impact on health care systems of the high burden of diseases such as HIV/AIDS and tuberculosis (Naidoo, 2012)
- challenges in terms of the social determinants of health.

Secondly, borders across Africa are porous. Migration due to socio-political and economic reasons is common and impacts health care planning, implementation and monitoring. Thirdly, the influences of linguistic and cultural diversity on seeking and delivering health care are arguably similar across the

African continent in terms of cultural beliefs and how illness is understood, as well as linguistic differences between patients, nurses and doctors.

This book is divided into three sections. The first two sections focus on the early detection of hearing impairment and EI, respectively. The third section considers factors that are significant to the South African context and how they influence EHDI, including family influences, the burden of disease, co-morbid conditions and ethical considerations.

EHDI is the gold standard for practising audiologists and the families of infants and children with hearing impairment. According to international guidelines, EHDI programmes aim to identify hearing impairment within one month of birth, diagnose by three months, and provide intervention to children with hearing impairment (as well as those at risk of hearing impairment) by six months of age to ensure that they develop and achieve in line with their hearing peers (Joint Committee on Infant Hearing [JCIH], 2007). Context-specific adjustments to these timelines have been made for South Africa: completion of hearing screening by six weeks of age, diagnosis by four months of age and commencement of intervention by eight months of age (HPCSA, 2018). These adjustments have taken the various South African screening platforms into account as well as other contextual factors such as home births, discharge timeframes and scheduled immunisation visits at the PHC level. The health care system in South Africa consists of both public and private health care. The public system is multi-tiered with primary, secondary and tertiary contexts offering different levels of care and service delivery. The feasibility of implementing EHDI programmes requires further deliberation in South Africa due to the country's unique health care context, as well as future plans for NHI and the re-engineering of PHC. The practicability and efficiency of newborn hearing screening (NHS) is discussed in chapter 4 of this book to ascertain feasibility within each level of service delivery. The chapter illustrates factors that may positively contribute to or impede early identification services, with clear recommendations for the South African context.

While international guidelines have been successfully achieved in studies from high-income countries (Ching, Dillon, Leigh, & Cupples, 2018; Fulcher et al., 2012; Fulcher, Purcell, Baker, & Munro, 2015), this is not so in sub-Saharan Africa. A retrospective review of the audiological management of children with hearing impairment, conducted at three public sector hospitals in South Africa's Gauteng province, found that the average age of diagnosis of hearing impairment is 23.65 months. Enrolment into an EI programme occurs at an average age of two years and five months (Khoza-Shangase & Michal, 2014). Similar findings were reported in the Western Cape and Free State provinces by Van der Spuy and Pottas (2008) and Butler et al. (2013). Delays in meeting the stipulated EHDI timeframes have been attributed to administrative challenges (such as procurement delays), lack of human resources, the busy schedules of speech-language therapists and audiologists in the public health care sector, and a lack of NHS services (Khoza-Shangase, Barratt, & Jonosky, 2010; Khoza-Shangase & Michal, 2014).

Early detection of hearing impairment

With regard to NHS services, significant focus has been placed on UNHS as the screening approach for early identification. While this approach is commonly practised in high-income countries, with well-established, standardised programmes and dedicated screeners outside of the profession of speech-language pathology and audiology, this is not the case for sub-Saharan Africa. Chapter 2 of this book explores the status of early identification services in sub-Saharan Africa, and highlights the status of these services in South Africa against the backdrop of the broader health care challenges and priorities in the country. The establishment of NHS services in higher-income countries has allowed for a shift in focus from hearing screening to diagnostic follow-up and intervention. However, South Africa and other countries in sub-Saharan Africa still appear to be at the infancy stages of implementing NHS programmes for early identification of hearing impairment. While the HPCSA guidelines are aimed at implementing UNHS, the benchmark for early identification, they are not necessarily currently applicable in all health care sectors in South Africa (HPCSA, 2018). Furthermore, they might not be adopted by other countries in the broader sub-Saharan African context. In fact, research from these contexts consistently indicates their state of unpreparedness to implement UNHS.

Early detection of hearing impairment continues to be a challenge throughout sub-Saharan Africa, for various reasons: the health care context; the focus on other, life-threatening health care priorities that are aimed at saving lives; and the challenges with social determinants of health. It is vital to understand the current status of early identification services, and the factors influencing their implementation in order to monitor progress and suggest realistic ways forward. Chapter 2 explores early detection services in sub-Saharan Africa with reference to health and health care and the availability of audiology and otolaryngology services, which are vital for implementing NHS programmes.

Despite UNHS being the gold standard that audiologists should strive to achieve, this approach to screening may not be feasible for some LAMI countries, where contextual challenges to implementation exist. These include a shortage of personnel and equipment, as well as associated costs. Chapter 5 explores the implementation of EHDI in South Africa. The author offers suggestions for EHDI service provision in this context, including the implementation of targeted NHS (TNHS) as an intermediate national approach.

Kanji (2018) asserts that all programmes need to have a starting point and go through their infancy stages and that doing something is better than doing nothing at all, particularly in contexts plagued by a lack of sufficient resources. NHS of high-risk neonates or infants through TNHS or risk-based programmes is a possible interim approach in such contexts. Chapter 3 discusses the feasibility of UNHS and TNHS as early identification methods in South Africa.

Should TNHS be the choice of approach, careful deliberation of the risk registry is required to assist in identifying children who need audiological screening and assessment. This is important in order to identify those requiring audiological or medical surveillance and to address the preventable risks associated with hearing impairment (JCIH, 2000; Kanji & Khoza-Shangase, 2018; Núñez-Batalla, Trinidad-Ramos, Sequí-Canet, De Aguilar, & Jáudenes-Casaubón, 2012; Olusanya, 2009). While risk registries in high-income countries are mainly used to identify children at risk for postnatal hearing loss and those in need of audiological monitoring and surveillance, they are useful tools in countries such as South Africa where a universal platform for NHS has not been established. The current high-risk registries have been compiled and revised by the Joint Committee on Infant Hearing (JCIH), based on evidence from developed world contexts (JCIH, 1982, 2000, 2007). The HPCSA has adapted these for the South African context (HPCSA, 2018). However, findings from international studies as well as some South African studies have indicated the need to continuously re-evaluate both the JCIH and the HPCSA risk registries and tailor them to the context (Beswick, Driscoll, & Kei, 2012; Beswick, Driscoll, Kei, Khan, & Glennon, 2013; Kanji & Khoza-Shangase, 2012). Chapter 6 reviews the key risk factors for hearing impairment used globally and evaluates their relevance to the South African context.

'Considering the realities of the South African healthcare context, and given that EHDI is vital for newborns and infants with hearing loss, we need to seriously consider how NHS services may be adapted to better meet these realities' (Kanji, 2018, p. 2). Following identification and diagnosis of hearing impairment, EI services need to be similarly evaluated and adapted to the realities of access to and availability of such services, as well as to the unique challenges that present within each of the relevant service delivery contexts.

Early intervention for hearing impairment

Diagnosed hearing impairment without adequate intervention may have long-term consequences for the affected individual. Besides affecting communication abilities, it can influence vocational performance and result in isolation and stigmatisation (Yoshinaga-Itano, 2004). Specific international principles and goals for EI for hearing impairment guide service provision. These principles and goals are discussed in chapters 7 and 11, which deal with approaches to EI and family-centred EHDI, respectively.

EI services are particularly important in children who are considered at risk for developmental delay. It is well documented that a lack of intervention may have negative consequences for development, school readiness, educational outcomes and vocational opportunities (World Health Organization [WHO], 2012; Yoshinaga-Itano, 2004). EI services may be provided at different sites or levels of service delivery, including health care clinics, hospitals, EI centres, rehabilitation centres, community centres, homes and schools (WHO, 2012). Exploring models of care in the various levels of service delivery in South Africa is important to ensure efficacious intervention that is contextually responsive and responsible. Chapter 8 looks at how specific communicative therapy approaches can be delivered to children with hearing impairment and their families. It considers contextual factors such as patient-to-professional ratios, as well as cultural and linguistic diversity issues that may influence these options and patient outcomes.

EI for hearing impairment is a multi-staged process that commences with the provision, fitting and adjustment of amplification devices followed by early communication intervention (McPherson, 2014; Peer, 2015). Most high-income countries have been able to access hearing health care through private and publicly funded aural (re)habilitation systems. However, many LAMI countries have not had these same opportunities for access despite the higher prevalence of childhood hearing impairment (McPherson, 2014; Stevens et al., 2011). The challenges to implementation are further influenced by the availability of and access to EI services. Chapter 7 highlights these challenges and discusses contextual considerations in terms of the cultural and linguistic diversity in South Africa. The chapter also explores various modes of communication and communicative therapy approaches to EI, and addresses the value and implementation of auditory verbal therapy in the South African context.

Ensuring continuity of care is important in the multifaceted process of EHDI, and requires the involvement of various stakeholders from different government sectors such as health, social development and education. Access to education is a key priority of the South African government. However, this access does not always practically translate into inclusivity in the educational sector for children with hearing impairment. Access has therefore not necessarily transformed into success in the educational setting for these learners. Addressing hearing impairment as a barrier to learning is vital to facilitate success, and to ensure maximal benefits from EHDI implementation. While chapter 7 highlights educational access for children with hearing impairment in sub-Saharan Africa, chapter 9 discusses EI in the South African basic education setting. It offers recommendations for inclusive education and explores telehealth in the form of tele-audiology as well as task shifting to facilitate this process.

Complexities of early hearing detection and intervention

To ensure contextually responsive practice in South Africa, clinicians and other stakeholders working in the EHDI field need to consider various complexities, including: EHDI in the context of other sensory impairments; EHDI in the context of family; EHDI in the context of HIV/AIDS; and ethical considerations for EHDI in the context of tele-audiology.

While the focus on hearing impairment and its influence on developmental outcomes, education and vocational attainment is vital, it is also important to recognise the possibility of additional sensory impairments in children with hearing deficits to ensure effective holistic assessment and management. Current studies have focused on the EHDI outcomes of children with hearing impairment only, with little to no consideration of any co-morbid conditions. This is a disservice to this cohort within a minority grouping of children. Chapter 10 explores this complexity, with a specific focus on deafblindness, and highlights the need for consideration of other co-morbid sensory impairments in the EHDI framework.

The primary member in an EI team is the family. Hence, EI programmes need to be responsive to the needs of the families of children with hearing impairment (HPCSA, 2018). The HPCSA guidelines specify that EI services following diagnosis of hearing impairment must be family-centred and tailored to cultural differences. The definitions, dynamics and compositions of families in an African context need to be considered, including their impact on health-seeking and intervention-adherence behaviours. Chapter 11 discusses family-centred EHDI in South Africa, with recognition of the cultural and linguistic aspects of a family. The chapter notes the complexities in defining family structures and functions in an African context, highlighting the influence of culture, migration and the burden of HIV/AIDS on families and thus on intervention outcomes.

Various reasons have been offered for the failure to successfully implement EHDI in South Africa. One of the most common reasons is linked to the burden of disease, specifically the HIV/AIDS pandemic. Besides the budgetary and resource burden linked to HIV/AIDS, this pandemic also results in auditory and otologic manifestations in those affected. Chapter 12 explores EHDI in the context of HIV/AIDS and highlights the implications for EHDI in this segment of the population.

Other common barriers to successful EHDI implementation include access to services and human resource shortages. These barriers have resulted in consideration of alternative models of service delivery, such as tele-audiology, to increase reach and access in resource-constrained environments. However, the core ethical aspects related to tele-audiology need to be taken into account, particularly given the lack of national regulations and guidelines. Chapter 13 looks at ethical and legal aspects and strategies to implement risk management and programme validation in the South African context.

Conclusion

International guidelines and research findings related to EHDI may not be easily transferable to clinical practice in Africa due to significant differences in context. This book is a research-driven intervention into the EHDI space and is aimed at providing current, contextually relevant and responsive evidence related to EHDI in LAMI countries, with a specific focus on the African context and South Africa in particular. The book covers all aspects of EHDI, with careful consideration of the complexities and challenges to implementation in South Africa. However, the findings may be applicable to other LAMI country contexts. After carefully engaging with local evidence, local context and local policies, the book offers possible solutions and recommendations for the challenges identified.

References

Beswick, R., Driscoll, C., & Kei, J. (2012). Monitoring for postnatal hearing loss using risk factors: A systematic literature review. *Ear and Hearing, 33*(6), 747–756.

Beswick, R., Driscoll, C., Kei, J., Khan, A., & Glennon, S. (2013). Which risk factors predict postnatal hearing loss in children? *Journal of the American Academy of Audiology, 24*(3), 205–213.

Butler, I., Basson, A., Britz, E., De Wet, R., Korsten, G. B., & Joubert, G. (2013). Age of diagnosis for congenital hearing loss at Universitas Hospital, Bloemfontein. *South African Medical Journal, 103*(7), 474–475.

Chetwood, J. D., Ladep, N. G., & Taylor-Robinson, S. D. (2015). Research partnerships between high and low-income countries: Are international partnerships always a good thing? *BMC Medical Ethics, 16*, 36–40.

Ching, T., Dillon, H., Leigh, G., & Cupples, L. (2018). Learning from the longitudinal outcomes of children with hearing impairment (LOCHI) study: Summary of 5-year findings and implications. *International Journal of Audiology, 57*(Suppl. 2), S105–S111.

Consultative Group on Early Childhood Care and Development. (2012). Placing early childhood on the global agenda: Positioning early childhood development in the post-2015 development framework. Retrieved from http://www.ecdgroup.com/pdfs/Positioning_ECD_on_the_Post_2015_Devt_Agenda_CG_Background_Paper_August%202012.pdf.

Fulcher, A., Purcell, A. A., Baker, E., & Munro, N. (2012). Listen up: Children with early identified hearing loss achieve age-appropriate speech/language outcomes by 3 years-of-age. *International Journal of Pediatric Otorhinolaryngology, 76,* 1785–1794.

Fulcher, A., Purcell, A. A., Baker, E., & Munro, N. (2015). Factors influencing speech and language outcomes of children with early identified severe/profound hearing loss: Clinician-identified facilitators and barriers. *International Journal of Speech-Language Pathology, 17*(3), 325–333.

Health Professions Council of South Africa (HPCSA). (2007). Early hearing detection and intervention programmes in South Africa, position statement year 2007. Retrieved from http://www.hpsca.co.za/hpcsa/default.aspx?id=137.

Health Professions Council of South Africa (HPCSA). (2018). Early hearing detection and intervention (EHDI) guidelines. Retrieved from http://www.hpcsa.co.za/Uploads/editor/UserFiles/downloads/speech/Early_Hearing_Detection_and_Intervention_(EHDI)_2018.pdf.

Joint Committee on Infant Hearing (JCIH). (1982). Position statement. Retrieved from http://www.jcih.org/JCIH1982.pdf.

Joint Committee on Infant Hearing (JCIH). (2000). Year 2000 position statement: Principles and guidelines for early hearing detection and intervention programs. *American Journal of Audiology, 9,* 9–29.

Joint Committee on Infant Hearing (JCIH). (2007). Year 2007 position statement: Principles and guidelines for early hearing detection and intervention programs. *Pediatrics, 120*(4), 898–921.

Kanji, A. (2016). Early hearing screening in South Africa – time to get real about context. *South African Journal of Child Health, 10*(4), 192.

Kanji, A. (2018). Early hearing detection and intervention: Reflections from the South African context. *South African Journal of Communication Disorders, 65*(1), 1–3.

Kanji, A., & Khoza-Shangase, K. (2012). The occurrence of high-risk factors for hearing loss in very low-birth-weight neonates: A retrospective exploratory study of targeted hearing screening. *South African Journal of Communication Disorders, 59,* 3–7.

Kanji, A., & Khoza-Shangase, K. (2018). In pursuit of successful hearing screening: An exploration of factors associated with follow-up return rate in a risk-based newborn hearing screening programme. *Iranian Journal of Pediatrics, 28*(4), 1–9.

Kennedy, C. R., McCann, D. C., Campbell, M. J., Law, C. M., Mullee, M., Petrou, S., . . . Stevenson, J. (2006). Language ability after early detection of permanent childhood hearing impairment. *New England Journal of Medicine, 354*(20), 2131–2141.

Khoza-Shangase, K., Barratt, J., & Jonosky, J. (2010). Protocols for early audiology intervention services: Views from early intervention practitioners in a developing country. *South African Journal of Child Health, 4*(4), 100–105.

Khoza-Shangase, K., & Michal, G. (2014). Early intervention in audiology: Exploring the current status from a developing country context. *British Journal of Medicine & Medical Research, 4*(11), 2238–2249.

Maphumulo, W. T., & Bhengu, B. R. (2019). Challenges of quality improvement in the healthcare of South Africa post-apartheid: A critical review. *Curationis, 42*(1), 1–9.

McPherson, B. (2014). Hearing assistive technologies in developing countries: Background, achievements and challenges. *Disability and Rehabilitation Assistive Technology, 9*(5), 360–364.

Moodley, S., & Störbeck, C. (2015). Narrative review of EHDI in South Africa. *South African Journal of Communication Disorders, 62*(1), 1–10.

Naidoo, S. (2012). The South African national health insurance: A revolution in healthcare delivery! *Journal of Public Health, 34*(1), 149–150. https://doi.org/10.1093/pubmed/fds008.

Neumann, K., Chadha, S., Tavartkiladze, G., Bu, X., & White, K. R. (2019). Newborn and infant hearing screening facing globally growing numbers of people suffering from disabling hearing loss. *International Journal of Neonatal Screening, 5*(7), 1–11.

Núñez-Batalla, F., Trinidad-Ramos, G., Sequí-Canet, J. M., De Aguilar, V. A., & Jáudenes-Casaubón, C. (2012). Risk factors for sensorineural hearing loss in children. *Acta Otorrinolaringológica Española, 63*(5), 382–390.

Olusanya, B. O. (2009). Newborns at risk of sensorineural hearing loss in low-income countries. *Archives of Disease in Childhood, 94*, 227–229.

Peer, S. (2015). Turning up the volume on hearing loss in South Africa. *South African Medical Journal, 105*(1), 31–32.

Republic of South Africa. (2015). National integrated early childhood development policy. Retrieved from https://unicef.org/southafrica/SAF_resources_integratedecd policy.pdf.

Rossetti, L. M. (2001). Communication intervention: Birth to three. In L. M. Rossetti (Ed.), *Populations at risk for communication delay* (2nd ed., pp. 1–45). San Diego, CA: Singular Thomson Learning.

Sininger, Y. S., Grimes, A., & Christensen, E. (2010). Auditory development in early amplified children: Factors influencing auditory-based communication outcomes in children with hearing loss. *Ear and Hearing, 31*(2), 166–185.

Stevens, G., Flaxman, S., Brunskil, E., Mascarenhas, M., Mathers, C. D., & Finucane, M. (2011). Global and regional hearing impairment prevalence: An analysis of 42 studies in 29 countries. *The European Journal of Public Health, 23*(11), 146–152.

Swanepoel, D., Delport, S. D., & Swart, J. G. (2004). Universal newborn hearing screening in South Africa - a first-world dream? *South African Medical Journal, 94*(8), 634–635.

Swanepoel, D., Hugo, R., & Louw, B. (2005). Infant hearing screening in the developing world. *Audiology Today, 17*(4), 16–19.

Tucci, D. L., Merson, M. H., & Wilson, B. S. (2010). A summary of literature in global hearing impairment: Current status and priorities for action. *Otology and Neurotology, 31*(1), 31–41.

Van der Spuy, T., & Pottas, L. (2008). Infant hearing loss in South Africa: Age of intervention and parental needs for support. *International Journal of Audiology, 47,* S30–S35.

World Health Organization (WHO). (2012). Early childhood development and disability: A discussion paper. Retrieved from http://apps.who.int/iris/bitstream/10665 /75355/1/9789241504065_eng.pdf?ua=1.

Yoshinaga-Itano, C. (2004). Levels of evidence: Universal newborn hearing screening (UNHS) and early hearing detection and intervention systems (EHDI). *Journal of Communication Disorders, 37,* 451–465.

2 Exploring Early Detection of Hearing Impairment in Sub-Saharan Africa

Amisha Kanji

Early detection of hearing impairment continues to be a challenge in the sub-Saharan African context, as well as in South Africa specifically. This challenge is due to a number of factors, including the health care context; other health care priorities that are the focus of the government; and a lack of resource allocation for successful, national implementation of newborn hearing screening (NHS). Another major challenge facing the region is linked to the social determinants of health.

This chapter explores early detection services in sub-Saharan Africa. It begins by describing the regional context, particularly health and health care and the availability of audiology and otolaryngology services, which are vital for the implementation of NHS programmes. The prevalence and incidence of hearing loss is presented, followed by a discussion of the principles for early detection of hearing impairment as defined by the Health Professions Council of South Africa's (HPCSA) early hearing detection and intervention (EHDI) guidelines. These guidelines are the only contextually relevant guidelines in the sub-Saharan context. Thereafter, a review of published evidence related to NHS in sub-Saharan Africa, and specifically South Africa, is presented. The chapter concludes with solutions and recommendations for early detection of hearing impairment in light of the challenges presented.

There are 49 countries in sub-Saharan Africa, of which seven are island states (Agyepong et al., 2018; Simkins, 2019). In 2017, the region had approximately 1.06 billion inhabitants (Statista, 2019). The population in sub-Saharan Africa continues to rise rapidly, and is expected to be the fastest-growing population of any of the world regions between 2015 and 2050 (Simkins, 2019). Given this context, access to equal and equitable health care remains a challenge (Chirwa, 2016).

Several factors contribute to inequality, inequity and poor-quality services in health care. Historically, access to health care has been a challenge for individuals of lower socio-economic status in sub-Saharan Africa. The reasons for this include: poor management of health care institutions; inadequate and insufficient health care personnel; physical and economic aspects related to access, especially when health care facilities are not located close to the population they serve; and financial constraints for patients who have to bear health care costs themselves (Olugbenga, 2017).

Health and health outcomes are not only affected by access to health care, but also by multiple, complex factors related to the social determinants of health (Ataguba, Day, & McIntyre, 2015). The social determinants of health are defined as the circumstances in which people are born, grow up, live, work and age, and the systems put in place to deal with illness (World Health Organization [WHO], 2017). Hence, the social determinants of health are influenced by social, political, economic, environmental and cultural factors, as well as those affecting human rights and gender equality (Ataguba et al., 2015). While these factors and the policies governing them do not directly impact health, they have a bearing on health and health equity (WHO, 2008). It is therefore vital to consider the impact of the social determinants of health when addressing health inequalities in specific countries or contexts. Scott, Schaay, Schneider, and Sanders (2017) propose an adapted conceptual framework for the determinants of health in South Africa. This framework describes biological and behavioural factors as having an immediate impact on health, socio-cultural factors as having an intermediate influence, and living and working conditions as well as structural factors (such as inadequate collaborative institutional and governance support and policies, resource distribution and inequity in political power) as having a distal or upstream influence. Khoza-Shangase discusses other contextual realities and challenges in the South African health care context in chapter 5. These need to be faced in order to contextualise EHDI in larger health care systems and against competing health care priorities.

Health priorities in sub-Saharan Africa

Health priorities and health performance have been monitored globally through the initial declaration of the Millennium Development Goals (MDGs) (Blumberg, Frean, & Moonasar, 2014). These eight goals, defined in 2000, are: 1) eradication of extreme poverty and hunger; 2) universal primary education; 3) gender equality; 4) reduction of child mortality; 5) improvement of maternal health; 6) combating HIV/AIDS, malaria and other diseases such as tuberculosis (TB); 7) ensuring environmental sustainability; and 8) developing a global partnership for development (Mayosi et al., 2012; WHO, 2015). Goals 4 to 6 are directly linked to health (Pillay & Barron, 2014).

Fifteen years later, the 2015 MDG report indicated that sub-Saharan Africa's performance in relation to the health goals was the poorest globally (United Nations, 2015). Maternal deaths were reported to be concentrated in sub-Saharan Africa and Southern Asia, which together accounted for 86 percent of such deaths globally in 2013. Similarly, sub-Saharan Africa was reported to be one of the two regions with the highest newborn mortality in the world. This is despite an overall reduction in the under-five mortality rate and a global increase in coverage of preventative care strategies such as measles vaccinations. Additionally, this region also accounts for a large proportion of individuals living with HIV and AIDS. East Africa and southern Africa are home to approximately 6.2 percent of the world's population and just over half of the total number of individuals living with HIV reside in these regions (Avert, 2019; UNAIDS, 2019). South Africa remains the epicentre of the pandemic, with 20 percent of all HIV-positive individuals and 4 500 newly infected individuals per week (Allinder & Fleischman, 2019).

The burden of disease in Africa has predominantly comprised acute and infectious diseases, such as malaria, TB and measles. However, over the last 25 years, both chronic communicable and non-communicable diseases such as HIV/AIDS, ischaemic heart disease, stroke and diabetes have become significant contributors to the burden of disease. This is coupled with weak health care systems as health expenditure, infrastructure and the number of skilled professionals relative to the population remain insufficient (Agyepong et al., 2018). South Africa faces a quadruple burden of disease: maternal, infant and child mortality; HIV/AIDS and TB; non-communicable diseases (NCDs); and injury and violence (Department of Health [DoH], 2011; Naidoo, 2012).

Despite some progress towards achieving the MDGs, major challenges persist in the MDG priority areas. These challenges need to be addressed if further progress is to be made in reducing maternal and child mortality, and in combating communicable diseases such as HIV/AIDS, TB and malaria (WHO, 2018). An expansion of focus on the global health agenda led to a shift from the MDGs to the development of 17 sustainable development goals (SDGs). These pay attention to a broader set of social determinants of health and are sensitive to equity, which could have a substantial effect on health (Scott et al., 2017). Goal 3 has a clear and detailed focus on health, with 10 other goals also concerned with health issues. More than 50 indicators have been agreed upon for the measurement of health outcomes, health provision and proximal determinants of health. These indicators are thematically grouped as follows (WHO, 2018):

- reproductive, maternal, newborn and child health
- infectious diseases
- NCDs and mental health
- injuries and violence
- universal health coverage and health systems
- environmental risks
- health risks and disease outbreaks.

The director-general of the WHO, Tedros Adhanom Ghebreyesus, emphasises that 'maintaining momentum towards the SDGs is only possible if countries have the political will and the capacity to prioritize regular, timely and reliable data collection to guide policy decisions and public health interventions' (WHO, 2018, p. v). Political will and commitment to the goal of universal health coverage should be expressed in legal mandates and translated into policies (Aregbeshola, 2017).

Health and health care in sub-Saharan Africa, where health spending is low, remain a global concern, and aid from the West has been increasingly targeted towards health (Deaton & Totora, 2015). Health spending by governments is generally the primary source of health funding globally. However, in sub-Saharan Africa, only about a third of health spending originates from government (Micah et al., 2019). A study examining government health spending and its determinants found variations in terms of spending across 46 countries in sub-Saharan Africa. Of these countries, South Africa has one of the highest levels of government health spending, thought to be associated with the high burden of HIV/AIDS in the country (Micah et al., 2019).

The growth in global health resources, in terms of government spending and development assistance for health, occurred during the same period as the MDGs (Micah et al., 2019). Since 2000, there has been an increase in foreign aid to low-income countries in order to facilitate their chances of meeting the MDGs (WHO, 2014). As of 2013, health expenditure made up between 20 and 69 percent of government spending in 26 of the least developed countries in sub-Saharan Africa (WHO, 2014). While there are debates regarding the effectiveness of foreign aid, findings from a study in Rwanda indicate positive associations with foreign aid and government spending in terms of service provision for maternal and child health, HIV, malaria and TB (Lu, Cook, & Desmond, 2017). The commitment to these aspects of the burden of disease and their link to the MDGs appear to have resulted in improved dedication and prioritisation of health from 2000 to 2015 (Micah et al., 2019). Within this framework of prioritising health, adequate human resources, such as health care workers, are needed for efficient health care service provision.

Health care and hearing health care services in sub-Saharan Africa

'Functioning health systems require a qualified health workforce that is available, equitably distributed and accessible by the population' (WHO, 2018, p. 8). Although the African continent has 25 percent of the global burden of disease, it has 3 percent of the world's health workers (Crisp, 2011). In many African countries, the primary health care (PHC) workforce has limited training, which results in primary care rarely being equipped to serve as a foundation for the health care system (Mash et al., 2018). However, countries such as Ghana, Botswana, Uganda, Kenya and Nigeria have established training programmes for family physicians, with Ethiopia and Malawi having implemented such training (Mash et al., 2018). In South Africa, family physicians are positioned at primary and district levels of health care. They require an extended range of procedural skills within a generalist environment, while providing support to the primary care platforms (Mash, Ogunbanjo, Naidoo, & Hellenberg, 2015).

Prevention and promotion are key aspects to service delivery in PHC platforms. Prevention and management of otolaryngology-related diseases require a team approach, with PHC delivered by professional nurses, clinical officers and general practitioners, and specialised care by ear, nose and throat (ENT) specialists, audiologists and other related specialities (Fagan, 2018).

Audiological and ENT services have been reported to be extremely poor in sub-Saharan Africa, with an inequitable distribution of services and limited training opportunities (Fagan & Jacobs, 2009). Hence, individuals requiring audiological and ENT services may not be able to effectively access them. Given the prevalence of hearing loss, this lack of availability of services raises concern for service provision. Furthermore, it risks leading to preventable auditory pathologies going undetected or untreated, which may result in hearing impairment, with a consequent negative impact on quality of life and economic productivity (Mulwafu, Ensink, Kuperd, & Fagan, 2017).

Mulwafu and colleagues (2017) report that there has been some improvement since 2009, with the establishment of six new ENT training programmes in sub-Saharan countries. Two new audiology and speech-therapy training programmes have been established in Ghana and Kenya, and new ENT training programmes in Rwanda, Zimbabwe and Ethiopia. In other countries, such as Malawi, Kenya, Mali, Togo and Cameroon, there has been little overall change in the number of qualifying ENT surgeons, audiologists and speech therapists per year (Mulwafu et al., 2017). In 2014, Zambia reportedly had five otolaryngologists and one audiologist in a population of 14 million (Mwamba, 2014).

A 2015 follow-up survey on services in sub-Saharan Africa indicated that in the 22 countries from which responses were obtained, there were a total of 847 ENT surgeons, 580 audiologists, 906 speech therapists and 264 ENT clinical officers (Mulwafu et al., 2017). When comparing these figures to those in 15 countries that participated in the 2009 survey (Fagan & Jacobs, 2009), results indicate an increase in the number of ENTs and audiologists. However, this increase needs to be viewed in relation to the overall increase in population size during this period, which may still reflect a significantly high patient-to-professional ratio, particularly in countries such as the Democratic Republic of Congo, Lesotho, Madagascar and Senegal (Mulwafu et al., 2017). Moreover, if data from South Africa,

Kenya and Sudan were to be excluded, the actual number of audiologists may be even lower (Mulwafu et al., 2017). This human resource disparity has serious implications for the implementation of EHDI in these regions, particularly if the prevalence and incidence of hearing impairment is on the rise, as estimated by the WHO.

Prevalence and incidence of hearing impairment

Globally, approximately 0.5 to 5 in every 1 000 neonates and infants present with congenital or early childhood onset hearing impairment that is severe to profound (WHO, 2010). More recent estimates indicate that 34 million of the 466 million individuals worldwide with disabling hearing loss are children, of whom 7.5 million are below five years of age (Neumann, Chadha, Tavartkiladze, Bu, & White, 2019). Within this global framework, prevalence rates have been reported to be higher in low and middle-income (LAMI) contexts, which are worst affected (Olusanya & Newton, 2007). These countries comprise 80 percent of the world's population, and are home to two-thirds of individuals with hearing impairment (Tucci, Merson, & Wilson, 2010). A review of population-based studies in 2011 estimated that 16 million children have a hearing impairment ≥35 decibel hearing level (Stevens et al., 2011). From this global estimate, prevalence rates were noted as being the highest in South Asia, sub-Saharan Africa and the Asia Pacific regions (Neumann et al., 2019; Stevens et al., 2011). Although these results are not specific to newborns and infants, prevalence rates in LAMI countries may be attributed to the higher prevalence of environmental risk factors for hearing impairment in these contexts (Olusanya & Newton, 2007). Such risk factors include infectious diseases; the use of ototoxic drugs; limited access to prenatal, perinatal and postnatal health care (Tucci et al., 2010); and pre- and postnatal infections such as rubella, measles and meningitis (Stevens et al., 2011). However, despite the estimated high incidence of hearing impairment in these countries, the causes have not been well documented.

The incidence of bilateral hearing impairment is estimated to be six or greater per 1 000 live births (Olusanya, Ruben, & Parving, 2006). This is in contrast to the lower incidence of bilateral, sensorineural hearing impairment, which is reported to be at a rate of two to four per 1 000 live births in high-income countries where NHS programmes are mostly well established (Tucci et al., 2010).

NHS pilot programmes in Nigeria have suggested a much higher prevalence of 28 per 1 000 live births. This rate is inclusive of all degrees of sensorineural hearing impairment and is thus by far the highest rate reported globally (Olusanya, 2011; WHO, 2010). In South Africa, it is estimated nationally that the prevalence of hearing impairment is four to six in every 1 000 live births in the public health care sector. This is approximately double the rate documented for the private health care sector, where a prevalence of three in every 1 000 has been estimated (Swanepoel & Störbeck, 2009). This higher estimated occurrence in the public health care sector highlights a greater need for audiological services in this sector in South Africa.

It is thus evident that prevalence rates differ within developing contexts and may be due to the differences in frequency of common risk factors for hearing impairment in each context, such as rubella, meningitis, measles and congenital cytomegalovirus. Risk factors like rubella, mumps and meningitis have become less common in some regions of the world, but have remained unchanged or increased in other regions (The Lancet, 2017). These differences in the incidence and prevalence of preventable conditions are probably due to a higher incidence of infections or diseases coupled with fewer maternal and child health programmes (Neumann et al., 2019). These risk factors highlight the importance of exploring preventative care and early detection of hearing impairment, which is key to facilitating the provision of timely diagnosis and intervention.

Preventative care in the context of EHDI

Preventative care comprises primary, secondary and tertiary prevention. Primary prevention refers to the elimination of exposure to certain conditions that may result in a specific health outcome. In the context of EHDI, primary prevention of newborn or infant hearing impairment can be achieved through addressing maternal exposure to environmental factors and other diseases or health conditions that may increase the risk of the unborn child developing a hearing impairment (Alvarez, 2008).

Secondary prevention refers to the use of measures that may lead to earlier diagnosis and treatment of conditions. In the context of EHDI, these initiatives may include early identification of hearing impairment through the provision of NHS prior to hospital discharge (Alvarez, 2008). Tertiary prevention refers to strategies that decrease the difficulties associated with disability. In terms of EHDI, this may relate to early intervention services (such as fitting of amplification, aural habilitation and culturally and linguistically appropriate communication interventions) that are provided to newborns and infants with confirmed hearing impairment, as well as intervention services for their families (Alvarez, 2008).

For EHDI programmes to yield positive outcomes, it is important that all three levels of prevention, particularly primary and secondary, are carefully considered and incorporated within the principles of early detection of hearing impairment.

Principles for early detection of hearing impairment

EHDI programmes are aimed at identifying and diagnosing hearing impairment in newborns and infants as soon as possible, as well as providing timely intervention to these individuals in order for them to reach their maximum potential (Joint Committee on Infant Hearing [JCIH], 2007). This objective is guided by a number of principles first outlined by the JCIH in 2000. In the sub-Saharan context, South Africa has taken the lead, with the HPCSA's Professional Board for Speech, Language and Hearing Professions developing and publishing a set of guidelines that clearly highlight the principles for early detection of hearing impairment (HPCSA, 2018). Of the six EHDI principles, five are specifically related to early identification of hearing impairment:

- Principle 1: All infants are afforded access to hearing screening through the use of physiological measures, with the initial hearing screening conducted by one month of age in hospital settings and six weeks of age in PHC clinic settings. Screening can be conducted in a variety of contexts such as the neonatal intensive care unit, high care ward, kangaroo mother care ward, well-baby nurseries, PHC clinics and midwife obstetric units (MOUs). The platform for screening is dependent on the health care system in each district.

- Principle 2: All infants should have access to an effective referral system if they do not pass the initial screen and any subsequent rescreen. The referral system should be efficient and prompt to ensure appropriate audiological and medical evaluations in order to confirm the presence of hearing impairment. Confirmation of hearing impairment should occur by three months of age in hospital programmes and no later than four months of age in clinic-based programmes.

- Principle 3: Infants who pass the initial hearing screening but present with any risk indicators for progressive, late-onset bilateral hearing impairment, other auditory disorders and/or speech and language delay should receive ongoing monitoring. This should be done by caregivers and/or primary care providers who are informed of the risks and the communication developmental milestones. Audiological monitoring protocols should be evidence-based.

- Principle 4: Infant and family rights should be guaranteed through upholding ethical practice in terms of informed choice and consent, and appropriate provision of audiological screening and assessment results that are in agreement with other health care and educational information.

- Principle 5: An integrated information system should be used to manage information related to hearing screening and/or any follow-up assessments. Efforts should be made to integrate this information.

These principles serve as a good foundation for ensuring the provision of efficient and integrated early detection programmes, and can also serve as a way of monitoring progress using the suggested ages for completing identification and diagnosis of hearing impairment. Their applicability to a variety of NHS contexts is key, especially for countries in sub-Saharan Africa where different levels of service delivery exist, and they can serve as a platform for early detection programmes.

Early detection of hearing impairment in sub-Saharan Africa

Published literature from sub-Saharan Africa has inconsistently reported on the aforementioned principles. Some studies have focused on aetiologies and degree of childhood hearing impairment (Banda et al., 2018; Gopal, Hugo, & Louw, 2001; Wonkam et al., 2013), while others have focused on NHS programmes for early detection of hearing impairment and the feasibility of telehealth to extend these screening services to larger populations (Ameyaw, Ribera, & Anim-Sampong, 2019). The exploration of telehealth is particularly useful in contexts where road networks, distance from health care facilities and transport costs preclude attendance or follow-up, but this does not come without challenges, including ethical dilemmas. Naudé and Bornman explore the ethical considerations of tele-audiology for EHDI in chapter 13.

Studies specifically focused on early detection through NHS have been documented in Nigeria, Côte d'Ivoire, Malawi and South Africa (Akinola, Onakoya, Tongo, & Lasisi, 2014; Brough, 2017; De Kock, Swanepoel, & Hall, 2016; Okhakhu, Ibekwe, Sadoh, & Ogisi, 2010; Tanon-Anoh, Sanogo-Gone, & Kouassi, 2010). NHS has been piloted in hospital settings as well as immunisation clinics in Nigeria. Although immunisation clinics received support from government and the mean age for the initial hearing screening was 10.55 days, the lack of electrophysiological measures for the second-stage screening, high infant mortality from infectious diseases and a poor follow-up return rate were reported challenges when implementing NHS in Benin, Nigeria (Okhakhu et al., 2010). Similar challenges were reported in another study conducted in a hospital context in Nigeria (Akinola et al., 2014).

Immunisation clinics in both PHC settings and the neonatal intensive care units in a hospital setting were explored as contexts for NHS in Côte d'Ivoire. A coverage rate of 87.4 percent was reported, with diagnosis of hearing impairment by 22 weeks of age. Despite both these contexts serving as feasible platforms for NHS, investment in equipment, staffing and efficient data management systems for follow-up were reported as being essential (Tanon-Anoh et al., 2010). A pilot project in Malawi explored various contexts for NHS, such as private maternity units, community-based immunisation clinics and kangaroo or special care units in a hospital setting (Brough, 2017). Screening in a hospital setting was found to be unfeasible due to the lack of follow-up. In addition, there were only two audiology departments equipped for diagnostic assessments. Despite the possible feasibility of immunisation clinics, adequate services for diagnostic assessments need to be carefully considered in this country prior to the expansion of NHS services.

Early detection of hearing impairment in South Africa

Detection of hearing impairment is not considered high on the priority list in South Africa due to the government's other health care priorities. South Africa faces a quadruple burden of disease with the health system struggling to cope with four major health issues: NCDs which are chronic diseases; communicable diseases, particularly HIV and TB; maternal and child health (morbidity and mortality rates); and death from injury and violence (DoH, 2014; Naidoo, 2012). The South African government is focused on health promotion aimed at combating diseases or reducing mortality rates, while increasing life expectancy and health system effectiveness (DoH, 2014). Specific challenges in the private health care sector include aspects related to NHS services not forming part of the birthing package or institutional policy. Early detection programmes in this sector have also not been supported by medical aid schemes (Meyer & Swanepoel, 2011), although Discovery, one of the largest schemes, started showing an interest in 2019 in funding screening programmes.

Programmes for early detection of hearing impairment in South Africa have not been standardised nationally, with documented differences existing between provinces as well as between the public and private health care sectors (Meyer & Swanepoel, 2011; Theunissen & Swanepoel, 2008). Overall, results from NHS studies in South Africa have revealed poor coverage rates and limited implementation of universal newborn hearing screening (UNHS) due to a number of context-specific challenges (Table 2.1).

The number of UNHS programmes implemented in the private health care sector has been limited. A UNHS programme conducted over a four-year period at a private health care hospital in South Africa reported a 75 percent coverage rate within the first 22 months when hearing screening was included in the hospital birthing package. This coverage rate decreased to 20 percent when parents were financially responsible for the NHS services (Swanepoel, Ebrahim, Joseph, & Friedland, 2007). A national survey conducted in the private health care sector in South Africa indicated that only 14 percent of obstetric units offer true UNHS (Meyer & Swanepoel, 2011).

Table 2.1 Summary of findings from studies related to early hearing detection in South Africa

Context	Province	Coverage rates	Age of identification of hearing impairment	Pros and cons	Study
MOUs	Western Cape	Not documented	Mean age at initial screening documented as 6.1 days	Well-trained and -managed screeners can be used successfully Good follow-up return rates for screening Loss to follow-up when referred for diagnostic assessment Variability in diagnostic assessment protocols	De Kock, Swanepoel, & Hall, 2016
MOUs	Gauteng	38 percent at initial screening	Not documented	Screening at the three-day MOU assessment clinic was more practical Time of discharge did not always coincide with audiologist's working hours Lack of staffing, equipment and resources Noise levels at the clinic were not ideal	Kanji, Khoza-Shangase, Petrocchi-Bartal, & Harbinson, 2018; Khoza-Shangase & Harbinson, 2015

continued

Context	Province	Coverage rates	Age of identification of hearing impairment	Pros and cons	Study
Hospital	Gauteng	17 percent over a two-year period	Not documented	Technical difficulties and/or equipment failure High patient-to-assessor ratio resulting in limited coverage Early discharge of neonates born without complications	Bezuidenhout, Khoza-Shangase, De Maayer, & Strehlau, 2018

A significant 47 percent of the private health care units included in the survey reported not performing NHS. Although risk-based or targeted newborn hearing screening (TNHS) may yield a greater coverage rate, more units (18 percent) reported conducting screening on request or referral in comparison to TNHS (Meyer & Swanepoel, 2011). This lack of UNHS programmes has also been documented in the public health care sector (Theunissen & Swanepoel, 2008).

Findings from an earlier national survey among public sector hospitals in eight of the nine South African provinces indicated that an estimated 7.5 percent of public sector hospitals provide some form of NHS, and less than 1 percent provide UNHS (Theunissen & Swanepoel, 2008). As a result, PHC clinics and MOUs were proposed as a platform for UNHS with the rationale that the PHC level provides an opportunity for improved coverage and follow-up return rates (HPCSA, 2007; Swanepoel, Hugo, & Louw, 2006). PHC has also been viewed as having a set of values and principles that support universal health care access and address the social determinants of health (Mash et al., 2018; Scott et al., 2017). A few studies in South Africa have explored or piloted early hearing detection programmes at different levels of service delivery (Bezuidenhout, Khoza-Shangase, De Maayer, & Strehlau, 2018; De Kock et al., 2016; Kanji, Khoza-Shangase, Petrocchi-Bartal, & Harbinson, 2018; Khoza-Shangase & Harbinson, 2015). Table 2.1 details findings from these studies.

Despite the various programmes piloted in different health care contexts in a few provinces in South Africa, early hearing detection programmes have not yet been implemented at a national level. There is a great need for resources in terms of staffing and equipment for screening and diagnostic assessment to ensure timely detection and diagnosis of hearing impairment. In chapter 4, Petrocchi-Bartal, Khoza-Shangase and Kanji explore the feasibility of implementing early detection programmes at various levels of service delivery in the South African context.

Solutions and recommendations

Audiologists should engage with EHDI guidelines or position statements where they exist in their countries. In the absence of these guidelines, LAMI countries in sub-Saharan Africa should consider using the South African guidelines as a foundation to contextualise EHDI in terms of key principles and benchmarks for their respective health care context(s). Provincial and national forums should be used as platforms to advocate for the mandating of existing EHDI guidelines by the DoH in South Africa, and by relevant structures in the rest of the continent.

In countries where audiologists or hearing health care services are limited or non-existent, South Africa could lead the way with sharing best practice and suggesting possible solutions for these contexts. One such solution may be to implement appropriate NHS services at different levels of service delivery. For example, UNHS at PHC level and TNHS at hospital level may increase coverage rates and facilitate the screening of both well babies and high-risk neonates. If and where possible, non-audiologists who have been adequately trained, with adherence to the United Nations task-shifting guidelines, may also be used to conduct NHS as this will address the evident human resource shortages. However, NHS programmes would still need to be managed by a qualified audiologist, as is regulated in the South African context.

PHC re-engineering in countries such as South Africa needs to be considered as a platform for early detection services, particularly as this strategy forms the cornerstone of addressing the social determinants of health (Scott et al., 2017). PHC also provides a commitment to universal health coverage and primary care, which are important when considering early detection of hearing impairment. In addition, there should be a key emphasis on health reforms in resource-constrained contexts such as South Africa, by ensuring the inclusion of not only curative but also preventative and promotive primary health services (Ataguba et al., 2015). Early detection of hearing impairment is thus important, particularly as it is a secondary prevention strategy within the PHC service delivery.

The SDGs include indicators related to maternal, newborn and child health, and universal coverage. Framing early hearing detection services within these indicators may facilitate support from government, and ensure that whatever initiatives are implemented have political backing and are therefore sustainable. Foreign aid and government health spending have reportedly increased during the period of the MDGs. Similarly, addressing SDGs will also require resources. Perhaps the use of foreign aid during the period of SDGs may be effective in supporting the implementation of UNHS services, if mandated by government.

Conclusion

Countries in sub-Saharan Africa face many health-related challenges, including access to health care as well as a high prevalence of communicable and non-communicable diseases, which are prioritised over hearing health care. This is despite some of these diseases, such as HIV/AIDS and TB, having possible audiological manifestations. In some countries, the overburdened health care system is further exacerbated by a shortage of ear and hearing health care professionals in relation to the population that needs to be served. These challenges influence the implementation of early hearing detection services and adherence to the early hearing detection principles, which are aimed at facilitating maximum potential in children presenting with hearing impairment. Hence, interim approaches to early detection of hearing impairment need to be explored in each context as health service delivery models may differ in each country. This exploration may include primary and middle-level workers in NHS as well as the use of PHC settings to ensure universal coverage. Effective data management systems and referral pathways for diagnostic assessment need to be established in order to reduce loss of follow-up, which may result in missed cases of hearing impairment.

References

Agyepong, I. A., Sewankambo, N., Binagwaho, A., Coll-Seck, A. M., Corrah, T., Ezeh, A., ... Piot, P. (2018). The path to longer and healthier lives for all Africans by 2030: The Lancet Commission on the future of health in sub-Saharan Africa. *The Lancet, 390*, 2803–2859.

Akinola, M. D., Onakoya, P. A., Tongo, O., & Lasisi, A. O. (2014). Neonatal hearing screening using transient evoked otoacoustic emission in a sub-urban population in Nigeria. *International Journal of Otolaryngology and Head & Neck Surgery, 3*, 205–211.

Allinder, S. M., & Fleischman, J. (2019). The world's largest HIV epidemic in crisis: HIV in South Africa. Retrieved from https://www.csis.org/analysis/worlds-largest-hiv-epidemic-crisis-hiv-south-africa.

Alvarez, A. E. (2008). An evaluation of the Virginia early hearing detection and intervention program. Retrieved from http://www.infanthearing.org/states/documents/evaluation_tools/Virginia%20VEHDIP_Evaluation_July2008.pdf.

Ameyaw, G. A., Ribera, J., & Anim-Sampong, S. (2019). Interregional newborn hearing screening via telehealth in Ghana. *Jounal of the American Academy of Audiology, 30*(3), 178–186.

Aregbeshola, B. S. (2017). Enhancing political will for universal health coverage in Nigeria. *MEDICC Review, 19*(1), 42–46.

Ataguba, J. E., Day, C., & McIntyre, D. (2015). Explaining the role of the social determinants of health on health inequality in South Africa. *Global Health Action, 8*, 1–11. https://doi.org/10.3402/gha.v8.28865.

Avert. (2019). Global information and education on HIV and AIDS. Retrieved from https://www.avert.org/professionals/hiv-around-world/sub-saharan-africa/overview.

Banda, F. M., Powis, K. M., Mokoka, A. B., Mmapetla, M., Westmoreland, K. D., David, T., & Steenhoff, A. P. (2018). Hearing impairment among children referred to a public audiology clinic in Gaborone, Botswana. *Global Pediatric Health, 5*, 1–8.

Bezuidenhout, J. K., Khoza-Shangase, K., De Maayer, T., & Strehlau, R. (2018). Universal newborn hearing screening in public healthcare in South Africa: Challenges to implementation. *South African Journal of Child Health, 12*(4), 154–158.

Blumberg, L., Frean, J., & Moonasar, D. (2014). Successfully controlling malaria in South Africa. *South African Medical Journal, 104*(3 Suppl. 1), 224–227.

Brough, H. (2017). Setting up a newborn hearing screening programme in a low-income country: Initial findings from Malawi. *International Journal of Neonatal Screening, 3*, 1–5.

Chirwa, D. M. (2016). Access to medicines and health care in sub-Saharan Africa: A historical perspective. *Maryland Journal of International Law, 31*(1), 21–43.

Crisp, N. (2011). Global health capacity and workforce development: Turning the world upside down. *Infectious Disease Clinics of North America, 25*, 359–367.

De Kock, T., Swanepoel, D., & Hall III, J. W. (2016). Newborn hearing screening at a community-based obstetric unit: Screening and diagnostic outcomes. *International Journal of Pediatric Otorhinolaryngology, 84*, 124–131.

Deaton, A. S., & Totora, R. (2015). People in sub-Saharan Africa rate their health and health care among lowest in world. *Health Aff (Millwood), 34*(3), 519–527.

Department of Health (DoH). (2011). National health insurance: Policy paper. Retrieved from http://www.bowman.co.za/FileBrowser/ContentDocuments/NHI.pdf.

Department of Health (DoH). (2014). The national health promotion policy and strategy. Retrieved from www.health.gov.za/index.php/2014-03-17-09-09-38/strategic-documents/category/229-2015str?download=936:doh-promotion-policy-and-strategy-printed-version.

Fagan, J. J. (2018). Workforce considerations, training, and diseases in Africa. *Otolaryngologic Clinics of North America, 51*(3), 643–650.

Fagan, J. J., & Jacobs, M. (2009). Survey of ENT services in Africa: Need for a comprehensive intervention. *Global Health Action, 2*, 1932.

Gopal, R., Hugo, S. R., & Louw, B. (2001). Identification and follow-up of children with hearing loss in Mauritius. *International Journal of Pediatric Otorhinolaryngology, 57*, 99–113.

Health Professions Council of South Africa (HPCSA). (2007). Early hearing detection and intervention programmes in South Africa, position statement year 2007. Retrieved from http://www.hpsca.co.za/hpcsa/default.aspx?id=137.

Health Professions Council of South Africa (HPCSA). (2018). Early hearing detection and intervention (EHDI) guidelines. Retrieved from http://www.hpcsa.co.za/Uploads/editor/UserFiles/downloads/speech/Early_Hearing_Detection_and_Intervention_(EHDI)_2018.pdf.

Joint Committee on Infant Hearing (JCIH). (2007). Year 2007 position statement: Principles and guidelines for early hearing detection and intervention programs. *Pediatrics, 120*(4), 898–921.

Kanji, A., Khoza-Shangase, K., Petrocchi-Bartal, B., & Harbinson, S. (2018). Feasibility of infant hearing screening from a developing country context: The South African experience. *Hearing Balance and Communication, 16*(4), 263–270.

Khoza-Shangase, K., & Harbinson, S. (2015). Evaluation of universal newborn hearing screening in South African primary care. *African Journal of Primary Health Care and Family Medicine, 7*(1), 1–12.

Lu, C., Cook, B., & Desmond, C. (2017). Does foreign aid crowd out government investments? Evidence from rural health centres in Rwanda. *BMJ Global Health, 2*(e000364). doi: 10.1136/bmjgh-2017-000364.

Mash, R., Howe, A., Olayemi, O., Makwero, M., Ray, S., Zerihun, M., ... Goodyear-Smith, F. (2018). Reflections on family medicine and primary healthcare in sub-Saharan Africa. *BMJ Global Health, 3*(e000662), 1–3. doi: 10.1136/bmjgh-2017-000662.

Mash, R., Ogunbanjo, G., Naidoo, S. S., & Hellenberg, D. (2015). The contribution of family physicians to district health services: A national position paper for South Africa. *South African Family Practice, 57*(3), 54–61.

Mayosi, B. M., Lawn, J. E., Van Niekerk, A., Bradshaw, D., Karim, S. S. A., & Coovadia, H. M. (2012). Health in South Africa: Changes and challenges since 2009. *The Lancet, 380*, 2029–2043.

Meyer, M. E., & Swanepoel, D. (2011). Newborn hearing screening in the private health care sector: A national survey. *South African Medical Journal, 101*(9), 665–667.

Micah, A. E., Chen, C. S., Zlavog, B. S., Hashimi, G., Chapin, A., & Dieleman, J. L. (2019). Trends and drivers of government health spending in sub-Saharan Africa, 1995–2015. *BMJ Global Health, 4*(e001159). doi: 10.1136/bmjgh-2018-001159.

Mulwafu, W., Ensink, R., Kuperd, H., & Fagan, J. (2017). Survey of ENT services in sub-Saharan Africa: Little progress between 2009 and 2015. *Global Health Action, 10*, 1–7.

Mwamba, A. (2014). Audiology in Zambia: Gaining strength in numbers. *The Hearing Journal, 67*(4), 34–37.

Naidoo, S. (2012). The South African national health insurance: A revolution in healthcare delivery! *Journal of Public Health, 34*(1), 149–150. https://doi.org/10.1093/pubmed/fds008.

Neumann, K., Chadha, S., Tavartkiladze, G., Bu, X., & White, K. R. (2019). Newborn and infant hearing screening facing globally growing numbers of people suffering from disabling hearing loss. *International Journal of Neonatal Screening, 5*(7), 1–11.

Okhakhu, A. L., Ibekwe, T. S., Sadoh, A. S., & Ogisi, F. O. (2010). Neonatal hearing screening in Benin City. *International Journal of Pediatric Otorhinolaryngology, 74*, 1323–1326.

Olugbenga, E. O. (2017). Workable social health insurance systems in sub-Saharan Africa: Insights from four countries. *Africa Development, 42*(1), 147–175.

Olusanya, B. O. (2011). Highlights of the new WHO report on newborn and infant hearing screening and implications for developing countries. *International Journal of Pediatric Otorhinolaryngology, 75*(6), 745–748.

Olusanya, B. O., & Newton, V. E. (2007). Global burden of childhood hearing impairment and disease control priorities in developing countries. *The Lancet, 369*, 1314–1317.

Olusanya, B. O., Ruben, R. J., & Parving, A. (2006). Reducing the burden of communication disorders in the developing world: An opportunity for the millenium development project. *The Journal of the American Medical Association, 296*, 441–444.

Pillay, Y., & Barron, P. (2014). Progress towards the millenium development goals in SA. *South African Medical Journal, 104*(3 Suppl. 1), 223.

Scott, V., Schaay, N., Schneider, H., & Sanders, D. (2017). Addressing social determinants of health in South Africa: The journey continues. *South African Health Review, 2017*(1),77–87.

Simkins, C. (2019). The coming demographic crisis in sub-Saharan Africa. Retrieved from https://www.politicsweb.co.za/opinion/the-coming-demographic-crisis-in-subsaharan-africa.

Statista. (2019). Sub-Saharan Africa: Total population from 2007 to 2017 (in million inhabitants). Retrieved from https://www.statista.com/statistics/805605/total-population-sub-saharan-africa/.

Stevens, G., Flaxman, S., Brunskil, E., Mascarenhas, M., Mathers, C. D., & Finucane, M. (2011). Global and regional hearing impairment prevalence: An analysis of 42 studies in 29 countries. *The European Journal of Public Health, 23*(11), 146–152.

Swanepoel, D., Ebrahim, S., Joseph, A., & Friedland, P. L. (2007). Newborn hearing screening in a South African private health care hospital. *International Journal of Pediatric Otorhinolaryngology, 71*, 881–887.

Swanepoel, D., Hugo, R., & Louw, B. (2006). Infant hearing screening at immunization clinics in South Africa. *International Journal of Pediatric Otorhinolaryngology, 70*(6), 1241–1249.

Swanepoel, D., & Störbeck, C. (2009). Early hearing detection and intervention services in South Africa. Retrieved from http://www.ehdi.co.za/UserFiles/File/EARLY%20 HEARING%202_final_pdf.

Tanon-Anoh, M. J., Sanogo-Gone, D., & Kouassi, K. B. (2010). Newborn hearing screening in a developing country: Results of a pilot study in Abidjan, Côte d'Ivoire. *International Journal of Pediatric Otorhinolaryngology, 74*, 188–191.

The Lancet. (2017). Hearing loss: Time for sound action. *The Lancet, 390*(10111), 2414.

Theunissen, M., & Swanepoel, D. (2008). Early hearing detection and intervention services in the public health care sector in South Africa. *International Journal of Audiology, 47*, S23–S29.

Tucci, D. L., Merson, M. H., & Wilson, B. S. (2010). A summary of literature in global hearing impairment: Current status and priorities for action. *Otology and Neurotology, 31*(1), 31–41.

UNAIDS. (2019). AIDSinfo. Retrieved from http://aidsinfo.unaids.org.

United Nations. (2015). The millennium development goals report. Retrieved from https://www.un.org/millenniumgoals/2015_MDG_Report/pdf/MDG%202015%20 rev%20(July%201).pdf.

Wonkam, A., Noubiap, J. J. N., Djomou, F., Fieggen, K., Njock, R., & Toure, G. B. (2013). Aetiology of childhood hearing loss in Cameroon (sub-Saharan Africa). *European Journal of Medical Genetics, 56,* 20–25.

World Health Organization (WHO). (2008). Social determinants of health: Key concepts. Retrieved from https://www.who.int/social_determinants/thecommission/ finalreport/key_concepts/en/.

World Health Organization (WHO). (2010). Newborn and infant hearing screening. Retrieved from http://www.who.int/blindness/publications/Newborn_and_Infant_ Hearing_Screening_Report.pdf.

World Health Organization (WHO). (2014). Global health expenditure database. Retrieved from http:// apps. who. int/nha/ database.

World Health Organization (WHO). (2015). Health in 2015: From MDGs, millennium development goals to SDGs, sustainable development goals. Retrieved from https://apps.who.int/iris/bitstream/handle/10665/200009/9789241565110_eng. pdf;jsessionid=397F198FC554290FFE116CE0DAC8BC71?sequence=1.

World Health Organization (WHO). (2017). Social determinants of health. Retrieved from http://www.who.int/social_determinants/sdh_definition/en/.

World Health Organization (WHO). (2018). *World health statistics 2018: Monitoring health for the SDGs.* Geneva, Switzerland.

3 Approaches to Early Detection of Hearing Impairment in Low and Middle-Income Countries

Amisha Kanji

Early detection of hearing impairment through newborn hearing screening (NHS) is the initial step to any early hearing detection and intervention (EHDI) programme. Universal newborn hearing screening (UNHS) is considered the gold standard worldwide. However, this approach may not initially be feasible for some developing contexts where contextual challenges to implementation exist. Targeted newborn hearing screening (TNHS) is a possible interim approach that may be implemented in such contexts. This chapter first discusses the different approaches to early detection of hearing impairment in South Africa, followed by the recommended approach for this context. The chapter concludes by suggesting possible solutions and recommendations for early detection of hearing impairment in South Africa and other low and middle-income (LAMI) countries that may not yet have early detection programmes in place.

Early detection of hearing impairment is conducted through NHS, and is usually followed by a comprehensive diagnostic audiological evaluation should a refer result be obtained from the screening. NHS has been used for over a century. Investigation of early detection of hearing impairment began in the 1800s with the use of subjective evaluation in the form of behavioural responses. It has now progressed to the use of objective measures in the form of otoacoustic emissions (OAEs) and the auditory brainstem response (Mencher & DeVoe, 2001), which are employed in NHS programmes globally. Similarly, risk-based hearing screening, commonly referred to as TNHS, was the first approach to early detection in the 1950s and 1960s, with the introduction of the high-risk register (HRR) to identify newborns and infants presenting with risk criteria for permanent congenital and early onset hearing impairment who require NHS (Mencher & DeVoe, 2001). Identification of infants at risk for permanent congenital and early onset hearing impairment based on established risk factors on the HRR was recommended by the Joint Committee on Infant Hearing (JCIH) in 1973. The use of this approach for early detection of hearing impairment gradually progressed toward the introduction of UNHS in 2000, which entails the screening of all newborns (JCIH, 2000, 2007).

Approaches to early detection

There are two main approaches to early detection of hearing impairment, namely UNHS and TNHS. UNHS is the recommended screening approach and has replaced TNHS, particularly in high-income countries (Olusanya et al., 2007). This choice is due to a considerable proportion of infants not having risk factors for hearing impairment in most developed contexts (Patel, Feldman, Canadian Paediatric Society, & Community Paediatrics Committee, 2011). NHS programmes from 46 countries were reviewed and evaluated against the JCIH (2007) recommendations (Tann, Wilson, Bradley, & Wanless, 2009). From the 26 high-income countries included in the review, 18 (69 percent) were recorded as having implemented UNHS. This is in comparison to the middle-income countries where UNHS was indicated for eight (44 percent) of the 18 countries, and low-income countries where no UNHS programmes were indicated at the time (Tann et al., 2009). In South Africa, the 2007 position statement and the 2018 EHDI guidelines by the Health Professions Council of South Africa (HPCSA) also recommend the use of UNHS as the preferred approach for the public health care sector (HPCSA, 2007, 2018).

Universal versus targeted newborn hearing screening

Despite the preferred approach to early detection, it is important to highlight the advantages and limitations of each approach in light of the context in which the NHS programme is to be implemented.

Implementation of UNHS has shown to decrease the age of diagnosis of hearing impairment (Durieux-Smith, Fitzpatrick, & Whittingham, 2008; Ghogomu, Umansky, & Lieu, 2014), which may in turn lead to earlier intervention and its associated positive outcomes in terms of early childhood development. UNHS further facilitates detection of hearing impairment in infants without risk factors who may otherwise be missed. Of the 709 children in the study by Durieux-Smith et al. (2008), 128 (of whom 124 presented with risk factors) had been identified through UNHS or TNHS programmes and the remaining 581 had been referred by a physician. Children who were screened through either of the NHS programmes were diagnosed significantly earlier (mean age of diagnosis at 6.3 months) than those with risk factors who were referred (mean age of diagnosis at 34.5 months). In comparison to the children without risk factors, those with risk factors were diagnosed earlier. Despite differences in ages at diagnosis, only 21 of the 128 children who underwent NHS had a confirmed diagnosis and received intervention by three and six months of age, respectively. Durieux-Smith and colleagues (2008) propose that this may be due to other medical conditions taking priority over the identification of hearing impairment in those admitted to the neonatal intensive care unit. Similar findings in terms of a significant decrease in the age of diagnosis of unilateral sensorineural hearing impairment were also reported in a retrospective record review conducted at a single site in Missouri in the United States (Ghogomu et al., 2014). Findings from this study indicated that the mean age of detection of hearing impairment decreased from 4.4 years to 2.6 years of age with an increase in the rate of detection from 3 percent to 26 percent by six months of age.

While the overall benefits of UNHS are evident, there are limitations to this approach as well. First, less severe congenital hearing impairment (less than 30–40dB) is often not detected in UNHS programmes. The second limitation is related to UNHS programmes using a two-step screening protocol in which low-risk infants with auditory neuropathy may not be detected by the use of OAEs as the only screening measure (Patel et al., 2011).

Similarly, one of the most commonly reported TNHS limitations is that it may result in missed cases of hearing impairment. Between 25 and 50 percent of infants with hearing impairment may not be identified if only TNHS is utilised, and babies without risk factors for hearing impairment may be at risk of being identified late (Durieux-Smith & Whittingham, 2000; Hyde, 2005; Kountakis, Skoulas, Phillips, & Chang, 2002). 'The percentage of babies missed may be due to the absence of hearing impairment in those with risk factors and the presence of hearing impairment in those without risk factors' (Kanji, 2016, p. 51). However, despite these limitations, it is important to consider the context in which TNHS is conducted, as the proportion of neonates or infants with risk factors may be greater in some contexts than in others. TNHS may be a beneficial, interim screening method in LAMI countries where the recommendation of UNHS appears rather overwhelming or is not yet feasible. The development of an appropriate and contextually relevant HRR documenting the risk factors for hearing impairment may also assist in highlighting the cases that require monitoring and follow-up (Johnson, 2002).

Irrespective of the choice of approach, there is cost involved in implementation:

> For NHS programmes, costs are incurred for all those screened, but the benefits are experienced by only a small percentage of neonates. The most important variables to include in such an analysis are the actual costs of the screening, the effectiveness of the screening, the prevalence of hearing impairment and the cost consequences associated with preventing, treating or managing hearing impairment. Assessment of benefits must then include both the health and economic benefits associated with preventing, treating or managing hearing impairment. (World Health Organization [WHO], 2010, p. 10)

The cost-effectiveness of UNHS and TNHS has been explored in eight different provinces in China (Huang et al., 2012) using the guidelines stipulated by the WHO (2010). UNHS was found to be more cost-effective when there was a good coverage rate in terms of the total number of newborns and infants screened, diagnosed and enrolled into an intervention programme. TNHS, on the other hand, was more feasible in provinces where all these rates were low. In order to improve TNHS in these provinces, Huang et al. (2012) recommended that pilot surveys be conducted to determine the context-specific risk factors for permanent congenital and early onset hearing loss. A systematic review by Colgan et al. (2012) suggested that the cost-effectiveness of UNHS can only be concluded if longer-term costs and outcomes associated with such programmes are accounted for.

A cost-effectiveness comparison of UNHS and selective screening (TNHS) of newborns with pre-specified risk factors was conducted by Burke, Shenton, and Taylor (2012) between a high-income and a LAMI country (United Kingdom and India). TNHS yielded a better positive predictive value (Burke et al., 2012). UNHS incurred more costs than TNHS as a result of a larger number of false positive findings. Costs may therefore be viewed as relative to the prevalence of hearing impairment in each region, with higher costs in regions with a lower prevalence as more infants need to be tested in order to detect those with hearing impairment (Burke et al., 2012). It may therefore be argued that the costs incurred in LAMI countries may be lower as that is where the prevalence of hearing impairment is reported to be higher in comparison to higher-income countries (Kanji, 2016).

Weighing up the options for South Africa

UNHS is a commonly practised approach to early detection in developed countries, with well-established, standardised programmes, and dedicated screeners outside of the profession of speech pathology and audiology. While these developed countries have established NHS programmes and are concerned with the diagnostic follow-up and intervention aspects, South Africa appears to be in the early stages of implementation of NHS services and programmes (Kanji, 2016). Research and conceptual papers related to EHDI in South Africa have acknowledged the impracticalities of attempting to implement developed world models of NHS in developing countries (Moodley & Störbeck, 2015; Swanepoel, Delport, & Swart, 2004; Swanepoel, Hugo, & Louw, 2005).

Both approaches to NHS have been explored in the South African context. Studies involving UNHS have looked at different health care contexts – private and primary health care, secondary level hospitals and midwife obstetric units (MOUs) – in the public sector in two provinces (Bezuidenhout, Khoza-Shangase, De Maayer, & Strehlau, 2018; De Kock, Swanepoel, & Hall, 2016;

Khoza-Shangase & Harbinson, 2015; Swanepoel, Ebrahim, Joseph, & Friedland, 2007).

A UNHS study conducted over a four-year period at a private hospital revealed a 75 percent coverage rate within the first 22 months when hearing screening was included in the hospital birthing package. However, the efficiency of the programme decreased to a 20 percent coverage rate during the following 26 months, when parents were responsible for payment of the NHS service (Swanepoel et al., 2007). Of the two studies conducted in the public health care sector, the study at a secondary level hospital included screening of 121 neonates out of a possible 2 704 births during the study period. Challenges to the implementation of UNHS included noise interference; vernix in the external auditory canal of neonates; human resource challenges due to a high patient-to-audiologist ratio, resulting in limited coverage; technical and equipment challenges; as well as early discharge of well babies (Bezuidenhout et al., 2018).

MOUs have been reported to serve as a useful platform for UNHS and follow-up with postnatal visits (De Kock et al., 2016). A study conducted over a 16-month period at three MOUs in the Western Cape revealed initial follow-up return rates to be high, with a decline for additional screening or diagnostic appointments (De Kock et al., 2016). The employment of dedicated non-professional screeners was reported to have positively influenced screening services, with quality training and regular supervision being vital to programme efficiency. While the HPCSA guidelines are geared toward UNHS and serve as the gold standard that audiologists in South Africa should aim to achieve, they are not necessarily applicable as the starting point in all health care sectors in the country.

Studies related to TNHS have been less frequently conducted in the South African context. However, findings from one study suggest the need to establish more context-specific risk factors in order to ensure effective implementation of TNHS programmes (Kanji, 2016). Results from this study indicate that the case history factors in the sample of high-risk neonates were not all present on the HRRs by the JCIH (2007) and HPCSA (2018). These differences in findings, along with those in Australian studies by Beswick, Driscoll, and Kei (2012), as well as Beswick, Driscoll, Kei, Khan, and Glennon (2013), highlight the need to specifically tailor risk factors to context. Kanji and Khoza-Shangase (2019) further highlight the importance of context itself as a risk indicator. These authors propose the concept of a quadruple influence on risk, which takes cognisance of the influence of the burden of disease, medical advancements, technological advancements and human advancements. The use of appropriate risk factors is further explored in chapter 6 of this book. It has also been suggested that TNHS be considered in contexts where UNHS is not yet feasible, particularly in hospital settings in the public health care sector, where high-risk neonates would be more likely to undergo follow-up and monitoring by paediatricians.

Table 3.1 Factors to consider when weighing up the approach to NHS

Factor	Details
Human resources	Availability of audiologists and whether non-professional personnel are available to conduct screening
Equipment	Availability of equipment for screening and/or diagnostic assessment Costs associated with maintenance of equipment
Data management	Availability of an effective and efficient data management and tracking system
Costs	Clinical assessment and management costs for newborns and infants with hearing impairment

The South African health care sector consists of a large public sector on which over 80 percent of the population is dependent (Naidoo, 2012). The Department of Health (DoH) focuses on other health priorities and specific health-related goals, such as the eradication of extreme hunger and poverty, the promotion of gender equality, reduction of child mortality, improvement in maternal health, and combating of HIV/AIDS, malaria and other major diseases (DoH, 2012).

Considering South Africa's health care context, and the importance of early detection of hearing impairment in newborns and infants, there is a need to seriously consider how early detection services may be adapted to better meet these realities (Kanji, 2018). A number of factors need to be considered when deciding on the most suitable approach to NHS, whether interim or long term (see Table 3.1). Khoza-Shangase explores the challenges and realities confronting the implementation of early detection services in South Africa in chapter 5.

Solutions and recommendations

Audiologists need to evaluate the contexts in which they work, and decide on the most suitable approach to early detection of hearing impairment. The evaluation needs to consider the costs involved with NHS, as well as the availability of equipment and human resources. This evaluation can be conducted using the needs assessment and planning guide in the HPCSA's EHDI guidelines. Audiologists could trial the use of non-audiologists as screening personnel following training as detailed in the curriculum suggested in the EHDI guidelines. The guidelines include a practical training and competency checklist which can be used to evaluate non-professional screeners (HPCSA, 2018).

Once the chosen approach is well established, there needs to be consideration of how to better develop the programme that is in place. This can only be done if it is evaluated regularly against key benchmarks specified in the guidelines, including: ages by which screening and confirmation of hearing impairment should take place in various levels of service delivery; evidence of an otologic evaluation in children diagnosed with hearing impairment; audiological and medical evaluations that are perceived as positive and supportive by families; and support to families in terms of appropriate provision of information and referrals for intervention (HPCSA, 2018).

Audiologists should also share key challenges and successes of the programmes at appropriate forums in order to develop such programmes at provincial and national levels. Differences between levels of service delivery also need to be explored and tiered approaches may need to be implemented to ensure the highest possible coverage rate. In chapter 4, Petrocchi-Bartal, Khoza-Shangase and Kanji explore implementation of early detection services at various levels of service delivery in the South African context. Audiologists need to record data accurately in order to monitor the efficiency of programmes, document prevalence and incidence rates for hearing impairment and use these data to motivate for funding for equipment.

As noted, careful consideration needs to be given to the possibility of training non-audiologists as screeners in order to overcome human resource shortages in developing contexts. In situations where TNHS is the chosen approach, audiologists need to screen newborns and infants in neonatal intensive care units and high care wards instead of using predetermined risk factors. All case history factors should be recorded in detail at the time of screening in order to facilitate retrospective, evidence-based research of risk factors associated with hearing impairment.

Conclusion

UNHS is the gold standard approach to early detection of hearing impairment. While this is the goal that LAMI countries such as South Africa need to strive towards, attention needs to be paid to specific and local needs of the context. This will ensure that the approach to early detection is contextually relevant, realistic, responsive and appropriate at any given time. It will further provide a beneficial start to service provision in terms of EHDI. 'As health care professionals we need to acknowledge the limitations but not allow it to preclude us from providing quality services within our means' (Kanji, 2018, p. 3).

References

Beswick, R., Driscoll, C., & Kei, J. (2012). Monitoring for postnatal hearing loss using risk factors: A systematic literature review. *Ear and Hearing, 33*(6), 747–756.

Beswick, R., Driscoll, C., Kei, J., Khan, A., & Glennon, S. (2013). Which risk factors predict postnatal hearing loss in children? *Journal of the American Academy of Audiology, 24*(3), 205–213.

Bezuidenhout, J. K., Khoza-Shangase, K., De Maayer, T., & Strehlau, R. (2018). Universal newborn hearing screening in public healthcare in South Africa: Challenges to implementation. *South African Journal of Child Health, 12*(4), 154–158.

Burke, M., Shenton, R. C., & Taylor, M. J. (2012). The economics of screening infants at risk of hearing impairment: An international analysis. *International Journal of Pediatric Otorhinolaryngology, 76*, 212–218.

Colgan, S., Gold, L., Wirth, K., Ching, T., Poulakis, Z., Rickards, F., & Wake, M. (2012). The cost-effectiveness of universal newborn screening for bilateral permanent congenital hearing impairment: Systematic review. *Academic Pediatrics, 12*(3), 171–180.

De Kock, T., Swanepoel, D., & Hall III, J. W. (2016). Newborn hearing screening at a community-based obstetric unit: Screening and diagnostic outcomes. *International Journal of Pediatric Otorhinolaryngology, 84*, 124–131.

Department of Health (DoH). (2012). Strategic plan for maternal, newborn, child and women's health (MNCWH) and nutrition in South Africa 2012–2016. Retrieved from www.doh.gov.za/docs/stratdocs/2012/MNCWHstratplan.pdf.

Durieux-Smith, A., Fitzpatrick, E., & Whittingham, J. (2008). Universal newborn hearing screening: A question of evidence. *International Journal of Audiology, 47*, 1–10.

Durieux-Smith, A., & Whittingham, J. (2000). The rationale for neonatal hearing screening. *Journal of Speech Language Pathology and Audiology, 24*, 59–67.

Ghogomu, N., Umansky, A., & Lieu, J. E. C. (2014). Epidemiology of unilateral sesorineural hearing loss with universal newborn hearing screening. *Laryngoscope, 124*(1), 295–300.

Health Professions Council of South Africa (HPCSA). (2007). Early hearing detection and intervention programmes in South Africa, position statement year 2007. Retrieved from http://www.hpsca.co.za/hpcsa/default.aspx?id=137.

Health Professions Council of South Africa (HPCSA). (2018). Early hearing detection and intervention (EHDI) guidelines. Retrieved from http://www.hpcsa.co.za/Uploads/editor/UserFiles/downloads/speech/Early_Hearing_Detection_and_Intervention_(EHDI)_2018.pdf.

Huang, L. H., Zhang, L., Tobe, R. G., Qi, F., Sun, L., Teng, Y., … Han, D. (2012). Cost-effectiveness analysis of neonatal hearing screening program in China: Should universal screening be prioritized?*BMC Health Services Research, 12*, 97.

Hyde, M. L. (2005). Newborn hearing screening programs: Overview. *Journal of Otolaryngology, 34*, S70–S78.

Johnson, C. D. (2002). Special populations. In J. Kats, R. F. Bukard, & L. Medwetsky (Eds.), *Handbook of clinical audiology* (5th ed., pp. 481–494). Baltimore, MD: Lippincott Williams & Wilkins.

Joint Committee on Infant Hearing (JCIH). (2000). Year 2000 position statement: Principles and guidelines for early hearing detection and intervention programs. *American Journal of Audiology, 9*, 9–29.

Joint Committee on Infant Hearing (JCIH). (2007). Year 2007 position statement: Principles and guidelines for early hearing detection and intervention programs. *Pediatrics, 120*(4), 898–921.

Kanji, A. (2016). Early detection of hearing loss: Exploring risk-based hearing screening within a developing country context. PhD thesis. University of the Witwatersrand, Johannesburg, South Africa.

Kanji, A. (2018). Early hearing detection and intervention: Reflections from the South African context. *South African Journal of Communication Disorders, 65*(1), 1–3.

Kanji, A., & Khoza-Shangase, K. (2019). Early detection of hearing impairment in high-risk neonates: Let's talk about the high-risk registry in the South African context. *South African Journal of Child Health, 13*(2), 53–55.

Khoza-Shangase, K., & Harbinson, S. (2015). Evaluation of universal newborn hearing screening in South African primary care. *African Journal of Primary Health Care and Family Medicine, 7*(1), 1–12.

Kountakis, S. E., Skoulas, I., Phillips, D., & Chang, C. Y. (2002). Risk factors for hearing loss in neonates: A prospective study. *American Journal of Otolaryngology, 23*(3), 133–137.

Mencher, G. T., & DeVoe, S. J. (2001). Universal newborn screening: A dream realized or a nightmare in the making?*Scandanavian Audiology, 30*(53), 15–21.

Moodley, S., & Störbeck, C. (2015). Narrative review of EHDI in South Africa. *South African Journal of Communication Disorders, 62*(1), 1–10.

Naidoo, S. (2012). The South African national health insurance: A revolution in healthcare delivery! *Journal of Public Health, 34*(1), 149–150. https://doi.org/10.1093/pubmed/fds008.

Olusanya, B. O., Swanepoel, D., Chapchap, M. J., Castillo, S., Habib, H., Mukari, S. Z., … McPherson, B. (2007). Progress towards early detection services for infants with hearing loss in developing countries. *BMC Health Services Research, 7*, 14–28.

Patel, H., Feldman, M., Canadian Paediatric Society, & Community Paediatrics Committee. (2011). Universal newborn hearing screening. *Paediatric Child Health, 16*(5), 301–305.

Swanepoel, D., Delport, S. D., & Swart, J. G. (2004). Universal newborn hearing screening in South Africa A first-world dream? *South African Medical Journal, 94*(8), 634–635.

Swanepoel, D., Ebrahim, S., Joseph, A., & Friedland, P. L. (2007). Newborn hearing screening in a South African private health care hospital. *International Journal of Pediatric Otorhinolaryngology, 71*, 881–887.

Swanepoel, D., Hugo, R., & Louw, B. (2005). Infant hearing screening in the developing world. *Audiology Today, 17*(4), 16–19.

Tann, J., Wilson, W. J., Bradley, A. P., & Wanless, G. (2009). Progress towards universal neonatal hearing screening: A world review. *Australian and New Zealand Journal of Audiology, 31*(1), 3–14.

World Health Organization (WHO). (2010). Newborn and infant hearing screening. Retrieved from http://www.who.int/blindness/publications/Newborn_and_Infant_Hearing_Screening_Report.pdf.

4 Implementing Early Hearing Detection in the South African Health Care Context

Luisa Petrocchi-Bartal, Katijah Khoza-Shangase and Amisha Kanji

This chapter explores the feasibility of implementing early detection of hearing impairment through infant hearing screening in various South African health care contexts, including both the public (primary, secondary and tertiary levels) and private health care sectors. These contexts and levels of service delivery are described, and the practicability and efficiency of implementing early hearing screening in each context discussed. Evidence indicates that: midwife obstetric units (MOUs) appear to be the most viable contexts for infant hearing screening; primary health care (PHC) immunisation clinics are appropriate platforms for screening, provided assets are fine-tuned and barriers formally addressed, especially regarding staffing; screening in the private hospital sector needs to be included as part of the birthing package, with full medical aid reimbursement; and aspects such as the availability of hearing screening space, ambient noise levels and discharge timing all influence the practicability and efficiency of screening in various health care contexts. The chapter illustrates that factors that facilitate or impede the feasibility of early hearing screening vary depending on the level of health care in South Africa. Finally, suggestions are made about how to maximise efficiency within each service delivery level.

When referring to early detection of hearing impairment as a component of child health care best practice, universal newborn hearing screening (UNHS) is regarded as the preferable means to do so (Kanji, Khoza-Shangase, Petrocchi-Bartal, & Harbinson, 2018). This is the first component of what is known as early hearing detection and intervention (EHDI), which has been implemented as best practice in many high-income countries, such as the United States of America, many European countries and China (Russ, White, Dougherty, & Forsman, 2010; World Health Organization [WHO], 2010). However, its implementation has significantly lagged behind in low and middle-income (LAMI) contexts such as Africa (Health Professions Council of South Africa [HPCSA], 2018). In South Africa, reasons for this include resource constraints (Kanji, Khoza-Shangase, Petrocchi-Bartal et al., 2018; Tandwa, 2017; World Bank, 2018), demand versus capacity challenges (Khoza-Shangase, 2019), poverty and inequality (Olusanya, 2005; World

Bank, 2018), as well as prioritisation of medical conditions where preservation of life is placed first (Kanji, Khoza-Shangase, Petrocchi-Bartal et al., 2018), such as tuberculosis (TB) and HIV/AIDS, which are highly prevalent (Day, Gray, & Ndlovu, 2018; Streefland, 2005; United Nations Children's Fund, 2013; World Bank, 2018). Hearing impairment is considered of secondary importance, as its issues relate more to quality of life than to survival. It is perhaps for these reasons that EHDI and UNHS have not become a legal requirement in South Africa.

The International Monetary Fund (IMF, 2018) describes South Africa as a middle-income economy with an emerging market. Despite significant post-apartheid progress in many spheres of the country's development, service delivery, especially regarding health care, has been done in pockets, with little integration between government and private health care sectors (Störbeck & Moodley, 2011). Part of this non-standardised approach relates to the application of EHDI in the South African context: it has not been mandated at a government level (Kanji, Khoza-Shangase, Petrocchi-Bartal et al., 2018), as in many high-income countries, and it appears that mostly non-systematic and non-standardised risk-based hearing screening occurs (Kanji & Khoza-Shangase, 2016). This takes place in a context of significant health care challenges, discussed by Khoza-Shangase in chapter 5. Besides lack of a government mandate for UNHS, these challenges include demand versus capacity issues, resource constraints, a high burden of disease with which EHDI has to compete, as well as poor social determinants of health. Chapter 5 sounds a call for a 'doing better with less' approach to ensure that EHDI occurs. This is a realistic approach to adopt in resource-constrained contexts as it is viewed as being cost-effective.

Evidence demonstrates that up to 50 percent of hearing impairment in infants is missed when a targeted newborn hearing screening approach is adopted (Kanne, Schaefer, & Perkins, 1999). Kanji argues in chapter 3 that this approach nevertheless needs to be adopted in South Africa as an interim measure, as no formalised national system is currently in place. This would take into account the HPCSA's (2018) recommendation for UNHS. Without EHDI and UNHS legislation, EHDI will continue to be relegated to secondary status and children with hearing impairment will be left to experience its negative consequences.

Hearing impairment has been shown to have a negative impact for the hearing-impaired individual on cognition (Olusanya, 2005), language development (Ching, 2015), literacy (DesJardin, Ambrose, Martinez, & Eisenberg, 2009), educational, social and emotional abilities (Northern & Downs, 1991; WHO, 2018), as well as vocational and financial outcomes (Olusanya, Ruben, & Parving, 2006; WHO, 2018). The negative consequences extend to the family of the hearing-impaired child, explored in more depth in chapter 11. These negative consequences emphasise EHDI's importance to individuals, their families and to society as a whole (Kanji, Khoza-Shangase, Petrocchi-Bartal et al., 2018), as governments will ultimately be required to deal with the long-term negative ramifications of hearing impairment, be it in terms of cost or support. Government plans should thus cater for EHDI with the application of contextually relevant and effective screening measures to identify those with hearing impairment as early as possible. As argued by Kanji and Khoza-Shangase (2018a, 2019), consideration of the South African context extends to the use of contextually relevant risk factors (see chapter 6). Once effective identification has taken place, and factors that influence follow-up return rate (Kanji & Khoza-Shangase, 2018b) and compromise EHDI service delivery (Khoza-Shangase, 2019) have been addressed, early intervention can be successfully implemented to maximise the hearing-impaired individual's potential at all levels of functioning. In high-income countries, it is recommended that post-diagnosis intervention is initiated by six months of age (Joint Committee on Infant Hearing [JCIH], 2000, 2007, 2019), while in South Africa it is by eight months of age (HPCSA, 2018).

The fastest, most cost-effective and simplest tool for hearing screening in the South African context is the use of otoacoustic emissions (OAEs), despite their known limitations (Kanji, Khoza-Shangase, Petrocchi-Bartal et al., 2018). These limitations include OAEs not being able to comprehensively assess hearing and the fact that they may be negatively affected by the external and middle ear status, such as the presence of vernix in the external auditory canal (Albuquerque & Kemp, 2001; Korres et al., 2003). Automated auditory brainstem responses (AABRs) may also be used as a hearing screening tool to better assess the auditory system and detect auditory neuropathy in this population (Kanji, Khoza-Shangase, Petrocchi-Bartal et al., 2018). Compared to OAEs, AABRs are, however, more expensive to conduct, take longer to administer (Choo & Meinzen-Derr, 2010) and require a greater level of expertise (Kanji & Khoza-Shangase, 2016). Depending on the specific health care context and the level of health care service delivery, such factors may impact hearing screening programme implementation.

South African health care structure

South Africa has progressed markedly since the democratic elections in 1994, which heralded equal rights for all citizens, including the right to health care (Delobelle, 2013). This is the key motivation for the national health insurance (NHI) plan reflected in the White Paper on NHI for South Africa (Department of Health [DoH], 2017a), which in 2019 became the NHI Bill. It justifies NHI for South Africa by stating that it is the 'right of citizens to have access to quality healthcare services' (DoH, 2017a, p. 1). NHI is based on principles of the right to access health care, described in the Constitution's Bill of Rights, initiated after the 1994 government changeover (DoH, 2017a).

The newly appointed post-apartheid government introduced its formalised health care reform in order to reduce the glaring discrepancies between South Africa's developing and industrialised world realities. This health care reform aimed to address the needs of previously neglected populations through provision of more equitable health care services for all (Government Communication and Information System [GCIS], 2009). A PHC approach was adopted, signalling a shift from a curative hospital-based structure to a cohesive and accessible community-based system at provincial level (GCIS, 2009; Maillacheruvu & McDuff, 2014). However, social inequalities and health care issues have persisted as a function of poverty (Delobelle, 2013). This is despite post-apartheid majority rule and the government's attempts to address the social and economic consequences of apartheid, as well as provide accessible health care services, particularly through its PHC and community-based initiatives (Maillacheruvu & McDuff, 2014). The NHI is touted as a significant approach to address health care access challenges. Khoza-Shangase argues in chapter 5 that the NHI has the potential to enhance EHDI. The White Paper on NHI for South Africa (DoH, 2017a, p. 1) and its 2019 Bill assert that 'good health is an essential value of the social and economic life of humans and is an indispensable prerequisite'. NHI aims to achieve a healthier nation, where people live longer and suffer less illness. This aim correlates very well with the goals of EHDI. NHI also aims to prevent illness and to ensure that patients receive treatment at an early stage of illness to avoid complications. This is consistent with the goals of early intervention for children with hearing impairment. Furthermore, NHI aims to have family health teams in all neighbourhoods providing preventive health services and home-based care, a strategy that improves access to health care services and would, for EHDI, be contextually relevant and responsive. Lastly, NHI encourages the expansion of PHC services, a model of health care that the South African government has adopted.

The South African health care system has been described as reasonably developed, with post-1994 public and private systems that run concurrently (Swanepoel, Störbeck, & Friedland, 2009). The less resourced public health care system is accessed by over 80 percent of the population for a minimal administration fee or for free (DoH, 2017b; Swanepoel et al., 2009). Accessing private health care is affordability based, and private health care expenditure is five times more per person than public health care spending (DoH, 2017b). The NHI proposes a homogeneous approach to health care, where citizens can access health services in both the public and private sectors at the expense of the NHI, regardless of their socio-economic status. It will run as a public, non-profit unit to render guaranteed, quality health care for all South African citizens (DoH, 2017b). This implies that the South African government aims to achieve universal health coverage and access to a high quality of care (Health Systems Trust, 2017).

Nationally, there are more than 400 public and 200 private hospitals (Britnell, 2015). This has clear implications for capacity versus demand. The larger hospitals are managed by provincial health departments, and districts manage the smaller hospitals and PHC clinics (Britnell, 2015). In terms of Treasury distribution of funds, health care sector funding, particularly at a provincial level, is determined according to specific contextual deliberations and service delivery needs (Motsepe, 2017). Funds are thus prioritised differently per province (Mailovich, 2019). This results in differing and non-standardised health care delivery, dependent on provincial priorities, with knock-on effects regarding intra- and intersectoral liaison approaches to health care. Consequently, this funding model tends to widen the apparent health care disparities between provinces when health care services are compared across regions. As such, standardisation is rendered superfluous. Furthermore, this occurs in the context of South Africa trying to attend to the long-term goal of addressing the social determinants of health, which vary between provinces, with some provinces such as Gauteng and the Western Cape being significantly better off than others. Addressing the social determinants of health in South Africa has been acknowledged as a long journey to improve 'the circumstances in which people grow, live, work and age, and the systems put in place to deal with illness' (Commission on the Social Determinants of Health, 2008, p. 3).

At present, the audiologist's role in detection and intervention for hearing impairment in the public health care system is formally tiered in a guideline compiled by the National Speech Therapy and Audiology Public Sector Forum (Health) and the Professional Board of the Speech, Language and Hearing Professions (n.d.), as depicted in Table 4.1.

Table 4.1 Audiology services at all levels of health care in South Africa

Level of care	Types of facilities	Audiology service provision
Primary	PHC clinics	• Development, monitoring and evaluation of ototoxicity, EHDI, ear and hearing care screening and intervention programmes • Management of referrals
	Community health centres	In addition to the listed services at PHC clinics: • Implementation and management of aural rehabilitation programmes • Earmould modifications and basic hearing aid trouble shooting

continued →

Level of care	Types of facilities	Audiology service provision
	District hospitals	• Development, monitoring and evaluation of intervention plans and programmes • Management of referrals • Cerumen management • Identification of neonates, paediatric and adults at risk and with established risk for hearing difficulties through EHDI and ototoxicity screening and monitoring programmes at inpatient and outpatient clinics • Diagnostic assessment of hearing • Management of hearing difficulties including aural rehabilitation post cochlear implantation and post bone-anchored hearing aid fitting • Ensure appropriate referrals for advanced diagnostic assessment to other levels of care • Collaboration with other team members including district health teams • Recommend school or vocational placement
Secondary	Regional hospitals	In addition to the listed services at primary and district levels: • Screening for vestibular disorders • Diagnostic hearing assessments which include visual reinforcement audiometry, immittance as well as electrophysiological measures such as OAEs, ABR and auditory steady state response • Hearing aid assessments and objective hearing aid verification • Hearing aid fitting • Recommendations and referrals to appropriate levels where necessary for surgical intervention, including cochlear implants
Tertiary	Provincial tertiary hospitals	In addition to the listed services at primary, district and regional levels: • Recommendations for surgical intervention, including cochlear implants • Provision of consultative clinics for cochlear implants, bone-anchored hearing aids, vestibular disorders, electrophysiology, complex disorders, auditory neuropathy spectrum disorder

EHDI contextualised

In order to minimise hearing impairment consequences, and improve the quality of life of children with hearing impairment, EHDI is key in order to capitalise on the child's period of maximal brain plasticity (Fulcher, Purcell, Baker, & Munro, 2015; HPCSA, 2018; Hutt & Rhodes, 2008; JCIH, 2007; Northern & Downs, 1991; WHO, 2018).

Globally, the JCIH, and locally, the HPCSA, advocate for culturally sensitive and contextually relevant EHDI to counter the negative consequences associated with hearing impairment (HPCSA, 2007, 2018; JCIH, 2000, 2007, 2013, 2019). Timeous intervention has been found to have similar communication outcomes for hearing-impaired individuals when compared with their non-hearing-impaired counterparts (Mehl & Thomson, 2002; Meyer, Swanepoel, & Le Roux, 2014; Moeller, 2000; Olusanya, 2005). Thus, the JCIH and HPCSA specify EHDI goals to include maximising outcomes pertaining to linguistic competence, literacy development and education while acknowledging cultural congruency (HPCSA, 2007, 2018; JCIH, 2000, 2007, 2013, 2019).

In order for EHDI to be successful, hearing screening, confirmation of hearing impairment through diagnostic assessment and appropriate intervention must be in place. The HPCSA (2018) further highlights the need for sustained surveillance of infants and toddlers, protection of infants and families, as well as adequate information infrastructure and quality monitoring. These components of EHDI not only emphasise timeous identification, intervention and programme sustainability to maximise communication outcomes (Harrington, Desjardin, & Shea, 2009; Yoshinaga-Itano, 2013), but also define early intervention as a primary determinant of a child's success in the wider world. Chapter 2 considers early hearing detection in sub-Saharan Africa, with a discussion of principles related to early detection of hearing impairment as outlined by the HPCSA (2018) guidelines.

To further contextualise early hearing detection, it is necessary to unpack EHDI timelines. International gold standards, defined as 1:3:6 (JCIH, 2007, 2019), specify that hearing screening is conducted by one month of age, diagnosis confirmed by three months of age and intervention provided by six months of age. Context-specific adjustments to timelines for South Africa specify hearing screening to be conducted by the latest six weeks of age, hearing impairment diagnosis confirmed by the latest four months of age and intervention provided by the latest eight months of age (HPCSA, 2018). In addition, early intervention must be family-centred, within the locus of community and culturally congruent (HPCSA, 2018; Louw & Avenant, 2002; Sass-Lehrer, Porter, & Wu, 2016; Swanepoel, Hugo, & Louw, 2006). Chapter 11 considers EHDI in the context of family, taking cognisance of cultural and linguistic factors. This contextualisation of EHDI allows for evidence-based best practice, and considers linguistic and cultural influences on health-seeking behaviours, health care and intervention adherence behaviours, as well as health outcomes. Khoza-Shangase and Mophosho (2018) argue for careful consideration of linguistic and cultural diversity in speech-language and hearing professions in South Africa to ensure that the country has better health outcomes. Globally, evidence indicates that these outcomes are worse in groups that do not form part of the dominant culture (Flood & Rohloff, 2018).

EHDI continues to demonstrate evidence-based value, but the challenges faced by LAMI countries derail the well-intentioned principles and goals. A paucity of South African evidence supporting EHDI precepts hinders elevating EHDI as a priority in the face of more serious health concerns and socio-economic demands in the country (Störbeck & Young, 2016). Research endeavours have focused mainly on early hearing detection, with early intervention services under-scrutinised (Störbeck & Young, 2016).

Early identification in different levels of health care service delivery

No formal, standardised newborn hearing screening (NHS) system currently exists at public hospitals across South Africa. According to Theunissen and Swanepoel's study (2008), only 27 percent of public health care hospitals at the time of their study had any form of NHS in place. Meyer and co-authors (2014) reported a marked delay in hearing impairment diagnosis and early intervention provision in their national survey of private health care. To date, South African EHDI studies have revealed a non-holistic approach to services rendered nationally (Moodley & Störbeck, 2015). This is in stark contrast to high-income countries such as the United States of America and the United Kingdom, where formalised screening and diagnostic and intervention systems are in place. However, some systems are complex, and numerous resources as well as financial support are required (Moodley & Störbeck, 2015).

As emphasised by the JCIH (2007, 2013, 2019) and the HPCSA (2007, 2018), context is key to EHDI's success. To better understand the South African setting, it is necessary to interrogate the practicability and efficiency of hearing screening at the various levels of care, as guided by published evidence in these contexts (see Table 4.2). The hearing screening contexts include public health care (primary, secondary and tertiary levels) and private health care:

- Level of care 1 (PHC):
    - Hearing screening at a community health care (CHC) centre or clinic using OAEs within six hours of birth

Table 4.2 Practicability and efficiency of NHS in various South African health care contexts

Context detail	Hearing screening age	Practicability and efficiency	Factors that may impact practicability and efficiency
Public health care sector, secondary level: CHC centre/clinic	≤6 hours post birth	• Low pass rate • Low patient yield (babies missed screening)	• Time of birth relative to discharge • Resources • Environmental factors • Referral rate increased
Public health care sector, secondary level: All neonatal wards	≤30 days post birth	• Pass rates affected by vernix caseosa, noise levels	• Staff availability • Equipment/resources • Environmental factors • Early discharge
Public health care sector, primary level: MOU	3 days post birth OAE (TEOAE, DPOAE)	• High pass rate • High patient yield/return rate	• Return rate for follow-up high • Referral rate decreased
	Mostly <14 days post birth (mean age 6 days)	• High pass rate • High patient yield/return rate	• Return rate for follow-up high • Refer rates decreased using AABR and two-stage screening protocol
Public health care sector, tertiary level: Neonatal intensive care unit (NICU) and/ or step-down wards when baby stable	Dependent upon baby's wellness level	• High bilateral refer rates for TEOAE, less for AABR • Dependent upon baby's wellness level • Well babies missed (approximately 50%) TEOAE	• Delays in EHDI timing strongly associated with infant's birth status and complexity of medical needs • Other factors – increased ambient noise levels, securing informed consent from parents may be difficult, aspects related to discharge

continued ⟶

Context detail	Hearing screening age	Practicability and efficiency	Factors that may impact practicability and efficiency
Public health care sector, tertiary level: Newborn follow-up clinic post discharge	1st newborn follow-up clinic post discharge	• Highest refer rates for DPOAE and AABR, lowest for TEOAE • Low patient yield/ return rate	• Low patient yield/ return rate
Public health care sector, primary level: PHC clinic	At 6-, 10- and/or 14-week immunisation clinic	• Assets: nurse willingness, high patient yield/ return rate • Barriers: space, equipment, environmental factors, high staff demands, prioritising other health conditions, lack of nurse awareness regarding hearing impairment, inconsistent record keeping	• Fine-tuning required to address barriers formally to improve feasibility • Dedicated screening staff can improve competency through experience and thus reduce false positives/over-refers; relieve already overburdened PHC staff who may prioritise other diseases • A screening coordinator can facilitate higher return rates through strategies such as telephonic appointment reminders and in-file visual rescreen reminders, facilitating consistent record keeping

continued
——————▶

Context detail	Hearing screening age	Practicability and efficiency	Factors that may impact practicability and efficiency
Private health care	Within 24 hours post birth	• High patient yield if hearing screening part of birthing package, otherwise coverage rates significantly less than 50% • Loss of patients to early discharge out of audiologist working hours • Difficulty tracking patients who have the option to choose the screening/ audiology service	• Parental education prior to birth to impart importance of hearing screening and facilitate consent • Structure screening as part of the birthing package to improve patient yield • Educate ward staff regarding the importance of hearing screening to ensure hearing screening before discharge • Ensure programme monitoring to improve programme efficiency and decrease refer rates • To improve quality control and accountable service provision, ensure appropriate data management and tracking

Sources: Bezuidenhout, Khoza-Shangase, De Maayer, & Strehlau, 2018; De Kock, Swanepoel, & Hall, 2016; Friderichs, Swanepoel, & Hall, 2012; Joubert & Casoojee, 2013; Kanji, Khoza-Shangase, Petrocchi-Bartal, & Harbinson, 2018; Meyer & Swanepoel, 2011; Swanepoel, Ebrahim, Joseph, & Friedland, 2007

Note: TEOAE = Transient evoked OAEs; DPOAE = Distortion product OAEs

- – Hearing screening using OAEs three days after birth at the MOU
- – Hearing screening using OAEs and AABR at mostly <14 days post birth at the MOU
- – Hearing screening at PHC immunisation clinics.
- Level of care 2 (secondary):
  - – Hearing screening at a secondary level hospital, using OAEs within 30 days of birth
  - – Hearing screening using OAEs and AABR at newborn follow-up visits after discharge for high-risk infants.
- Level of care 3 (tertiary): Hearing screening at tertiary level health care using OAEs and AABR in neonatal intensive care units and/or step-down wards.
- Private health care: Hearing screening at private health care facilities.

As Table 4.2 indicates, hearing screening at CHC centres/clinics is possible prior to hospital discharge within six hours of birth, but it comes with significant challenges in the South African context (Khoza-Shangase & Harbinson, 2015). These challenges include the possibility of low patient capture, despite the babies being inpatients. This may be a result of staff availability. For example, audiologists are employed during standard daytime working hours, but babies' arrivals cannot be timed to fit in with these hours – they may be born at night or over the weekend and discharged before their hearing is screened. Some births in South Africa also take place at home (Bezuidenhout, Khoza-Shangase, De Maayer, & Strehlau, 2018; Khoza-Shangase & Harbinson, 2015). Likewise, in many other LAMI countries (Olusanya & Somefun, 2009) a large number of infants are born outside hospital settings. Community-oriented NHS must thus be emphasised, particularly in these contexts (Kanji, Khoza-Shangase, Petrocchi-Bartal et al., 2018). In addition, hearing screening pass rates in these contexts may be low because of vernix caseosa (Albuquerque & Kemp, 2001; Korres et al., 2003), which may result in a hearing screening refer due to obstruction in the external auditory canal. This higher hearing screening refer rate, not as a result of a hearing issue per se, is thus a factor that raises challenges with cost-effectiveness and parental psycho-emotional status management in an already vulnerable system.

At secondary level hospitals where UNHS was attempted on neonates within 30 days of birth in all wards, significant challenges were identified: reduced staffing, resource issues (lack of back-up equipment due to resource constraints) and factors that further impede testing, such as ambient noise levels in wards. Furthermore, as noted, additional findings were the presence of vernix caseosa as well as babies being missed due to discharge during audiologists' non-working hours (Bezuidenhout et al., 2018). Bezuidenhout and colleagues (2018) suggest that hearing screening should be conducted at the three-day MOU visit in order to overcome the challenges raised by early discharge and vernix caseosa during screening. The fact that there are not enough audiologists available to screen all neonates may be resolved by training non-audiologists to conduct the screening, as recommended by the HPCSA (2018), with audiologists serving as managers of the screening programmes. This strategy would also allow for 24-hour access to screening services which are currently impeded by audiologists' limited working hours.

At three-day MOU clinics, where scheduled appointments are made, patient capture rates are markedly improved and return rates are reported to be high when hearing screening coincides with the postnatal general medical check-up (Kanji, Khoza-Shangase, Petrocchi-Bartal et al., 2018; Khoza-Shangase & Harbinson, 2015). Capture rates are high because infants tend not to be missed due to off-duty staff factors and home births. High return rates suggest that babies born outside medical facilities are brought to the three-day follow-up clinic. Moreover, hearing screening pass rates are reported to be high because factors such as the negative influence of vernix in the external auditory canal have mostly been minimised by this stage (Bezuidenhout et al., 2018). Hearing screening protocol selection (OAEs versus AABRs) is therefore important to reduce the number of refers, although the importance of obtaining accurate results as early as possible remains paramount (De Kock, Swanepoel, & Hall, 2016).

Thus, while hearing screening may be possible within six hours postpartum, it is more efficient and practical to screen infant hearing at the MOU assessment clinic, particularly the three-day appointment post birth. This setting maximises patient capture rates relative to other contexts, and significantly reduces false positive rates. Time of birth in relation to discharge, environmental aspects, resource availability, referral rates and return for follow-up rates have all been identified as possible factors that impact the practicability and efficiency of screening in specific contexts. Ng, Hui, Lam, Goh, and Yeung (2004) report similar findings where newborns were missed in terms of hearing screening because of time of birth and discharge out of normal working hours. However, contrary to these findings, evidence also indicates highest coverage to take place for screening before discharge in non-South African contexts where discharge occurs after six hours post birth (Adelola, Papanikolaou, Gormley, Lang, & Keogh, 2010; Lim & Daniel, 2008). These factors underscore the importance of EHDI coordinators being mindful of circumstances which may cause infants to be overlooked within the particular NHS system.

In South Africa, the importance of investigating alternative avenues for contextually appropriate hearing screening is also emphasised. Such screening may need to be included in the scheduling of other medical visits. According to Theunissen and Swanepoel (2008), the most frequently reported reasons for shortages of NHS programmes in South Africa are the lack of appropriate hearing screening equipment and the relatively small number of audiologists in the country, within whose remit hearing screening mainly falls. Chan and Leung (2004), as well as Olusanya, Wirz, and Luxon (2008), suggest using nurses and community health workers for NHS. The HPCSA (2018) advocates that with appropriate training, the use of non-audiologist staff may help to optimise time and resources at all levels of service delivery. This would require compliance with the HPCSA's minimum standards of training to ensure quality.

A clear caution is the prospect of false positive results before discharge, when a hearing impairment is not present but the infant does not pass the hearing screening (Herrero & Moreno-Ternero, 2005). This has been documented as a major NHS concern (Kanji, Khoza-Shangase, & Moroe, 2018; Korres et al., 2005; Lam, 2006).

In NICU and step-down wards such as the kangaroo mother care ward, timing of NHS is dependent upon the newborns' level of wellness, ranging up to 62 days post birth (Kanji, Khoza-Shangase, Petrocchi-Bartal et al., 2018), as well as other medical conditions in the high-risk neonatal population that may impede timely hearing screening as per JCIH (2013, 2019) and HPCSA (2007, 2018) guidelines (Kanji, Khoza-Shangase, Petrocchi-Bartal et al., 2018). This is confirmed by Chapman et al. (2011), who purport that EHDI process delays are strongly associated with the infant's medical status at and post birth. Delays for babies with concomitant health issues are on average 25 days later for hearing screening and 2.5 months later for hearing impairment diagnosis. Initial NICU screening in the South African context may also demonstrate high referral rates (Kanji, Khoza-Shangase, Petrochhi-Bartal et al., 2018), which is in agreement with reports by Chen et al. (2012) and Colella-Santos, Hein, De Souza, Do Amaral, & Casali (2014). Refer rates tend to decrease with an increase in the infant's age, reflecting that the longer the interim period between the initial and the rescreen, the lower the refer rate (Akinpelu, Peleva, Funnell, & Daniel, 2014; Kanji & Khoza-Shangase, 2018a). Practicability and efficiency in the South African NICU context may be further negatively affected by high ambient noise levels in wards, difficulty obtaining informed consent for hearing screening because of caregiver absence from the NICU, and, where discharge dates are not clearly detailed in patient files, the unanticipated discharge of the patient prior to screening (Kanji, Khoza-Shangase, Petrocchi-Bartal et al., 2018). The latter factor may necessitate booking the neonate for the outpatient rescreen on the same day as the next follow-up visit (Kanji, Khoza-Shangase, Petrocchi-Bartal et al., 2018).

Return rates may decrease at the first newborn follow-up clinic appointment, which usually takes place six weeks post discharge (Kanji, Khoza-Shangase, Petrocchi-Bartal et al., 2018). This does not bode well for NHS test–retest protocols, as neonates and infants may be lost to follow-up, compromising NHS programme quality (Vos, Lagasse, & Levêque, 2014). It is thus important to consider follow-up rates in general and screening contexts.

Tables 4.3 and 4.4 indicate assets and barriers to hearing screening in PHC immunisation clinics in South Africa.

Table 4.3 Assets facilitating the efficiency of hearing screening at PHC immunisation clinics

DoH policy assets	DoH funding assets	Logistics assets	Other factors/assets
• PHC immunisation policies and strategies • Infant record documentation • Referrals	• Otoscope supply	• Patient return rates for immunisations • Immunisation days available • Methods prompting infant returns for follow-up appointments • Infant record documentation systems	• Parental awareness, education and willingness, regarded as mostly surmountable through education • Ongoing surveillance by caregivers • Disability policy

Source: Kanji, Khoza-Shangase, Petrocchi-Bartal, & Harbinson, 2018, p. 5

Table 4.4 Barriers influencing the practicability of hearing screening at PHC immunisation clinics

DoH policy liabilities	DoH funding liabilities	Other factors/liabilities

The nursing scope of practice delineates rudimentary hearing screening techniques such as:
• PHC package protocols, including: Road to Health Card assessments
• Integrated management of childhood illness (IMCI) protocols, including: Hearing assessments framed predominantly within the context of otitis media
	• Inconsistent otoscope usage
	• Lack of formal objective equipment
	• Clinic infrastructure, e.g. lack of space available for hearing screening
	• Staff complement and work distribution
	• Funding inequity between districts
	• Staff training, where:
	  – IMCI protocols are emphasised
	  – Funding needs assessment in terms of added hearing screening specific training
		• Burden of disease
		• Staff currently working at capacity
		• Staff knowledge base pertaining to hearing loss in general

Source: Kanji, Khoza-Shangase, Petrocchi-Bartal, & Harbinson, 2018, p. 6

Clear PHC immunisation policies at a government level are key. These policies should facilitate the practicability of NHS in the PHC context. As far as assets in this context are concerned, they should include, firstly, immunisation day guidelines and positive approaches to prompt infant follow-up returns for immunisations (DoH, 2001). High hearing screening coverage is anticipated as a consequence, given that return rates for infant immunisation are reportedly between 90 and 100 percent (Day & Gray, 2008; DoH, 2009). Hearing screening that coincides with clinic schedules for infant immunisation, as recommended by the HPCSA (2018), is thus strategic in achieving high screening coverage. Secondly, assets should include generalised documentation pertaining to infant record keeping. Electronic databases are already in place in certain regions (Kanji, Khoza-Shangase, Petrocchi-Bartal et al., 2018). DoH policies advocate for accountable infant record documentation, especially with respect to otitis media (DoH, 2005). Such databases are promising for the practical and efficient addition of hearing screening data, and this is already being implemented in some levels of service delivery in provinces such as Gauteng.

Thirdly, acceptable continuity of care is facilitated by adequate resources for referrals. The capacity to refer infants for diagnosis and intervention appears to be generally satisfactory in provinces such as Gauteng and North West (Kanji, Khoza-Shangase, Petrocchi-Bartal et al., 2018). As such, hearing impairment diagnosis by four months of age with intervention by eight months, as promulgated by the HPCSA (2007, 2018), appears practicable, dependent upon demand versus capacity at secondary and tertiary facilities (Bezuidenhout et al., 2018; Kanji, Khoza-Shangase, Petrocchi-Bartal et al., 2018).

Lastly, information about hearing impairment can be incorporated into existing caregiver health education programmes, such as the Vitamin A supplementation programme (DoH, 2001). Khoza-Shangase (2019) highlights the importance of engaging and involving caregivers as key stakeholders in EHDI programmes. She documents various factors compromising early intervention, as reported by caregivers in the South African context. These include long distances between the few EHDI services that are available and the places of residence of service users; significant costs linked to the services; limited skills and knowledge of professionals regarding hearing impairment; inconsistent and conflicting professional opinions about the child's diagnosis and treatment; as well as limited community awareness about hearing impairment and services available for hearing-impaired children (Khoza-Shangase, 2019).

In terms of barriers at PHC immunisation clinics, a lack of funding may underpin logistical issues regarding the identification of hearing impairment (Kanji, Khoza-Shangase, Petrocchi-Bartal et al., 2018). The practicability of hearing screening in the South African context can be improved by

addressing factors such as the lack of specialised hearing screening equipment (Kanji, Khoza-Shangase, Petrocchi-Bartal et al., 2018). Barriers also
include rudimentary hearing screening techniques, where non-audiometric
or non-evoked potential hearing screening techniques are delineated by the
scope of practice for nurses who are the frontline professionals employed in
South Africa's immunisation clinics (HPCSA, 2018).

Adherence to screening techniques appears to be inconsistent, which
may be the result of protocol ambiguity between central and district levels,
with district autonomy prevailing (DoH, 2009). This may also be influenced
by differences in district and provincial funding (Day & Gray, 2008; DoH,
2009). Another barrier to hearing screening in South Africa is the increased
burden of disease, resulting in priority being given to life-threatening conditions rather than hearing impairment (Olusanya, 2005).

Friderichs, Swanepoel, and Hall (2012) propose training and assigning
dedicated screening staff to the immunisation clinics as a possible solution. By so doing, hearing screening competency through experience can
be improved and false positives and high refer rates reduced. These authors
explain that dedicated hearing screening staff can also relieve already overburdened PHC staff, who may prioritise conditions such as HIV/AIDS and
TB (Friderichs et al., 2012). Moreover, a screening coordinator can facilitate
higher return rates through applying strategies such as caregiver telephonic
appointment reminders and in-file visual rescreen reminders, facilitating
consistent record keeping and using tele-audiology. Joubert and Casoojee
(2013) identified inconsistency in record keeping as a challenge, specifically with regard to recording hearing screening results. This is despite the
presence of electronic databases in some regions (Kanji, Khoza-Shangase,
Petrocchi-Bartal et al., 2018).

These findings accentuate the importance of fine-tuning assets and
addressing barriers to prepare the HPCSA clinic-based PHC platform for
EHDI actualisation (Kanji, Khoza-Shangase, Petrocchi-Bartal et al., 2018).
Only in this way can the practicability and efficiency in the PHC context be
improved to enable feasible hearing screening for infants.

In the private health care sector, high screening coverage has occurred
when hearing screening has been included as part of the birthing package
(Swanepoel, Ebrahim, Joseph, & Friedland, 2007). Running screening programmes outside the birthing package is the most frequently recorded challenge to hearing screening implementation in the private sector (Meyer &
Swanepoel, 2011). Practicability and efficiency would thus be dramatically
improved if hearing screening were included in the birthing package (Meyer
& Swanepoel, 2011). To facilitate improved parental involvement, parental
education prior to birth regarding the importance of hearing screening is recommended to facilitate consent (Swanepoel et al., 2007). Additionally, because
caregivers in the private health care system have the liberty to consult with

their preferred service provider, patient tracking becomes difficult. As such, data management and tracking solutions are key to improving quality control (Swanepoel et al., 2007). Lastly, challenges relating to unethical business practice have been raised around screening in the private sector and need to be addressed.

Conclusion

A significant quota of hearing-impaired children in South Africa will continue to have their rights denied until EHDI is incorporated as a cohesive, systematic and comprehensive nationalised health care strategy that is contextually responsive and relevant. Health care practitioners bear the ethical responsibility to facilitate the realisation of the rights of the hearing impaired to actualise their potential through EHDI (Petrocchi-Bartal, 2011).

Due consideration of factors influencing NHS practicability and efficiency is necessary. As Kanji, Khoza-Shangase, Petrocchi-Bartal et al. (2018) state, the level of health care influences the factors that manifest, and these factors may facilitate or inhibit NHS.

In the South African context, current evidence supports the MOU three-day assessment clinic as the most accessible and efficient context for hearing screening programme implementation (Kanji, Khoza-Shangase, Petrocchi-Bartal et al., 2018). Inclusion of these findings in NHI planning is important to ensure hearing screening as part of the re-engineered PHC services. However, Kanji (2016) suggests consideration of a two-tiered approach involving early hearing screening of high-risk babies in the hospital setting, with screening of well babies at clinic level. There should be continued reassessment of the South African contexts for hearing screening and the associated assets and barriers regarding practicability and efficiency. Although other health care contexts such as in-hospital clinics and PHC clinics demonstrate potential for viable hearing screening settings, barriers to successful NHS programme implementation must be addressed before hearing screening can be practicably and efficiently implemented in the ever-changing health care landscape (Kanji, Khoza-Shangase, Petrocchi-Bartal et al., 2018). Only in this way can hearing screening as promulgated by the HPCSA (2007, 2018) be accommodated in this dynamic process.

References

Adelola, O. A., Papanikolaou, V., Gormley, P., Lang, J., & Keogh, I. J. (2010). Newborn hearing screening: A regional example for national care. *Irish Medical Journal, 103*, 146–149.

Akinpelu, O. V., Peleva, E., Funnell, W. R. J., & Daniel, S. J. (2014). Otoacoustic emissions in newborn hearing screening: A systematic review of the effects of different protocols on test outcomes. *International Journal of Pediatric Otorhinolaryngology, 78,* 711–717.

Albuquerque, W., & Kemp, D. T. (2001). The feasibility of hospital-based universal newborn hearing screening in the United Kingdom. *Scandinavian Audiology, 53,* 22–28.

Bezuidenhout, K. J., Khoza-Shangase, K., De Maayer, T., & Strehlau, R. (2018). Universal newborn hearing screening in public healthcare in South Africa: Challenges to implementation. *South African Journal of Child Health, 12*(4), 159–163. doi: 10.7196/SAJCH.2018.v12i4.1522.

Britnell, M. (2015). *In search of the perfect health system.* London: Palgrave.

Chan, K. Y., & Leung, S. S. L. (2004). Infant hearing screening in maternal and child health centres using automated otoacoustic emission screening machines: A one-year pilot project. *Hong Kong Journal of Paediatrics, 9,* 118–125.

Chapman, D. A., Stampfel, C. C., Bodurtha, J. N., Dodson, K. M., Pandya, A., Lynch, K. B., & Kirby, R. S. (2011). Impact of co-occurring birth defects on the timing of newborn hearing screening and diagnosis. *American Journal of Audiology, 20,* 132–139.

Chen, G., Yi, X., Chen, P., Dong, J., Yang, G., & Fu, S. (2012). A large-scale newborn hearing screening in rural areas in China. *International Journal of Pediatric Otorhinolaryngology, 76,* 1771–1774.

Ching, T. (2015). Is early intervention effective in improving spoken language outcomes of children with congenital hearing loss? *American Journal of Audiology, 24,* 345–348.

Choo, D., & Meinzen-Derr, J. (2010). Universal newborn hearing screening in 2010. *Current Opinion in Otolaryngology & Head and Neck Surgery, 18,* 399–404. doi: 10.1097/MOO.0b013e32833d475d.

Colella-Santos, M. F., Hein, T. A. D., De Souza, G. L., Do Amaral, M. I. R., & Casali, R. L. (2014). Newborn hearing screening and early diagnostic in the NICU. *BioMed Research International, 2014,* Article ID 845308, 1–11. doi: 10.1155/2014/845308.

Commission on the Social Determinants of Health (CSDH). (2008). Closing the gap in a generation: Health equity through action on the social determinants of health. *Final Report of the Commission on Social Determinants of Health.* Geneva, Switzerland: World Health Organization. Retrieved from https://apps.who.int/iris/bitstream/handle/10665/43943/9789241563703_eng.pdf;jsessionid=0DBA3E46A7358C1C5506BECC269A826C?sequence=1.

Day, C., & Gray, A. (2008). Indicators: Health and related indicators. In P. Barron & J. Roma Reardon (Eds.), *South African Health Review 2008* (pp. 239–395). Durban, South Africa: Health Systems Trust.

Day, C., Gray, A., & Ndlovu, N. (2018). Health and related indicators. In L. C. Rispel & A. Padarath (Eds.), *South African Health Review 2018* (pp. 139–250). Durban, South Africa: Health Systems Trust.

De Kock, T., Swanepoel, D., & Hall, J. (2016). Newborn hearing screening at a community-based obstetric unit: Screening and diagnostic outcomes. *International Journal of Pediatric Otorhinolaryngology, 84,* 124–131. doi: 10.1016/j.ijporl.2016.02.031.

Delobelle, P. (2013) The health system in South Africa: Historical perspectives and current challenges. In C. C. Wolhuter (Ed.), *South Africa in focus: Economic, political and social issues* (pp. 159–205). New York, NY: Nova Science Publishers.

Department of Health (DoH). (2001). The primary health care package for South Africa: A set of norms and standards. Retrieved from http://ww.doh.gov.za/docs/policy/norms/full-norms.html.

Department of Health (DoH). (2005). Hearing guidelines. Retrieved from www.doh.gov.za: http://www.doh.gov.za/docs/fact-sheets/guidelines/hearing.pdf.

Department of Health (DoH). (2009). Strategic plan 2009/10–2011/12. Retrieved from http://www.doh.gov.za/department/strategic%20plan.html.

Department of Health (DoH). (2017a). National health insurance for South Africa: Towards universal health coverage. Retrieved from http://www.health.gov.za/index.php/nhi?download=2257:white-paper-nhi-2017.

Department of Health (DoH). (2017b). National health insurance: Healthcare for all South Africans, understanding national health insurance. Retrieved from https://www.hst.org.za/publications/NonHST%20Publications/Booklet%20-%20Understanding%20National%20Health%20Insurance.pdf.

DesJardin, J., Ambrose, S., Martinez, A., & Eisenberg, L. (2009). Relationships between speech perception abilities and spoken language skills in young children with hearing loss. *International Journal of Audiology, 48*, 248–259.

Flood, D., & Rohloff, P. (2018). Indigenous languages and global health: Comment. *The Lancet, 6*, e134–135.

Friderichs, N., Swanepoel D., & Hall, J. W. (2012). Efficacy of a community-based infant hearing screening program utilising existing clinic personnel in Western Cape, South Africa. *International Journal of Pediatric Otorhinolayngology, 76*, 552–559.

Fulcher, A., Purcell, A., Baker, E., & Munro, N. (2015). Factors influencing speech and language outcomes of children with early identified severe/profound hearing loss: Clinician-identified facilitators and barriers. *International Journal of Speech-Language Pathology, 17*(3), 325–333.

Government Communication and Information System (GCIS). (2009). Health. In D. Burger (Ed.), *S.A. yearbook 2008/2009* (pp. 310–331). Pretoria, South Africa: GCIS. Retrieved from https://www.gcis.gov.za/sites/default/files/docs/resourcecentre/yearbook/2009/chapter12.pdf.

Harrington, M., Desjardin, J. L., & Shea, L. C. (2009). The relationship between early childhood factors and school readiness skills in young children with hearing loss. *Communication Disorders Quarterly, 32*(1), 50–62.

Health Professions Council of South Africa (HPCSA). (2007). Early hearing detection and intervention programmes in South Africa position statement year 2007. Retrieved from http://www.hpcsa.co.za/hpcsa/UserFiles/Files/Speech%20language%20and%20hearing/EHDI5position%20statement%20(HPCSA%2007).pdf.

Health Professions Council of South Africa (HPCSA). (2018). Early hearing detection and intervention (EHDI) guidelines year 2018. Retrieved from http://www.hpcsa.co.za/Uploads/editor/UserFiles/downloads/speech/Early_Hearing_Detection_and_Intervention_(EHDI)_2018.pdf.

Health Systems Trust. (2017). South African Health Review 2017 *(20th ed.)*. Retrieved from https://www.hst.org.za/publications/South%20African%20Health%20Reviews/HST%20SAHR%202017%20Web%20Version.pdf.

Herrero, C., & Moreno-Ternero, J. D. (2005). Hospital costs and social costs: A case study of newborn hearing screening. *Investigaciones Económicas, 29*, 203–216.

Hutt, N., & Rhodes, C. (2008). Post-natal hearing loss in universal neonatal hearing screening communities: Current limitations and future directions. *Journal of Pediatrics and Child Health, 44*, 87–91.

International Monetary Fund (IMF). (2018). IMF country report No.18/247. South Africa selected issues July 2018. International Monetary Fund. African Department. Retrieved from https://www.imf.org/en/Publications/CR/Issues/2018/07/30/ South-Africa-Selected-Issues-46133.

Joint Committee on Infant Hearing (JCIH). (2000). Year 2000 position statement: Principles and guidelines for early hearing detection and intervention programs. *Pediatrics, 106*(4), 798–817.

Joint Committee on Infant Hearing (JCIH). (2007). Year 2007 position statement: Principles and guidelines for early hearing detection and intervention programs. *Pediatrics, 120*, 898–921.

Joint Committee on Infant Hearing (JCIH). (2013). Supplement to the JCIH position statement: Principles and guidelines for early intervention after confirmation that a child is deaf or hard of hearing. *Pediatrics, 131*, e1324–e1349.

Joint Committee on Infant Hearing (JCIH). (2019). Year 2019 position statement: Principles and guidelines for early hearing detection and intervention programs. *The Journal of Early Hearing Detection and Intervention, 4*(2), 1–44.

Joubert, J., & Casoojee, A. (2013). Hearing-screening record-keeping practices at primary healthcare clinics in Gauteng. *South African Journal of Communication Disorders, 60*, 27–30. doi: 10.7196/SAJCD.233.

Kanji, A. (2016). Early hearing screening in South Africa: Time to get real about context. *South African Journal of Communication Disorders, 10*(4), 192.

Kanji, A., & Khoza-Shangase, K. (2016). Feasibility of newborn hearing screening in a public hospital setting in South Africa: A pilot study. *South African Journal of Communication Disorders, 63*(1), a142. https://doi.org/10.4102/sajcd.v63i1.150.

Kanji, A., & Khoza-Shangase, K. (2018a). Objective hearing screening measures: An exploration of a suitable combination for risk-based newborn hearing screening. *Journal of American Academy of Audiology, 29*(6), 495–502. doi: 10.3766/jaaa.16155.

Kanji, A., & Khoza-Shangase, K. (2018b). In pursuit of successful hearing screening: An exploration of factors associated with follow up return rate in a risk-based newborn hearing screening programme. *Iranian Journal of Pediatrics, 28*(4). doi: 10.5812/ijp.56047.

Kanji, A., & Khoza-Shangase, K. (2019). Early detection of hearing impairment in high risk neonates: Let's talk about the high-risk registry in the South African context. *South African Journal of Child Health, 13*(2), 53–55.

Kanji, A., Khoza-Shangase, K., & Moroe, N. (2018). Newborn hearing screening protocols and their outcomes: A systematic review. *International Journal of Pediatric Otorhinolaryngology*, (*115*), 104–109.

Kanji, A., Khoza-Shangase, K., Petrocchi-Bartal, L., & Harbinson, S. (2018). Feasibility of infant hearing screening from a developing country context: The South African experience. *Hearing, Balance and Communication*, *16*(4), 263–270. doi: 10.1080/21695717.2018.1519144.

Kanne, T. J., Schaefer, L., & Perkins, J. A. (1999). Potential pitfalls of initiating a newborn hearing screening programme. *Archives of Otolaryngology Head Neck Surgery*, *125*(1), 28–32. doi: 10.1001%2Farchotol.125.1.28.

Khoza-Shangase, K. (2019). Early hearing detection and intervention: Exploring factors compromising service delivery as expressed by caregivers. *International Journal of Pediatric Otorhinolaryngology*, *118*, 73–78. doi: 10.1016/j.ijporl.2018.12.021.

Khoza-Shangase, K., & Harbinson, S. (2015). Evaluation of universal newborn hearing screening in South African primary care. *African Journal of Primary Health Care Family Medicine*, *7*, 1–12.

Khoza-Shangase, K., & Mophosho, M. (2018). Language and culture in speech-language and hearing professions in South Africa: The dangers of a single story. *South African Journal of Communication Disorders*, *65*(1), a594. doi: 10.4102/sajcd.v65i1.594.

Korres, S., Nikolopoulos, T., Ferekidis, E., Gotzamanoglou, Z., Georgiou, A., & Balatsouras, D. G. (2003). Otoacoustic emissions in universal hearing screening: Which day after birth should we examine the newborns? *Journal Oto-Rhino-Laryngology and Its Related Specialities*, *65*, 199–201. https://dx.doi. org/10.1159/000073114.

Korres, S., Nikolopoulos, T. P., Komkotou, V., Balatsouras, D., Kandiloros, D., Constantinou, D., & Ferekidis, E. (2005). Newborn hearing screening: Effectiveness, importance of high-risk factors, and characteristics of infants in the neonatal intensive care unit and well-baby nursery. *Otology and Neurotology*, *26*, 1186–1190.

Lam, B. C. C. (2006). Newborn hearing screening in Hong Kong. *Hong Kong Medical Journal*, *12*, 212–218.

Lim, S., & Daniel, L. M. (2008). Establishing a universal newborn hearing screening programme. *Annals Academy of Medicine Singapore*, *37*, 63–65.

Louw, B., & Avenant, C. (2002). Culture as context for intervention: Developing a culturally congruent early intervention program. *International Pediatrics*, *17*(3), 145–150.

Maillacheruvu, P., & McDuff, E. (2014). South Africa's return to primary care: The struggles and strides of the primary health care system. *The Journal of Global Health*. Retrieved from https://www.ghjournal.org/south-africas-return-to-primary-care-the-struggles-and-strides-of-the-primary-health-care-system/.

Mailovich, C. (2019). Budget 2019: Provinces: Sort out your books … or else, spending and budgetary performances may be improving—but there's still a long way to go. *Financial Mail*. Retrieved from https://www.businesslive.co.za/fm/special-reports/2019-02-21-provinces-sort-out--your-books--or-else/.

Mehl, A., & Thomson, V. (2002). The Colorado newborn hearing screening project, 1992–1999: On the threshold of effective population-based universal newborn hearing screening. *Pediatrics*, *109*(1), E7.

Meyer, M. E., & Swanepoel, D. (2011). Newborn hearing screening in the private health care sector: A national survey. *South African Medical Journal, 101*, 665–667.

Meyer, M. E., Swanepoel, D., & Le Roux, T. (2014). National survey of paediatric audiology services for diagnosis and intervention in the South African private health care sector. *South African Journal of Communication Disorders, 61*(1), Art. #62, 8 pages.

Moeller, M. P. (2000). Early intervention and language development in children who are deaf and hard of hearing. *Pediatrics, 106*, 1–9.

Moodley, S., & Störbeck, C. (2015). Narrative review of EHDI in South Africa. *South African Journal of Communication Disorders, 62*(1), 1–10.

Motsepe, T. (2017). Budget speech 2017: Budgeting at the height of inequality. Retrieved from http://www.politicsweb.co.za/archive/budgeting-at-the-heigh-of-inequality--.equal-educat.

National Speech Therapy and Audiology Public Sector Forum (Health) & the Professional Board of the Speech, Language and Hearing Professions (PBSLH–HPCSA). (n.d.). A guideline for planning STA services at all levels of health care. Retrieved from https://www.hpcsa.co.za/Uploads/editor/UserFiles/downloads/speech/guidelines/guideline_planning_STA_services_at_all_levels_health%20care.pdf.

Ng, P. K., Hui, Y., Lam, B. C., Goh, W. H., & Yeung, C. Y. (2004). Feasibility of implementing a universal neonatal hearing screening programme using distortion product otoacoustic emission detection at a university hospital in Hong Kong. *Hong Kong Medical Journal, 10*(1), 6–13.

Northern, J. L., & Downs, M. P. (1991). *Hearing in children* (4th ed.). Baltimore, MD: Williams and Wilkins.

Olusanya, B. (2005). Can the world's infants with hearing loss wait? *International Journal of Pediatric Otorhinolaryngology, 69*, 735–738.

Olusanya, B., Ruben, R., & Parving, A. (2006). Reducing the burden of communication disorders in the developing world: An opportunity for the millennium development project. *Journal of the American Medical Association, 296*, 441–444.

Olusanya, B. O., & Somefun, A. O. (2009). Place of birth and characteristics of infants with congenital and early-onset hearing loss in a developing country. *International Journal of Pediatric Otorhinolaryngology, 73*, 1263–1269.

Olusanya, B. O., Wirz, S. L., & Luxon, L. M. (2008). Hospital-based universal newborn hearing screening for early detection of permanent congenital hearing loss in Lagos, Nigeria. *International Journal of Pediatric Otorhinolaryngology, 72*, 991–1001.

Petrocchi-Bartal, L. (2011). *Clinic based hearing screening protocols: The feasibility of implementing the health professions council of South Africa Year 2007 guidelines* (Master's dissertation). Retrieved from http://wiredspace.wits.ac.za/handle/10539/10134.

Russ, S. A., White, K., Dougherty, D., & Forsman, I. (2010). Preface: Newborn hearing screening in the United States: Historical perspective and future directions. *Pediatrics, 126*, S3–S6.

Sass-Lehrer, M., Porter, A., & Wu, C. L. (2016). Families: Partnerships in practice. In M. Sass-Lehrer (Ed.), *Early intervention for deaf and hard-of-hearing infants, toddlers, and their families: Interdisciplinary perspectives* (pp. 65–104). New York, NY: Oxford University Press.

Störbeck, C., & Moodley, S. (2011). ECD policies in South Africa: What about children with disabilities? *Journal of African Studies and Development, 3*(1), 1–8.

Störbeck, C., & Young, A. (2016). The HI HOPES data set of deaf children under the age of 6 in South Africa: Maternal suspicion, age of identification and newborn hearing screening. *BMC Pediatrics, 16*, 1–10. https://doi.org/10.1186/s12887-016-0574-1.

Streefland, P. (2005). Public health care under pressure in Sub-Saharan Africa. *Health Policy, 71*, 375–382.

Swanepoel, D., Ebrahim, S., Joseph, A., & Friedland, P. (2007). Newborn hearing screening in a South African private health care hospital. *International Journal of Pediatric Otorhinolaryngology, 71*(6), 881–887.

Swanepoel, D., Hugo, R., & Louw, B. (2006). Infant hearing screening at immunisation clinics in South Africa. *International Journal of Pediatric Otorhinolaryngology, 70*(7), 1241–1249.

Swanepoel, D., Störbeck, C., & Friedland, P. (2009). Early hearing detection and intervention in South Africa. *International Journal of Pediatric Otorhinolaryngology, 73*, 783–786.

Tandwa, L. (2017). Education gets largest chunk of Gauteng budget. Retrieved from https://www.news24.com/SouthAfrica/News/education-gets-largest-chunk-of-gauteng-budget-20170307.

Theunissen, M., & Swanepoel, D. (2008). Early hearing detection and intervention services in the public health sector in South Africa. *International Journal of Audiology, 47*(Suppl. 1), S23–S29.

United Nations Children's Fund. (2013). The state of the world's children 2013: Children with disabilities. Retrieved from https://www.unicef.org/sowc2013/files/SWCR2013_ENG_Lo_res_24_Apr_ 2013.pdf.

Vos, B., Lagasse, R., & Levêque, A. (2014). Main outcomes of a newborn hearing screening program in Belgium over six years. *International Journal of Pediatric Otorhinolaryngology, 78*, 1496–1502.

World Bank. (2018). South Africa—Systematic country diagnostic: An incomplete transition—overcoming the legacy of exclusion in South Africa. Retrieved from http://documents.worldbank.org/curated/en/815401525706928690/South-Africa-Systematic-country-diagnostic-an-incomplete-transition-overcoming-the-legacy-of-exclusion-in-South-Africa.

World Health Organization (WHO). (2010). Newborn and infant hearing screening. Retrieved from http://www.who.int/blindness/publications/Newborn_and_Infant_Hearing_Screening_Report.pdf.

World Health Organization (WHO). (2018). Deafness and hearing loss. Retrieved from https://www.who.int/news-room/fact-sheets/detail/deafness-and-hearing-loss.

Yoshinaga-Itano, C. (2013). Principles and guidelines for early intervention after confirmation that a child is deaf or hard of hearing. *Journal of Deaf Studies and Deaf Education, 19*(2), 143–175.

5 Confronting Realities to Early Hearing Detection in South Africa

Katijah Khoza-Shangase

Implementation of early hearing detection and intervention (EHDI) is a significant challenge in the South African context, despite its documented benefits. South Africa, like other low and middle-income (LAMI) countries, is confronted with specific contextual realities. These include the lack of a government mandate for universal newborn hearing screening (UNHS), major resource constraints, a high burden of disease with which EHDI has to compete, and significantly poor social determinants of health. This chapter deliberates on the various issues plaguing early detection in South Africa. It begins by describing the South African health care context and its challenges. This is followed by a more detailed and focused review of literature on the challenges around demand versus capacity and resources, the burden of disease, as well as research evidence on newborn hearing screening (NHS) in South Africa. A call for a 'doing better with less' approach is presented. Lastly, possible solutions and recommendations for hearing detection initiatives in the South African context are offered.

The former South African health minister, Aaron Motsoaledi (2012), pronounced 'a long and healthy life' as a motto guiding the ministry's health strategy for the country during his tenure. This motto is supported by a key motivation for the national health insurance (NHI) plan reflected in the White Paper on NHI (Department of Health [DoH], 2017) and its subsequent National Health Insurance Bill of 2019. NHI is justified for the country because South Africa believes that access to health care is a human right. NHI is based on the following principles: the right to access health care, as outlined in the Bill of Rights, Section 27 of the Constitution of the Republic of South Africa (Act 108 of 1996); social solidarity, which relies on cross-subsidisation between the young and old, rich and poor as well as the healthy and the sick; equity; health care as a public good and not a commodity of trade; affordability, which implies reasonable cost as well as the sustainability of health care within the country's available resources; efficiency with regard to value for money; effectiveness, which means that expected outcomes are obtained and acceptable standards of quality exist; and, lastly, appropriateness to the context and various levels of care (DoH, 2017).

The White Paper on NHI (DoH, 2017, p. 1) asserts that 'good health is an essential value of the social and economic life of humans and is an indispensable prerequisite'. NHI aims to achieve a healthier nation, where people live longer and suffer less illness. This aim correlates with the goals of EHDI. NHI also aims to prevent illness and to ensure that patients receive treatment at an early stage of illness to avoid complications. Again, this is consistent with the goals of early intervention for children with hearing impairment. Furthermore, NHI aims to have family health teams in all neighbourhoods providing preventive health services and home-based care – strategies that improve access to health care services and would, for EHDI, be contextually relevant and responsive. Lastly, NHI encourages the expansion of primary health care (PHC) services, a model of health care that the South African government has adopted.

The South African hospital sector has distinct divisions between old historical divides and new developments, as well as between public and private health sectors. The public health sector services over 80 percent of South African citizens, who are not privately funded. The NHI proposes a harmonised approach to health care where citizens can access health services in both the public and private sectors at the NHI's cost, irrespective of their socio-economic status. This indicates the South African government's intention to achieve universal health coverage (UHC) and access to a high quality of care (Ranchod et al., 2017). However, this needs to occur in the context of the country attending to the long-term goal of tackling the social determinants of health. This has been acknowledged as a long journey where 'the circumstances in which people are born, grow up, live, work and age, and the systems put in place to deal with illness are enhanced' (Commission on the Social Determinants of Health [CSDH], 2008, p. 2). I believe that this approach should also carefully consider the risks and benefits of any initiative adopted to address health challenges in this resource-constrained context. This would require consideration of potential harms and positive effects of all audiology clinical initiatives, such as EHDI interventions and programmes adopted by the country. These would need to be checked for contextual relevance, responsiveness and accountability. Interventions and programmes should be systematic, comprehensive, have a strategic plan behind them, and involve audiologists in all stages, from their development to implementation and monitoring.

The World Health Organization's (WHO) director-general, Tedros Adhanom Ghebreyesus (2017), asserts that all roads lead to UHC, highlighting that this is the goal. He acknowledges that countries adopt different paths to achieving UHC, whether public or private, but emphasises that countries 'need to know where they stand on UHC, benchmarked against others' (Ghebreyesus, 2017, e839). Furthermore, he stresses that UHC is not an end in itself, but allows realisation of other health-related sustainable development goals. Together with the World Bank, the WHO has furnished guidance on tracking progress towards UHC in the form of the UHC service coverage index (Hogan, Stevens, Hosseinpoor, & Boerma, 2018; WHO, 2017).

South Africa is nowhere close to achieving UHC. Although NHI plans continue, final implementation dates have not been given. There are numerous challenges to achieving UHC in the near future in the country (Petersen & Ramma, 2015). These implementation challenges raise serious implications for attaining EHDI goals. Health financing remains a major challenge for the South African government. State spending on health is expected to grow by 7.8 percent per annum between 2017/18 and 2020/21. This is lower than the expected growth in spending on 'learning and culture' (8.5 percent) and social development (9.2 percent) (National Treasury, 2018, pp. 56–61). Consolidated government expenditure on health for the 2018/19 financial year was expected to be R191.685 billion, growing to R205.448 billion, R222.046 billion and R240.297 billion in the medium term. Noting that 'provinces face substantial spending pressures in health and education', Treasury indicated that the health sector is 'working with provincial treasuries on a three-year turnaround plan' (National Treasury, 2018, p. 72). A major challenge remains that of managing the public sector wage bill while simultaneously confronting increasing demands for health care services from an already overextended public health sector. The increasing demands for health care services arise in the context of insufficient capacity when it comes to health care professionals. Although this is a global phenomenon, the challenge is significantly greater in LAMI countries like South Africa, where the burden of disease is also much higher.

Demand versus capacity and resources

Globally, it is predicted that there will be a net shortage of 15 million health care workers by 2030, with middle-income countries unable to meet their own demand (Wilford et al., 2018). Wilford and colleagues (2018) advise that in order to boost efficiency, all health systems will need to explore task shifting and upskilling, making best use of community health workers (CHWs). In the case of EHDI, I suggest training PHC nurses. It has been argued that CHWs are central to integrated HIV and tuberculosis (TB) care and cover important gaps in maternal and child services (Wilford et al., 2018). Such strategies are important now in the developing world, and not just for 2030. Decentralising and professionalising certain aspects of service delivery, such as screening, as part of preventative care requires increased attention in order for the PHC approach to be successful in South Africa. Task sharing, task shifting and role release are important considerations given the human resource predicament the country finds itself in. This includes training nurses, volunteers and CHWs. Clear minimum standards for training non-professionals would need to be established, and clear and specific scopes of practice promulgated. This would ensure protection of the public and prevent malpractice claims, which are a significant expenditure and undesirable in a resource-constrained context like South Africa. The National Treasury (2018) has acknowledged the impact on provincial health budgets of the contingent liabilities for malpractice claims. It noted that the 'value of claims against health departments grew from R43.1 billion in 2016 to R56.3 billion in 2017', and, while acknowledging that 'some of these claims relate to serious errors in clinical practice or hospital management ... others appear to be unjustified or excessive' (National Treasury, 2018, p. 75).

As far as scopes of practice are concerned, role ambiguity and conflict are important impediments to the effective implementation of decentralised services. For example, implementation of district-based clinical specialist teams in South Africa is reportedly significantly impacted by role ambiguity and conflict (Oboirien, Harris, Goudge, & Eyles, 2018). It has been argued that having family physicians on the staff of both community health centres and district hospitals would lead to improved care. However, this has not been found to be true in the South African context, where the results have been mixed (Von Pressentin et al., 2018). Staff retention at this level of care was challenging. In a survey of 514 health care professionals (including doctors, dentists, dental therapists, pharmacists, physiotherapists and radiographers) employed at public sector district hospitals in KwaZulu-Natal, findings showed that 87 percent had worked in such settings for five years or less, while 65 percent planned to leave in the near future (29 percent at the end of the year in which the survey was conducted) (Ross, Gumede, & Mianda, 2017). Staff retention challenges are linked to limited career paths; budgetary constraints, including poor salaries; as well as the increasing pressure to accommodate ever-larger numbers of interns and community service practitioners (Health Systems Trust, 2018). These challenges apply equally in the speech-language and hearing (SLH) professions, and have significant implications for the provision of SLH services, including EHDI implementation.

According to the *South African Health Review* (Health Systems Trust, 2018), although over 80 percent of the South African population depends entirely on public health facilities, only 30 percent of specialists work in that sector. Only 3 out of every 10 doctors on the professional register work in public hospitals and clinics; 1 in 10 registered dentists works in a public hospital or clinic; 4 in 10 registered professional nurses work in public health facilities, with half of enrolled nurses employed in the public health sector; only 1 in 10 registered pharmacists works in a public hospital or clinic; fewer than 2 in 10 registered physiotherapists work in public facilities; and about 1 in 20 registered psychologists works in the public sector. Figure 5.1 and Table 5.1 depict numbers of SLH professionals registered

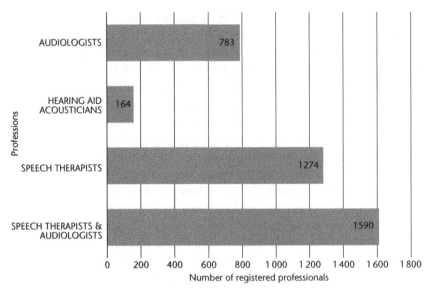

Figure 5.1 SLH professionals registered with the HPCSA nationally, January 2020
Source: Based on data obtained from the HPCSA registration department (HPCSA, 2018a)

Table 5.1: SLH professionals registered with the HPCSA in January 2020 by province

	SLH category			
	Aud	**HAA**	**ST**	**STA**
Eastern Cape	33	16	51	40
Free State	15	4	33	33
Gauteng	233	61	363	949
KwaZulu-Natal	273	25	278	131
Limpopo	23	11	15	107
Mpumalanga	47	5	55	88
North West	7	8	17	35
Northern Cape	11	6	22	10
Western Cape	141	28	440	197
Total	**783**	**164**	**1274**	**1590**

Source: Based on data obtained from the HPCSA registration department (HPCSA, 2018a)

Note: Aud = audiologist; HAA = hearing aid acoustician; ST = speech therapist; STA = speech therapist and audiologist with the Health Professions Council of South Africa (HPCSA) by January 2020, for the entire South African population, clearly highlighting the demand–capacity challenge. The lack of staffing norms for the SLH professions in the South African context complicates this scenario, as lobbying for posts becomes challenging.

State health spending in South Africa is challenging at a time of low economic growth and fiscal constraint (Blecher et al., 2017), with R183 billion having been spent in the public sector alone in 2017/18 (United Nations Children's Fund [UNICEF], 2017). This lack of adequate funding has led to the health sector responding in various ways, with implications for EHDI implementation: personnel numbers have been reduced and various posts frozen when vacated; there is a focus on greater savings on medicine tenders; the establishment of ministerial non-negotiable budget items; budget cuts on administration and expenditure as well as on buildings and medical equipment; budget cuts on capital projects and equipment purchases; and increased emphasis on PHC (Blecher et al., 2017). Currently, the public health sector is in a well-documented staff crisis (Akintola, Gwelo, Labonté, & Appadu, 2016; Bateman, 2007), with the quality of care compromised and remaining staff overextended. These challenges affect health care initiatives, particularly those aimed at issues that are not considered life threatening, such as hearing impairment. It is therefore a challenge to implement EHDI in South Africa as it has to compete for attention with highly prevalent life-threatening communicable diseases such as HIV/AIDS and TB.

Burden of disease

HIV is the greatest contributor to the burden of disease in South Africa and uses most of the health budget. Health resources and the budget are geared towards curbing mortality, with insufficient attention being given to other health issues. The country in fact faces a quadruple burden of disease: maternal, newborn and child health; HIV/AIDS and TB; non-communicable diseases; and violence and injury. This quadruple burden, HIV/AIDS in particular, results in an increased workload for SLH professions. Thus, increased HIV infection rates raise implications for EHDI implementation, as detailed in chapter 11.

The most recent Joint United Nations Programme on HIV/AIDS (UNAIDS, 2019) estimates are that there were 37.9 million people living with HIV by the end of 2018, of whom 1.7 million were children. There were 1.7 million new HIV infections globally in 2018, with 160 000 being children aged 15 years or younger. Around 770 000 people worldwide died of AIDS-related deaths in

2018, with a 33 percent decline in AIDS-related mortality since 2010 (UNAIDS, 2019). South Africa, a developing middle-income country, is reported to have among the highest HIV/AIDS prevalence rates in the world, with 7.7 million people living with HIV in 2018, including approximately 320 000 children under the age of 14 (UNAIDS, 2019). National figures for South Africa reflected 240 000 new infections and 71 000 AIDS-related deaths in that year (UNAIDS, 2019). The 2018 UNAIDS *Global AIDS Update* reported on progress towards the 90-90-90 targets, which aim to ensure that 90 percent of people living with HIV know their status, that 90 percent of those who know their status are on treatment, and that 90 percent of people on treatment are virally suppressed. In 2018, globally, 79 percent of people living with HIV knew their status, 62 percent were reported to be accessing treatment, with 53 percent virally suppressed. In the same period, figures for South Africa reflect that 90 percent knew their status, 62 percent were on treatment and 54 percent were virally suppressed (UNAIDS, 2019). The 2019 UNAIDS report indicates a major milestone in the 90-90-90 targets, with 62 percent of all people living with HIV reported to be accessing antiretroviral therapy (ART). Improved access to ART resulted in 1.72 million fewer HIV-related deaths in adults from 2000 to 2014 than would have occurred otherwise (Johnson et al., 2017). In addition to reduced mortality and a reduction in the transmission of HIV, improved access has also had a measurable impact on the global workforce.

These are some of the realities that EHDI has to confront in the South African health care context, as they do not exist in isolation from other challenges in the paediatric population. HIV not only takes up the lion's share of the budget, but it also contributes to the burden of hearing impairment, which increases the workload for audiologists, including for early hearing detection and intervention (Khoza-Shangase & Anastasiou, 2020).

Newborn hearing screening contextualised

NHS programmes are an important step towards early detection of hearing impairment and the provision of early intervention. These programmes require careful examination and planning in each context. The HPCSA (2018b) recommended specific contexts in which to actualise EHDI application. Numerous studies, detailed in chapter 2, indicate that South Africa is far from achieving what is advocated by the HPCSA position statement (Bezuidenhout, Khoza-Shangase, De Maayer, & Strehlau, 2018; Friderichs, Swanepoel, & Hall, 2012; Kanji & Khoza-Shangase, 2019; Kanji, Khoza-Shangase, Petrocchi-Bartal, & Harbinson, 2018; Khoza-Shangase & Harbinson, 2015). Studies exploring the feasibility and current status of EHDI implementation in the South African health care context at various levels (primary, secondary and tertiary) have found a lack of formal, standardised and systematic EHDI implementation (Kanji, Khoza-Shangase, & Moroe, 2018; Swanepoel, Störbeck, & Friedland, 2009; Theunissen & Swanepoel, 2008). Various reasons are proposed for this: insufficient knowledge, lack of equipment, budgetary constraints and human resource challenges. Regardless of the level of care and varied resource allocations and levels of specialisation, EHDI implementation as advocated by the HPCSA in its 2018 position statement currently does not seem feasible, unless the barriers identified are addressed and NHS is mandated by the South African government. Findings from these studies also highlight the need to ensure that context-specific studies in EHDI are conducted. This is necessary to ensure that national position statements are sensitive to contextual challenges and allow for evidence-based practice. This is particularly important in South Africa, where resource constraints dictate the success or failure of a programme, no matter how well intended.

The HPCSA (2018b) guidelines and principles for EHDI are primarily based on guidelines from developed contexts, with slight contextual adaptations in terms of the timeframes for screening and diagnosis. These guidelines are geared towards UNHS and serve as the gold standard that audiologists in South Africa should aim to achieve. However, they may not be applicable in all health care sectors in the country, particularly the public health care sector. Kanji (2016) presents evidence from a research review of studies related to EHDI in South Africa. She notes the impracticalities of attempting to implement developed world models of NHS in LAMI countries, where contexts are very different. Kanji argues that the current status of NHS, coupled with human resources challenges, suggests that UNHS is currently not applicable in this country. The majority of registered audiologists in South Africa work in the private health care sector. There is thus a demand for personnel in the public health care sector given the higher prevalence rate of infant hearing impairment in that sector. Moreover, there is currently no established mid-level worker programme in audiology to facilitate hearing screening by personnel other than audiologists. These issues influence the ability of audiologists in South Africa to effectively implement UNHS and EHDI. Kanji (2016) argues for an interim approach to early detection of hearing impairment to identify affected newborns and infants who would ordinarily be missed given the absence of an NHS programme.

With hearing impairment in four to six of every 1 000 live births in the public sector, and three in 1 000 in the private sector in South Africa (Swanepoel et al., 2009, p. 783), there is a pressing need for systematic EHDI services. Progress is being made in offering NHS and studies have been conducted to document these processes in South Africa (Bezuidenhout et al., 2018; Friderichs et al., 2012; Kanji & Khoza-Shangase, 2018a, 2018b, 2019;

Moodley & Störbeck, 2015; Petrocchi-Bartal & Khoza-Shangase, 2014). However, due to the lack of a national and holistic overview of EHDI services to date, an accurate picture of the current status of EHDI is required. Moodley and Störbeck (2015) conducted a narrative review of EHDI in South Africa in order to document and profile what had been published in the field. Their findings revealed extensive knowledge related to paediatric hearing screening and intervention services. However, this evidence comes from studies mostly located in the provinces of Gauteng and the Western Cape (Friderichs et al., 2012). Furthermore, studies pertaining to the diagnosis of hearing impairment revealed that, although much has been written on the scientific aspects of the tools used, there is a lack of comprehensive information on diagnostic protocols and procedures (Kanji & Khoza-Shangase, 2018a; Moodley & Störbeck, 2015). Moodley and Störbeck (2015) note that despite the clear progress made in South Africa, comprehensive studies on protocols and procedures used in diagnosing paediatric hearing impairment are needed, with an expansion of focus beyond Gauteng and the Western Cape.

According to Petrocchi-Bartal and Khoza-Shangase (2014), there is a need for context-relevant research aimed at facilitating the efficacious provision of EHDI services in South Africa. Their findings illustrate that although South Africa is pushing the PHC agenda as its health strategy, PHC clinics in at least two provinces (one being the better-resourced Gauteng) did not provide formalised newborn or infant hearing screening and none of the facilities had the equipment to do so. Most sites attributed the lack of formalised hearing screening to budgetary and human resource issues, staff training in particular. Existing non-formalised hearing screening protocols demonstrated inconsistencies in application across districts and none complied with HPCSA clinic guidelines or any international guidelines. This is in addition to their lack of sensitivity and specificity. Petrocchi-Bartal and Khoza-Shangase (2014) conclude that unless assets and barriers to EHDI implementation are identified in the South African context, EHDI will remain an international goal that cannot be locally attained. They argue that it is important to establish what existing protocols are in use, and to review their implementation and effectiveness before national plans are recommended.

Petrocchi-Bartal and Khoza-Shangase (2014) found that the deprivational index did not influence their findings on screening procedures and protocols used at PHCs in South Africa. They suggest that this has implications for forward planning in PHC. The main reasons for the lack of formalised hearing screening – budgetary and human resource constraints, with staff training in particular being important – should be considered when planning for EHDI.

The ideal hearing screening measure is yet to be defined, with various NHS protocols currently being recommended for different contexts.

Such diverse recommendations create challenges where resources have to be negotiated and rationalised. No standardised protocol has been adopted in South Africa, hence Kanji and Khoza-Shangase's (2018a) call for further exploration and definition of feasible and context-specific protocols, as well as careful deliberation around high-risk registries (Kanji & Khoza-Shangase, 2019). Based on findings from their study, Kanji and Khoza-Shangase (2018a) recommend the use of a two-stage automated auditory brainstem response (AABR) protocol or transient evoked otoacoustic emission/AABR protocol in resource-stricken contexts, where the availability of all screening measure options may not be feasible.

'Doing better with less' approach

The implementation of risk-based or targeted newborn hearing screening (TNHS) programmes by trained volunteers or nurses seems to be the most feasible initial step while resources are procured for comprehensive UNHS. Bezuidenhout et al. (2018) highlight the fact that in South Africa, TNHS has not been formally and systematically implemented as the intermediate, small step towards a larger UNHS programme. Kanji (2016) suggests careful consideration of a number of factors for effective implementation of TNHS in South Africa, including the choice of screening measures and how they are employed in a screening protocol. This should occur while taking into account contextually relevant and established risk factors for hearing impairment in the various levels of service delivery in the South African health care system. Kanji and Khoza-Shangase (2019) extend the argument of contextualising risk factors by introducing the idea of always considering the quadruple influences on risk factors for hearing impairment in South Africa.

The currently used high-risk factors for hearing impairment stipulated by the HPCSA (2018b) are based on position statements from developed contexts and have been adapted to include two conditions that are considered unique to the South African context. While research findings from higher-income developed contexts may be of value, they are difficult to implement in practice in LAMI countries as they are contextually incongruent and often focus on non-communicable diseases that are prevalent in developed contexts. There is therefore a tendency to neglect the specific, local needs of lower-income or developing countries. This is a serious challenge, particularly in LAMI countries where the social determinants of health are vastly different to those in developed contexts. It is important to identify and contextualise risk factors for hearing impairment. Infants displaying any of these factors in their neonatal history have a greater chance of presenting with hearing impairment (Colella-Santos, Hein, De Souza, Do Amaral, & Casali, 2014;

Kanji & Khoza-Shangase, 2018b). Therefore, contextual research is imperative in guiding relevant clinical practice.

A variety of health care contexts need to be explored as possible platforms for the establishment and provision of NHS services, particularly TNHS as an interim approach. This is important as the context may influence coverage rates and follow-up return rates, two key determinants of effective and successful NHS programmes (Kanji, 2016). PHC clinics in South Africa have been proposed as a platform for conducting NHS in order to ensure optimal coverage and follow-up return rates. A study in Gauteng revealed that a significant number of well neonates were missed because of early discharge soon after birth and some babies were born at home, making it difficult to coordinate screening (Bezuidenhout et al., 2018; Khoza-Shangase & Harbinson, 2015). Kanji (2016) is of the view that a two-tiered approach may be appropriate, involving early hearing screening of high-risk babies in the hospital setting, with screening of well babies at clinic level. This would ensure a more comprehensive coverage of babies, regardless of their health status, or time or place of birth. This requires coordinated and systematic planning by audiologists, who need to play an active role in piloting, planning, implementing and managing TNHS programmes in the South African public health care context.

The challenges outlined in this chapter are not unique to South Africa. Kumar, Kolethekkat, and Kurien (2015) studied the age of suspicion, confirmation and amplification of hearing handicap in children, and assessed the burden of parental delay in the evaluation of hearing loss in South India. They found significantly delayed ages of detection and intervention, with clear indications of EHDI not being feasible in their developing country context. They argue that these EHDI implementation challenges are due to lack of parental knowledge about the handicap and its identification, a dearth of hearing health care professionals, as well as resource constraints. They acknowledge that setting up EHDI through UNHS is a challenge in developing countries, although an unavoidable strategy. Hence, cost-effective national policies with well-structured scientific educational programmes that have community support should be considered in order to enhance the linguistic, psychological and social development of hearing-impaired children. Based on their research in Sudan, Ahmed, Hajabubker, and Satti (2017) recommend the early screening of neonates and infants with risk factors by introducing an NHS programme, the safe administration of drugs, activation of primary health programmes, as well as the establishment of audiological units throughout the country.

EHDI challenges in the South African context include poor follow-up return rates. This is especially problematic because follow-up appointments ensure that benchmarks are met and that no child with suspected hearing loss is left unidentified. Kanji and Krabbenhoft (2018) identified factors influencing audiological follow-up of high-risk infants in a risk-based NHS programme in South Africa. Their findings reveal that the most common contributors facilitating participants' attendance at follow-up appointments are friendly audiologists, a clear line of communication between caregiver and audiologist, and a reminder of the appointment. The most significant perceived challenge that participants described in returning for the follow-up appointment was living far away from the hospital. Kanji and Krabbenhoft (2018) conclude that demographic, socio-economic and interpersonal factors influence follow-up return rates. They recommend implementing an all-inclusive appointment day for the South African population in order to resolve this challenge. They further caution that it is not only important to look at what is being done to improve the follow-up return rate, but also how it should be done in terms of professional-to-patient communication and interactions. Findings from this study are supported by those of Kanji and Khoza-Shangase (2018b) in the same context, and those of Scheepers, Swanepoel, and Roux (2014). In Kanji and Khoza-Shangase's (2018b) study, the return rate decreased significantly, to below 50 percent, for follow-up diagnostic assessment. Reasons for non-attendance varied from change of residential location (the most common) to maternal age. The mean maternal age of mothers who returned with their newborns for diagnostic assessment was significantly higher than for those who did not return. The authors conclude that reasons for follow-up default are influenced by contextual challenges, but may be improved by aligning appointments with other medical follow-up services.

Solutions and recommendations

Because NHS has become the standard of care internationally, with sufficient evidence proving its efficacy, South Africa needs to plan strategically in order to be able to implement successful EHDI programmes. In the framework of an intersectoral approach, each of the country's nine provinces needs to put in place an EHDI programme responsible for establishing, maintaining and improving the system of services needed to serve children with hearing impairment and their families. This needs to take place at the various levels of health care to ensure increased access, and within the proposed NHI system. Furthermore, improved coordination is called for between the departments of health, education and social development.

There is a need for audiologists to adopt an advocacy role to promote NHS/EHDI. This can be in the form of public–private partnerships, as well as government–non-government organisation collaborations, such as that with HI HOPES (Home intervention: Hearing and language opportunities parent education services). This should take place while adhering to ethical conduct, HPCSA regulations around screening, and the protection of personal information. Such advocacy should include ensuring the sustainability of EHDI services in this context.

While there have been some developments in recent years, significant challenges to NHS, follow-up and early intervention still exist. The HPCSA SLH Board constituted an EHDI task team to put together national guidelines to be implemented in the public and private sectors. These guidelines require provinces to host national strategic planning activities to identify EHDI programme coordinators. These coordinators will in turn identify ways to implement the guidelines through the use of a SWOT (strengths, weaknesses, opportunities, threats) analysis framework. A SWOT analysis and subsequent TOWS (threats, opportunities, weaknesses, strengths) matrix analysis are commonly used methods of strategic planning, and are a strategy recommended by White and Blaiser (2011). Such strategic planning should include deliberations around the use of tele-audiology as a complementary approach to deal with the demand–capacity challenges around the availability of audiologists in the country.

Tele-audiology, a subset of telehealth, was established primarily to deliver audiological care in areas with limited access to health care due to a shortage of resources. Krupinski (2015) describes telehealth as the use of telecommunication technologies to reach out to patients, reduce barriers to optimal care in underserved areas, improve user satisfaction and accessibility to specialists, decrease professional isolation in rural areas, help medical practitioners expand their practice reach, and save patients from having to travel or be transported to receive high-quality care. An obvious advantage of tele-audiology is that it may help overcome common barriers to early identification of hearing impairment and obtaining hearing aids, such as cost and distance from service providers (Schweitzer, Moritz, & Vaughan, 1999).

In LAMI countries such as South Africa, many people continue to experience barriers to accessing health care services. While multiple factors contribute to these barriers (Khoza-Shangase & Mophosho, 2018), the establishment of tele-audiology was inspired by the extreme shortages of audiologists, speech-language pathologists and ear, nose and throat specialists (Fagan & Jacobs, 2009; Mulwafu, Ensink, Kuper, & Fagan, 2017). The health professionals that are available are often located in health centres in big cities and private practices, where many people cannot access their services. The situation is made worse for UNHS by the limited working hours of audiologists, who miss babies born during off hours, and babies born and discharged when audiologists are attending to other work responsibilities. Therefore, tele-audiology could become an alternative model of service delivery, with audiologists serving as programme managers or directors while trained screeners or nurses perform the screening services. However, South Africa has not made significant strides in its progress for health technology assessment (HTA). A legal and policy landscape analysis reveals that no specific provision in the National Health Act for HTA exists, and HTA is narrowly and incompletely defined. Siegfried, Wilkinson, and Hofman (2017) put out a call for the National Department of Health to host an HTA summit, and hopefully resolutions from this summit will positively impact tele-audiology.

Tele-audiology in EHDI can use computer-based technology and internet connectivity to screen all babies requiring screening, and not just those with risk factors. This can be done in a variety of ways, either synchronous or asynchronous. Synchronous tele-audiology requires the audiologist to be present during the session, though in a different location to the baby, for example through video-conferencing and remote programming of hearing aids (Steuerward, Windmill, Scott, Evans, & Kramer, 2018). Hughes, Sevier, and Choi (2018) found that this method is useful for programming hearing technologies such as cochlear implants. However, given capacity versus demand issues, such as too few audiologists for the number of patients requiring audiology services, as well as challenges around network connectivity, the implementation of synchronous tele-audiology may not yet be feasible in South Africa.

The asynchronous telehealth method can be used in the absence of an audiologist, and would thus be ideal for implementing EHDI programmes in South Africa, where the services of audiologists are not readily available. Screeners or nurses can be trained to conduct certain audiological tests, save the results and forward them to the audiologist managing the programme. Studies have demonstrated the accuracy of asynchronous tele-audiology when compared to traditional face-to-face diagnosis by qualified professionals (Biagio, Adeyemo, Hall, & Vinck, 2013; Biagio, Swanepoel, Laurent, & Lundberg, 2014). I recommend using both synchronous and asynchronous tele-audiology in EHDI programmes, given the challenges around network connectivity, particularly in rural and peri-urban areas, as well as the shortage of audiologists. Swanepoel et al. (2010) believe that the asynchronous method is more feasible for the South African context, especially in school settings. This has been confirmed in the education sector, where findings demonstrate that asynchronous telehealth-based automated hearing testing in the school context can be used to facilitate early identification of hearing impairment (Govender & Mars, 2018).

If non-audiologists such as screeners and nurses are to be involved in NHS, they must be well trained and minimum standards must be adhered to. Because nurses are the backbone of PHC, and PHC is the first point of contact with the health system for at least 85 percent of the South African population (Khan, Joseph, & Adhikari, 2018), it is important to ensure that this level of care is adequately equipped and resourced to implement NHS. Khan and colleagues (2018) investigated PHC nurses' experiences, practices and beliefs regarding hearing impairment in infants in KwaZulu-Natal, South Africa. Their findings revealed that at least one-third of PHC nurses had never screened a child for hearing impairment, and most clinics did not have access to basic hearing screening equipment or materials. Only 49 percent of nurses had access to an otoscope, while 31 percent used the Road to Health development screener to check for hearing impairment. None of the clinics had access to an otoacoustic emission screener or the Swart questionnaire, a case history questionnaire that was used in the Western Cape at clinic level as part of the prevention of hearing impairment due to otitis media. Although nurses reported that they would refer to audiology services for some of the risk factors, as indicated on the Joint Committee on Infant Hearing (JCIH, 2007) list, they were less likely to refer if the child was in a neonatal intensive care unit (NICU) for longer than five days, had neurodegenerative disorders, meningitis, hyperbilirubinaemia requiring blood transfusion or was undergoing chemotherapy. Less than a third of nurses always referred if the child displayed additional non-JCIH risk factors or those pertinent to the South African context. Approximately 38 percent reported that communities believed that hearing impairment could have spiritual or supernatural causes. These findings are similar to those at PHC clinics in Gauteng and Limpopo provinces (Kanji et al., 2018; Khoza-Shangase, Kanji, Petrocchi-Bartal, & Farr, 2017; Petrocchi-Bartal & Khoza-Shangase, 2014, 2016). Such findings demonstrate that hearing screening and referral practices at PHC clinics need to be strengthened for successful EHDI implementation, through imparting knowledge and skills to nurses. Knowledge dissemination would need to be extended to include educating parents about risk factors and hearing impairment.

Studies have supported the need for parental education in order to enhance EHDI implementation in South Africa. Govender and Khan (2017) describe the knowledge (including cultural beliefs) of mothers in Durban regarding risk factors for hearing impairment in infants and their awareness of audiology services. Their findings reveal that just over half of the sampled mothers were aware of risk factors, such as middle ear infections, ototoxic medication and consumption of alcohol during pregnancy. However, two-thirds did not know which professional to seek help from. Seventy percent were unaware that NICU/mechanical ventilation for more than five days, prematurity, rubella and jaundice are considered risk factors for hearing impairment, highlighting the need for health education in this population. The cultural beliefs around causes of hearing impairment found in this study call for careful consideration of cultural diversity and its potential impact on EHDI implementation. Sixty percent of the mothers believed that bewitchment and ancestral curses can cause hearing impairment. This finding cannot be ignored as it has significant implications for health-seeking behaviours in South Africa. Evidence on global health indicates that groups that do not form part of the dominant culture have worse health outcomes than dominant populations (Flood & Rohloff, 2018). EHDI initiatives must therefore take into consideration cultural influences if they are to be successful.

Success in programme implementation also relies on a proper data management system that allows for tracking of identified infants as well as coordinated referral pathways within a migration-aware health care system, which South Africa encourages (Vearey, Modisenyane, & Hunter-Adams, 2017). Data management includes data collection, storage, analysis and interpretation to guide the future planning, implementation and evaluation of EHDI programmes. A migration-aware health system calls for a response to migration and health that acknowledges that people move internally within South Africa, which has implications for EHDI nationally. Moodley and Störbeck (2017) investigated data management for EHDI in South Africa. They found that there was no uniform data management system in use nationally, and no consistent shared system in the public or private sectors. The majority of respondents in their study (44 percent) used a paper-based system for data recording. No public or private hospitals were using data management systems that enabled sharing of information with other medical professionals. These findings indicate a significant barrier to successful EHDI implementation in the country. Moodley and Störbeck (2017) argue that data management and tracking of the pathway from screening to diagnosis to intervention need careful attention in South Africa to ensure quality care and outcomes for children identified with hearing impairment. Lack of uniform and adequate data, poor record keeping and referrals practices, and lack of tracking present significant barriers to EHDI service provision and monitoring. This needs to be addressed.

Conclusion

South Africa has made strides in growing the knowledge base in the field of EHDI, and has recognised and tried to overcome challenges in the implementation of EHDI services by researching and identifying alternative forums for screening, parent reasons for refusing screening, and the availability of early intervention services. However, studies have mainly been conducted in Gauteng and the Western Cape. Additionally, a large portion of the research is focused on the screening process, although some have looked at the usefulness of Auditory Steady State Response as a diagnostic tool and record reviews related to diagnostic procedures. The research has shown that South Africa lacks a nationally agreed battery of tests and protocols for diagnosing hearing impairment in infants and babies. Although the HPCSA (2018b) EHDI guidelines have been published, no process has yet been put in place to ensure their implementation by the Department of Health. Studies looking at the development of universal screening, diagnosis and intervention across both the public and private health care systems will provide much-needed information on all aspects of EHDI in a developing world context. This will make EHDI implementation in South Africa contextually relevant, responsive and responsible.

Given that EHDI is key for newborns and infants with hearing impairment, it is important to consider the realities of the South African health care context to ensure better implementation. As far as early detection is concerned, Kanji's (2018) recommendation that South Africa seriously consider targeted NHS as a starting point or interim approach, particularly in a hospital setting, should be carefully considered. Inclusion of NHS at the first follow-up visit at midwife obstetric units is recommended for all babies, including those without risk factors and those who were born at home. This approach respects both the documented evidence of established risk factors for hearing impairment, and the contextual challenge of resource constraints. It also responds to questions raised by Kanji (2018, p. 2) when she argues for a 'doing better with less' approach. She asks: 'As a profession in South Africa, what should we be advocating as standard care in the quest for the ideal? Are we attempting to digest the elephant as a whole instead of piecemeal as a logical step?' Targeted NHS can be argued to be a smaller logical step towards achieving the bigger UNHS target. This 'doing better with less' approach acknowledges that effective and quality health care is not only dependent on professionals but also involves using other stakeholders (Moyakhe, 2014), such as volunteers and nurses as screeners. It is only when such a strategic approach is adopted that the goals of EHDI in eradicating the negative impact of hearing impairment can be achieved.

This chapter addressed the challenges to EHDI implementation in South Africa. The issues around EHDI implementation are multidimensional, multilayered and complex. The chapter suggested that any response by South African stakeholders must be cohesive, comprehensive and integrated into existing service delivery platforms in an effort to 'do better with less'. An overview was provided of the South African context and the realities that need to be confronted when considering EHDI non-implementation in relation to competing priorities, such as the high burden of disease, resource limitations and the generally poor socio-economic status of the country. The chapter described relevant legislation and threats to the progressive realisation of the right to health care in South Africa, including EHDI. While in favour of UNHS, it was argued that it may not be immediately feasible given contextual limitations. Thus, contextually relevant risk-based screening should be implemented and the reasons for poor return rates explored. The chapter provided an evidence-based perspective in the South African context while acknowledging global trends, and concluded by offering suggestions for hearing detection initiatives that are contextually relevant.

References

Ahmed, S., Hajabubker, M. A., & Satti, S. A. (2017). Risk factors and management modalities for Sudanese children with hearing loss or hearing impairment done in Aldwha and Khartoum ENT hospitals, Sudan. *Annals of Tropical Medicine and Public Health, 10*, 357–361.

Akintola, O., Gwelo, N. B., Labonté, R., & Appadu, T. (2016). The global financial crisis: Experiences of and implications for community-based organizations providing health and social services in South Africa. *Critical Public Health, 26*(3): 307–321. doi: 10.1080/09581596.2015.1085959.

Bateman, C. (2007). Slim pickings as 2008 health staff crisis looms. *South African Medical Journal, 97*(11): 1020–1024.

Bezuidenhout, K. J., Khoza-Shangase, K., De Maayer, T., & Strehlau, R. (2018). Universal newborn hearing screening in public health care in South Africa: Challenges to implementation. *South African Journal of Child Health, 12*(4), 159–163. doi: 10.7196/SAJCH.2018.v12i4.1522.

Biagio, L., Adeyemo, A., Hall, J. W., & Vinck, B. (2013). Asynchronous video-otoscopy with a telehealth facilitator. *Telemedicine and e-Health, 19*(4), 252–258.

Biagio, L., Swanepoel, D. W., Laurent, C., & Lundberg, T. (2014). Paediatric otitis media at a primary healthcare clinic in South Africa. *South African Medical Journal, 104*(6), 431–435.

Blecher, M., Daven, J., Kollipara, A., Maharaj, Y., Mansvelder, A., & Gaarekwe, O. (2017). Health spending at a time of low economic growth and fiscal constraint. In A. Padarath & P. Barron (Eds.), *South African Health Review 2017*. Durban, South Africa: Health Systems Trust. Retrieved from http://www.hst.org.za/publications/south-african-health-review-2017.

Colella-Santos, M. F., Hein, T. A. D., De Souza, G. L., Do Amaral, M. I. R., & Casali, R. L. (2014). Newborn hearing screening and early diagnostic in the NICU. *BioMed Research International, 2014*, Article ID 845308, 1–11. doi: 10.1155/2014/845308.

Commission on the Social Determinants of Health (CSDH). (2008). Closing the gap in a generation: Health equity through action on the social determinants of health. Final *Report of the Commission on Social Determinants of Health*. Geneva, Switzerland: World Health Organization. Retrieved from https://apps.who.int/iris/bitstream/handle/10665/43943/9789241563703_eng.pdf;jsessionid=0DBA3E46A7358C1C5506BECC269A826C?sequence=1.

Department of Health (DoH). (2017). National health insurance for South Africa: Towards universal health coverage. Retrieved from http://www.health.gov.za/index.php/nhi?download=2257:white-paper-nhi-2017.

Fagan, J. J., & Jacobs, M. (2009). Survey of ENT services in Africa: Need for a comprehensive intervention. *Global Health Action, 2.* doi: 10.3402/gha.v2i0.1932.

Flood, D., & Rohloff, P. (2018). Indigenous languages and global health: Comment. *The Lancet, 6,* e134–135.

Friderichs, N., Swanepoel, D., & Hall, J. W. (2012). Efficacy of a community-based infant hearing screening program utilizing existing clinic personnel in Western Cape, South Africa. *International Journal of Pediatric Otorhinolaryngology, 76*(4), 552–559.

Ghebreyesus, T. A. (2017). All roads lead to universal health coverage. *Lancet Global Health, 5*(9), e839–e840.

Govender, S. M., & Khan, N. B. (2017). Knowledge and cultural beliefs of mothers regarding the risk factors of infant hearing loss and awareness of audiology services. *Journal of Public Health in Africa, 8*(1), 557. doi: 10.4081/jphia.2017.557.

Govender, S. M., & Mars, M. (2018). Assessing the efficacy of asynchronous telehealth-based hearing screening and diagnostic services using automated audiometry in a rural South African school. *South African Journal of Communication Disorders, 65*(1), a582. https://doi.org/10.4102/sajcd.v65i1.582.

Health Professions Council of South Africa (HPCSA). (2018a). Registrations department. Pretoria, South Africa.

Health Professions Council of South Africa (HPCSA). (2018b). Early hearing detection and intervention (EHDI) guidelines. Retrieved from http://www.hpcsa.co.za/Uploads/editor/UserFiles/downloads/speech/Early_Hearing_Detection_and_Intervention_(EHDI)_2018.pdf.

Health Systems Trust. (2018). *South African Health Review 2018 (21st ed.).* Retrieved from https://www.hst.org.za/publications/South%20African%20Health%20Reviews/SAHR%202018.pdf

Hogan, D. R., Stevens, G. A., Hosseinpoor, A. R., & Boerma, T. (2018). Monitoring universal health coverage within the sustainable development goals: Development and baseline data for an index of essential health services. *The Lancet Global Health, 6*(2), e152–e168.

Hughes, M. L., Sevier, J. D., & Choi, S. (2018). Techniques for remotely programming children with cochlear implants using pediatric audiological methods via telepractice. *American Journal of Audiology, 27,* 385–390.

Johnson, L. F., May, M. T., Dorrington, R. E., Cornell, M., Boulle, A., Egger, M., & Davies, M.-A. (2017). Estimating the impact of antiretroviral treatment on adult mortality trends in South Africa: A mathematical modelling study. *PLoS Med, 14*(12), e1002468.

Joint Committee on Infant Hearing (JCIH). (2007). Year 2007 position statement: Principles and guidelines for early hearing detection and intervention programs. *Pediatrics, 120*(4), 898–921.

Kanji, A. (2016). Early hearing screening in South Africa: Time to get real about context. *South African Journal of Child Health, 10*(4), 192.

Kanji, A. (2018). Early hearing detection and intervention: Reflections from the South African context. *South African Journal of Communication Disorders, 65*(1), a581. https://doi.org/10.4102/sajcd.v65i1.581.

Kanji, A., & Khoza-Shangase, K. (2018a). Objective hearing screening measures: An exploration of a suitable combination for risk-based newborn hearing screening. *Journal of American Academy of Audiology, 29*(6), 495–502. https://doi.org/10.3766/jaaa.16155.

Kanji, A., & Khoza-Shangase, K. (2018b). In pursuit of successful hearing screening: An exploration of factors associated with follow-up return rate in a risk-based newborn hearing screening programme. *Iranian Journal of Pediatrics, 28*(4), e56047. doi: 10.5812/ijp.56047.

Kanji, A., & Khoza-Shangase, K. (2019). Early detection of hearing impairment in high risk neonates: Let's talk about the high-risk registry in the South African context. *South African Journal of Child Health, 13*(2), 53–55. doi: 10.7196/SAJCH.2019.v13i2.1675.

Kanji, A., & Krabbenhoft, K. (2018). Audiological follow-up in a risk-based newborn hearing screening programme: An exploratory study of the influencing factors. *South African Journal of Communication Disorders, 65*(1), e1–e7. doi: 10.4102/sajcd.v65i1.587.

Kanji, A., Khoza-Shangase, K., & Moroe, N. (2018). Newborn hearing screening protocols and their outcomes: A systematic review. *International Journal of Pediatric Otorhinolaryngology, 115*, 104–109.

Kanji, A., Khoza-Shangase, K., Petrocchi-Bartal, L., & Harbinson, S. (2018). Feasibility of infant hearing screening from a developing country context: The South African experience. *Hearing, Balance and Communication, 16*(4), 263–270. https://doi.org/10.1080/21695717.2018.1519144.

Khan, N., Joseph, L., & Adhikari, M. (2018). The hearing screening experiences and practices of primary health care nurses: Indications for referral based on high-risk factors and community views about hearing loss. *African Journal of Primary Health Care & Family Medicine, 10*(1), a1848. https://doi.org/10.4102/phcfm.v10i1.1848.

Khoza-Shangase, K., & Anastasiou, J. (2020). An exploration of recorded otological manifestations in South African children with HIV/AIDS: A pilot study. *International Journal of Pediatric Otorhinolaryngology, 133*. https://doi.org/10.1016/j.ijporl.2020.109960.

Khoza-Shangase, K., & Harbinson, S. (2015). Evaluation of universal newborn hearing screening in South African primary care. *African Journal of Primary Health Care and Family Medicine, 7*(1), 1–12.

Khoza-Shangase, K., Kanji, A., Petrocchi-Bartal, L., & Farr, K. (2017). Infant hearing screening in a developing-country context: Status in two South African provinces. *South African Journal of Child Health, 11*(4), 159–163. doi: 10.7196/sajch.2017.v11i4.1267.

Khoza-Shangase, K., & Mophosho, M. (2018). Language and culture in speech-language and hearing professions in South Africa: The dangers of a single story. *South African Journal of Communication Disorders, 65*(1), 594.

Krupinski, E. (2015). Innovations and possibilities in connected health. *Journal of American Academy of Audiology, 26*, 761–767.

Kumar, S., Kolethekkat, A. A., & Kurien, M. (2015). Challenges in the detection and intervention of childhood deafness: Experience from a developing country. *International Journal of Biomedical Research, 6*(01), 40–45.

Moodley, S., & Störbeck, C. (2015). Narrative review of EHDI in South Africa. *South African Journal of Communication Disorders, 62*(1), 126. doi: 10.4102/sajcd.v62i1.126.

Moodley, S., & Störbeck, C. (2017). Data management for early hearing detection and intervention in South Africa. *South African Journal of Information Management, 19*(1), 6.

Motsoaledi, A. (2012). Department of Health budget vote speech 2012/13 by Minister of Health Aaron Motsoaledi, National Assembly, Cape Town. Retrieved from http://cegaa.org/resources/docs/Knowledge_Centre/Policy_Docs/SA_Dept_of_Health_Budget_Vote_Speech_2012.pdf.

Moyakhe, N. P. (2014). Quality healthcare: An attainable goal for all South Africans? *South African Journal of Bioethics and Law, 7*(2), 80–83.

Mulwafu, W., Ensink, R., Kuper, H., & Fagan, J. (2017). Survey of ENT services in sub-Saharan Africa: Little progress between 2009 and 2015. *Global Health Action, 10*(1), Art. #1289736. doi: 10.1080/16549716.2017.1289736.

National Treasury. (2018). *Budget review 2018*. Pretoria, South Africa: National Treasury.

Oboirien, K., Harris, B., Goudge, J., & Eyles, J. (2018). Implementation of district-based clinical specialist teams in South Africa: Analysing a new role in a transforming system. *BMC Health Services Research, 18*(1), 600. https://doi.org/10.1186/s12913-018-3377-2.

Petersen, L., & Ramma, L. (2015). Screening for childhood hearing impairment in resource constrained settings: Opportunities and possibilities. *South African Medical Journal, 105*(11), 901–902.

Petrocchi-Bartal, L., & Khoza-Shangase, K. (2014). Hearing screening procedures and protocols in use at immunisation clinics in South Africa. *South African Journal of Communication Disorders, 61*(1), Art. #66, 9 pages. http://dx.doi.org/10.4102/sajcd.v61i1.66.

Petrocchi-Bartal, L., & Khoza-Shangase, K. (2016). Infant hearing screening at primary health care immunization clinics in South Africa: The current status. *South African Journal of Child Health, 10*(2), 139–143. doi: 10.7196/SAJCH.2016.v10i2.1114.

Ranchod, S., Adams, C., Burger, R., Carvounes, A., Dreyer, K., Smith, A., ... Van Biljon, C. (2017). South Africa's hospital sector: Old divisions and new developments. In A. Padarath & P. Barron (Eds.), *South African Health Review 2017* (pp. 101–110). Durban, South Africa: Health Systems Trust. Retrieved from http://www.hst.org.za/publications/south-africanhealth-review-2017.

Ross, A., Gumede, D., & Mianda, S. (2017). Staffing levels at KwaZulu-Natal district hospitals: Is the University of KwaZulu-Natal training for the needs of the province? *South African Family Practice, 60*(2), 58–62.

Scheepers, L. J., Swanepoel, D. W., & Roux, T. L. (2014). Why parents refuse newborn hearing screening and default on follow-up rescreening: A South African perspective. *International Journal of Pediatric Otorhinolaryngology, 78*(4), 652–658.

Schweitzer, C., Moritz, M. S., & Vaughan, N. (1999). Perhaps not by prescription – but by perception. In S. Kochkin & K. E. Strom (Eds.), *High performance hearing solutions, Vol. 3. Hearing Review, 6*(1) [suppl], 58–62.

Siegfried, N., Wilkinson, T., & Hofman, K. (2017). Where from and where to for health technology assessment in South Africa? A legal and policy landscape analysis. In A. Padarath & P. Barron (Eds.), *South African Health Review 2017* (pp. 41–48). Durban, South Africa: Health Systems Trust. Retrieved from http://www.hst.org.za/publications/south-african-health-review-2017.

Steuerward, W., Windmill, I., Scott, M., Evans, T., & Kramer, K. (2018). Stories from the webcams: Cincinnati children's hospital medical center audiology telehealth and pediatric auditory device services. *American Journal of Audiology, 27*, 391–402.

Swanepoel, D. W., Clark, J. L., Koekemoer, D., Hall, J. W., Krumm, M., & Ferrari, D. V. (2010). Telehealth in audiology: The need and potential to reach underserved communities. *International Journal of Audiology, 49*, 195–202.

Swanepoel, D., Störbeck, C., & Friedland, P. (2009). Early hearing detection and intervention services in South Africa. *International Journal of Pediatric Otorhinolaryngology, 73*(6), 783–786.

Theunissen, M., & Swanepoel, D. (2008). Early hearing detection and intervention services in the public health care sector in South Africa. *International Journal of Audiology, 47*, S23–S29.

UNAIDS. (2018). *Global AIDS update 2018: Miles to go – closing gaps, breaking barriers, righting injustices.* Geneva, Switzerland: UNAIDS.

UNAIDS. (2019). UNAIDS data 2019. Retrieved from https://www.unaids.org/sites/default/files/media_asset/2019-UNAIDS-data_en.pdf.

United Nations Children's Fund (UNICEF). (2017). Health budget South Africa 2017/2018. Retrieved from https://www.unicef.org/esaro/UNICEF_South_Africa_--_2017_--_Health_Budget_Brief.pdf.

Vearey, J., Modisenyane, M., & Hunter-Adams, J. (2017). Towards a migration-aware health system in South Africa: A strategic opportunity to address health inequality. In A. Padarath & P. Barron (Eds.), *South African Health Review 2017* (pp. 89–98). Durban, South Africa: Health Systems Trust. Retrieved from http://www.hst.org.za/publications/south-african-health-review-2017.

Von Pressentin, K. B., Mash, R. J., Baldwin-Ragaven, L., Botha, R. P. G., Govender, I., Steinberg, W. J., & Esterhuizen, T. M. (2018). The influence of family physicians within the South African district health system: A cross-sectional study. *Annals of Family Medicine, 16*(1), 28–36.

White, K. R., & Blaiser, K. M. (2011). Strategic planning to improve EHDI programs. *Volta Review, 111*(2), 83–108.

Wilford, A., Phakathi, S., Haskins, L., Jama, N. A., Mntambo, N., & Horwood, C. (2018). Exploring the care provided to mothers and children by community health workers in South Africa: Missed opportunities to provide comprehensive care. *BMC Public Health, 18*(1), 171.

World Health Organization (WHO). (2017). *Tracking universal health coverage: 2017 global monitoring report.* Geneva, Switzerland: World Health Organization & World Bank.

6 Contextualisation of Risk Factors for Hearing Impairment

Jane Fitzgibbons, Rachael Beswick and Carlie J. Driscoll

The introduction of universal newborn hearing screening (UNHS) programmes has changed the purpose of risk factor registries. Most developed nations with established UNHS programmes primarily use risk factors to identify children who may be at risk of developing postnatal hearing loss and require hearing surveillance throughout childhood. However, for countries without a universal platform, continued use of a risk factor registry is recommended to identify children who require audiological assessment for congenital hearing loss. This chapter reviews the key risk factors used in programmes globally for their relevance in the South African context. The chapter concludes with programme-level recommendations, as well as risk factors to be considered for a South African programme.

Risk factor registries have been used for many decades to identify infants and children at risk of permanent childhood hearing loss (PCHL). In 1973, the Joint Committee on Infant Hearing (JCIH) first published a list of five factors signalling increased risk of PCHL and recommended regular hearing evaluations for affected infants. Since then, ongoing discussion and emerging evidence has led to the development and release of five JCIH risk factor registry revisions. The most recent version, the JCIH 2007 position statement, identified 11 risk factors associated with PCHL, with eight of these marked as greater concern for delayed onset hearing loss (see JCIH, 2007).

Risk factor registries were initially developed as a primary screening tool to identify infants at risk of PCHL for diagnostic assessment and monitoring purposes (JCIH, 1973). During this time, risk factor registries were arguably the most effective method for identifying at-risk infants and were used routinely in developed nations. However, it became increasingly evident through review of established programmes that risk factor registries were not a sensitive method of screening as they only identified 50–60 percent of children with congenital hearing loss, with the remaining infants with PCHL having no identifiable risk factor(s) (Thompson et al., 2001).

For universal detection of congenital hearing loss, the use of risk factor registries in isolation has become less common and has been replaced by UNHS programmes. Universal screening was originally recommended in 1993 at the National Institutes of Health Consensus Development Conference on Early Identification of Hearing Impairment in Infants and Young Children. More than 20 years on, UNHS is a standard of care for newborns in developed countries worldwide (Hyde, 2005), but continues to be a challenge in some developing countries (Krishnan & Donaldson, 2013).

The advent of UNHS has modified the purpose of collecting risk factors for some programmes, as children with congenital hearing loss typically refer on the newborn hearing screen. In regions where UNHS is well established, risk factor registries are now used to identify children at risk of developing a postnatal hearing loss. Despite passing the newborn hearing screen, if children are identified with risk factors, they should receive follow-up diagnostic evaluation by 24 to 30 months of age (JCIH, 2007). However, in regions where UNHS has not been established, the JCIH continues to recommend the use of risk indicators to identify infants who should receive audiological evaluation to detect congenital hearing loss (JCIH, 2007).

Infant hearing screening in South Africa

In response to the JCIH (2000) position statement advocating for UNHS, in 2002 the Health Professions Council of South Africa (HPCSA) released a hearing screening position statement supporting targeted, risk-based screening as an interim step while working towards a goal of 98 percent UNHS coverage by 2010 (HPCSA, 2002). This proved to be overly optimistic, with neither targeted nor universal newborn hearing screening programmes established systematically across South Africa within this timeframe, nor by the present day (Khoza-Shangase, Kanji, Petrocchi-Bartal, & Farr, 2017).

A 2008 survey revealed only 7.5 percent of South African public hospitals had implemented any form of newborn hearing screening, with less than 1 percent offering a universal programme (Theunissen & Swanepoel, 2008). By 2011, 53 percent of private sector hospitals with obstetric units reported newborn hearing screening activities, but only 14 percent offered a true universal screen (Meyer & Swanepoel, 2011). Research continues to suggest that around 90 percent of South African newborns are not screened for hearing loss (Khoza-Shangase et al., 2017; Meyer & Swanepoel, 2011; Theunissen & Swanepoel, 2008).

Given the absence of hearing screening progress, the more recent HPCSA (2007, 2018) position statements proposed disregarding previous recommendations of risk-based screening in favour of UNHS. However, this refocus contradicts advice from the World Health Organization (2010, cited in Olusanya, 2011a) that unless UNHS is immediately practicable, high-risk infants should be selectively targeted for hearing screening. More recently, Kanji (2018) reiterated that conducting targeted or risk-based newborn hearing screening as an interim measure provides good foundations, and establishing a well-structured targeted approach using risk factors is better than no action.

Prior to establishing a risk factor registry, the target population and condition need to be defined to maximise the effectiveness of the registry. For example, risk factors present in all hearing losses (including conductive and unilateral) may differ to congenital bilateral hearing loss. Similarly, risk factors to be included in a programme post UNHS (that is, for postnatal hearing loss) may be different to those used to triage for detection of congenital hearing loss. Nonetheless, whether South Africa moves forward with targeted or universal newborn hearing screening, a risk factor registry specific to the South African context will be required, either for screening or for surveillance purposes.

Need for contextualisation

The JCIH risk factor registry is frequently adopted or adapted for infant hearing screening programmes internationally. However, JCIH recommendations may not be fully applicable for developing countries. Factors to consider when developing a risk factor registry specific for the local context are outlined below.

Risk factor prevalence

Risk factor prevalence can vary regionally, may differ between developing and developed nations and may change over time. For example, consanguinity is associated with non-syndromic hearing loss (Bener, Eihakeem, & Abdulhadi, 2005) but is not included in the JCIH's 2007 risk registry. Although less common in western nations, marrying a cousin or blood relation remains part of cultural practice in specific religious and ethnic groups (Bittles & Black, 2010) and should be considered if relevant to the programme.

Risk factor identification

This can prove challenging in certain contexts due to resource issues and cultural beliefs. For example, resource-poor countries may lack diagnostic resources for detection of some risk factors, such as birth asphyxia and hyperbilirubinaemia (Olusanya, 2011b). Additionally, parental concern about hearing ability, family history of hearing loss or maternal infections may go unmentioned due to embarrassment, social stigma or cultural beliefs about spiritual causes of hearing loss (Graham, Seeley, Gina, & Saman, 2019; Khan, Joseph, & Adhikari, 2018; Olusanya, 2011b).

Risk factor yield

This also needs to be considered before a risk factor is included in the local registry. A risk factor has most utility in detecting infant hearing loss when a high proportion of infants with that risk factor are born with or develop hearing loss. In a resource-limited context, risk factors with lower yields of hearing loss will place extra demand on screening resources, particularly when there is a high prevalence of that risk factor in the general infant population.

Alternative or additional risk factors

Alternative or additional risk factors to those recommended by the JCIH may emerge as flags for hearing loss in specific contexts. For example, in Nigeria, the lack of a skilled attendant at birth was highlighted as the most significant predictor of neonatal hearing loss, followed by neonatal jaundice requiring exchange transfusion. Targeting screening to only children who presented with these indicators would have enabled detection of permanent hearing loss in 77 percent of the study cohort (Olusanya, Wirz, & Luxon, 2008). Very low birth weight (VLBW), while not a cause of hearing loss per se, has high concurrence with factors listed in the HPCSA's risk registry and could be an easily measurable means of enlisting infants with relevant risk factors into hearing screening and surveillance (Kanji & Khoza-Shangase, 2012).

JCIH risk factor registry

The following sections review the JCIH (2007) risk factors and their relevance to the South African context. Additional risk factors specific to South Africa, including those in the HPCSA registry, are also discussed. Risk factors marked with an asterisk (*) are those specified by the JCIH and the HPCSA as having greater potential for progressive or postnatal hearing loss.

Caregiver concern regarding hearing, speech, language or developmental delay*

Evidence

Parental or caregiver concern is often not effective in detecting neonatal or early onset hearing loss as caregivers may not be alerted to possible hearing loss until early childhood when delays in speech and language are noted (Störbeck & Young, 2016; Watkin, Baldwin, & Laoide, 1990). Conversely, caregiver concern is often the first flag for postnatal hearing losses (Dedhia, Kitsko, Sabo, & Chi, 2013). Although caregivers may have delayed awareness of possible hearing problems in their children, if concern is raised, hearing screening is warranted.

Contextualisation

South African research has indicated gaps in caregiver knowledge about hearing loss, with variations noted in awareness of risk factors, developmental implications and importance of early intervention (Swanepoel & Almec, 2008; Swanepoel, Hugo, & Louw, 2005). In some cases, diagnosis may be delayed when parents prefer prayer or traditional healing for their child's hearing issues rather than seeking conventional medical advice (Graham et al., 2019).

There is also evidence that the health system may contribute to delays in diagnosis where parental concern exists. Although South Africa's Road to Health booklet contains a checklist of developmental milestones that primary health care nurses discuss with caregivers, only 31 percent of primary health care nurses use this to check for hearing concerns (Khan et al., 2018). A shortage in South Africa of audiologists and other professionals typically involved in diagnosis, medical management and early intervention for hearing-impaired children may also contribute to health system delays (Fagan & Jacobs, 2009).

A study by Störbeck and Young (2016) reported that although 81 percent of parents suspected a hearing loss, there was still on average a 10-month delay between suspicion of the hearing loss (18 months) and hearing loss confirmation (28 months). Whether the delay was due to parental inaction or inadequacies in the health system was unclear.

Improving caregiver awareness of normal developmental milestones, signs of hearing loss and importance of early intervention, consistent use of developmental checklists in primary health care settings, plus timely and ready access to hearing screening and diagnostic services where parental concern is noted may mitigate delays in detection of PCHL.

*Family history of permanent childhood hearing loss**

Evidence

Family history of hearing loss is commonly reported in infants and children with PCHL in developed nations. Reported prevalence of family history among cohorts of infants with congenital hearing loss ranges from 7 percent (Driscoll, Beswick, Doherty, D'Silva, & Cross, 2015) to over 20 percent (Adachi, Ito, Sakata, & Yamasoba, 2010; Cone-Wesson et al., 2000). Despite this, the evidence for including this risk factor on a risk factor registry is mixed, particularly if the purpose is for hearing monitoring post newborn screen (Driscoll et al., 2015). The downfall of this risk factor is that it generates a high referral rate. However, once hearing loss is detected, a large proportion will have family history as their only risk factor (Driscoll et al., 2015).

Contextualisation

Family history has been reported in 11–28 percent of South African infants and children with permanent hearing loss (Sellars & Beighton, 1983; Swanepoel,

Johl, & Pienaar, 2013), which mirrors prevalence data from developed nations. Given the high prevalence of hearing loss in South Africa (Ramma & Sebothoma, 2016), referral rates in this context would be high. Therefore, the HPCSA (2018) has introduced tighter criteria than the JCIH (2007) recommendations to include only 'first cousin or closer to baby'. This risk factor could be tightened further to specifically exclude hearing losses acquired through trauma, infection, ototoxic medication and other non-genetic causes, which would place less burden on screening resources.

'Family history' may also be currently under-reported as notification relies largely on parental report. Consideration needs to be given to how to elicit this information sensitively to avoid the potential social stigma around conditions such as hearing loss (Olusanya, 2011b).

Neonatal intensive care of more than five days or any of the following: extracorporeal membrane oxygenation (ECMO), assisted ventilation, exposure to ototoxic medications or loop diuretics, and hyperbilirubinaemia that requires exchange transfusion*

Evidence

Health conditions and medical interventions prevalent in the neonatal intensive care unit (NICU) may place infants at risk of permanent hearing loss. Reasons for higher prevalence of hearing loss in NICU graduates are not yet fully known. However, there is some evidence to suggest hypoxia, hyperbilirubinaemia, congenital infections and the individual or synergistic effects of ototoxic medication and noise exposure as potential causes (Berg, Spitzer, Towers, Bartosiewicz, & Diamond, 2005; Pourarian, Khademi, Pishva, & Jamali, 2012; Roizen, 2003; Williams, Van Drongelen, & Lasky, 2007).

Prevalence of hearing loss varies depending on the conditions surrounding the infant's stay in NICU. For example, in developed nations, permanent hearing loss (congenital and postnatal) has been reported in 16.7 percent of ECMO survivors (Lasky, Wiorek, & Becker, 1998) and in 37 percent of infants with persistent pulmonary hypertension of the newborn (Walton & Hendricks-Munoz, 1991). Permanent hearing loss has also been identified in 13 percent of infants with a history of hyperbilirubinaemia at levels indicating exchange transfusion (Amin et al., 2017). In this study, hearing impairment was either sensorineural or auditory neuropathy spectrum disorder (ANSD) and mostly detectable following resolution of hyperbilirubinaemia, although there were some cases of delayed onset hearing loss.

Hearing loss prevalence in NICU graduates can also depend on survival rates, which have changed over time and can also differ within and between countries (Roizen, 2003). In addition, medications with known ototoxic potential (aminoglycoside antibiotics, loop diuretics) are used in NICU to treat potentially life-threatening conditions. Regardless of the conditions, hearing loss in NICU graduates is markedly more prevalent than in well, full-term infants (Roizen, 2003).

Contextualisation

NICU admittance has been identified as a significant risk factor for hearing impairment in South Africa, with research indicating this risk factor as the most prevalent in children with a profound hearing loss (Le Roux, Swanepoel, Louw, Vinck, & Tshifularo, 2015). In this study, 28.1 percent had NICU stay as a risk factor, of which 90 percent exceeded five days. Neonatal hyperbilirubinaemia at levels requiring exchange transfusion has also been identified as a key risk indicator, as this condition was identified in 50 percent of a small cohort of South African children with ANSD (Swanepoel et al., 2013). Neonatal hyperbilirubinaemia is reported to be more common in low and middle-income countries due to late presentation at appropriate treatment facilities and prolonged suboptimal phototherapy (Olusanya, Ogunlesi, & Slusher, 2014).

In a resource-limited setting such as South Africa, infants who would be admitted to NICU in a developed nation may not always have access to full tertiary support. Therefore, alternative neonatal facilities outside of NICUs may warrant further investigation to understand the full impact of the above conditions (Khoza-Shangase et al., 2017).

In-utero infections such as cytomegalovirus (CMV), herpes simplex virus, syphilis, rubella and toxoplasmosis*

CMV
Evidence
Congenital CMV infection (cCMV) is the leading non-genetic cause of PCHL, with worldwide estimates of cCMV incidence varying from 0.3–2.0 percent (Barkai et al., 2014; Fowler et al., 2017; Leruez-Ville et al., 2017). Approximately 10–15 percent of infants with cCMV are symptomatic, of which one in three will experience hearing loss. The other 85–90 percent are asymptomatic, of which one in ten will experience hearing loss (Goderis et al., 2014). CMV-related hearing loss is typically sensorineural, often with postnatal onset, with severity highly variable (Cohen, Durstenfeld, & Roehm, 2014).

Contextualisation
Given the high prevalence of CMV in Africa, a significant proportion of pregnant women have already been exposed to CMV (Bates & Brantsaeter, 2016). Despite this, reinfection or reactivation during pregnancy can occur, which can lead to cCMV in the infant (Cannon, Schmid, & Hyde, 2010; Goderis et al., 2014). cCMV incidence rates have been reported between 2.5–6.0 percent (Pathirana et al., 2019; Tshabalala et al., 2018). While there is strong evidence

to include CMV as a risk factor, identification of cCMV may prove challenging in South Africa as CMV screening during pregnancy and post birth is uncommon (Momberg & Geerts, 2016) and infants may be asymptomatic at birth.

Herpes simplex virus (HSV) and syphilis
Evidence
While there are case reports of sensorineural hearing loss in children with HSV and syphilis, systematic reviews have concluded that there is insufficient evidence to define the incidence of hearing loss in these conditions (Chau, Atashband, Chang, Westerberg, & Kozak, 2009; Westerberg, Atashband, & Kozak, 2008). Despite this, these reviews concluded with the recommendation to continue hearing surveillance for affected neonates due to the lack of conclusive evidence for or against these congenital infections.

Contextualisation
HSV prevalence is high (30–80 percent) in sub-Saharan African women (Paz-Bailey, Ramaswamy, Hawkes, & Geretti, 2007), with congenital HSV infection affecting 15.4 per 100 000 live births (Looker et al., 2017). This rate is higher than that reported in Europe and Asia. Additionally, HSV infection is almost exclusively HSV-2 (genital, as opposed to HSV-1, orolabial), where case reports for hearing loss have been confirmed (Westerberg et al., 2008).

Prevalence rates for maternal syphilis are the highest in the world in the African region, with congenital syphilis estimated in 1 119 per 100 000 live births (Korenromp et al., 2019). Despite the higher rates of both infections in South Africa, more evidence is required to clarify the relevance of these risk factors in the South African context. In addition, as cultural factors may limit the disclosure of these infections, culturally sensitive communication with parents about the importance of accurate reporting of these risk factors to generate onward referrals is required (Swanepoel et al., 2005).

Rubella
Evidence
Maternal rubella infection has serious sequelae and may lead to foetal death or congenital anomalies (Banatvala & Peckham, 2007). Congenital rubella syndrome (CRS) occurs in 80–85 percent of infants where primary maternal infection is contracted in the first trimester. Infants may be symptomatic at birth and present with a characteristic 'blueberry muffin' rash. However, diagnosis of CRS may also occur at a later age, due to presentation of autism, or learning or behavioural problems (Banatvala & Peckham, 2007).

Hearing loss is a significant risk in maternal rubella acquired up to the fourth month of gestation. However, beyond this time point the risk is negligible. Hearing loss occurs in 70–90 percent of infants with CRS and is typically sensorineural, either bilateral or unilateral, and may be congenital, progressive or late onset, and of any degree (Banatvala & Peckham, 2007).

Contextualisation

Rubella vaccination is not currently part of South Africa's standard immunisation schedule and is widespread in South Africa, with a large proportion of the population exposed at a young age (Motaze et al., 2018). Reports indicate that more than 600 infants are born with CRS in South Africa annually (Schoub, Harris, McAnerney, & Blumberg, 2009). Therefore, for the South African context, rubella should be considered as a risk factor for a local registry.

Toxoplasmosis
Evidence

Congenital toxoplasmosis is associated with a range of potentially devastating complications including intracranial calcification, chorioretinitis and hydrocephalus. While most (85 percent) affected infants are asymptomatic at birth (Montoya & Liesenfeld, 2004), symptoms may present within the first two or three months (Khan & Khan, 2018). There is a moderate level of evidence to include congenital toxoplasmosis as a risk factor for congenital hearing loss, as studies have reported sensorineural hearing loss ranging from mild to profound in up to 30 percent of affected infants (De Castro Corrêa, Maximino, & Weber, 2018). However, a systematic literature review identified no conclusive cases of progressive or postnatal hearing loss associated with congenital toxoplasmosis (Brown, Chau, Atashband, Westerberg, & Kozak, 2009).

Contextualisation

Africa has high toxoplasmosis seroprevalence (Hammond-Aryee, Esser, & Van Helden, 2014). Differences in seroprevalence between cultural groups in southern Africa may be related to varying hygiene and dietary practices (Jacobs & Mason, 1978). Of people worldwide with HIV infection, those in sub-Saharan Africa have the highest rate (87.1 percent) of toxoplasmosis (Wang et al., 2017). Challenges in diagnostic confirmation of toxoplasmosis infection in resource-limited contexts (Hammond-Aryee et al., 2014), along with the high proportion of maternal and congenital infections that are asymptomatic, may hinder identification of this risk factor.

Craniofacial anomalies including those that involve the pinna, ear canal, ear tags, ear pits and temporal bone anomalies

Evidence

The risk factor 'craniofacial anomalies' is a broad category used to describe anatomical anomalies of the head and face, and includes cleft lip and/or palate, microtia, atresia, facial asymmetry or dysmorphia, microcephaly, hydrocephaly and others. The risk factor may occur in isolation or may be associated with a syndrome. Children with craniofacial anomalies are at increased risk of congenital and postnatal hearing loss, and middle ear pathology, with approximately 50 percent of infants with craniofacial anomalies presenting with some form of hearing loss (Cone-Wesson et al., 2000; De Jong, Toll, De Gier, & Mathijssen, 2011; Hayes, 1994). Given the different anatomical structures involved, type, degree and time course will vary (Beswick & Driscoll, 2013). Although neither the JCIH (2007) nor the HPCSA (2018) flags craniofacial anomalies as placing a child at risk of developing a postnatal hearing loss, evidence suggests these children are 2.6 times more likely than others to develop a postnatal hearing loss. Therefore, ongoing surveillance beyond the newborn period may be warranted for these children (Beswick, Driscoll, Kei, Khan, & Glennon, 2013).

Contextualisation

There is limited information regarding the relationship between craniofacial anomalies and hearing loss in the South African context. Despite this, prevalence data for some conditions provide insight into the relevance of including craniofacial anomalies in a risk factor registry. One area that has received some attention is cleft lip and palate, with a reported incidence of 0.3 per 1 000 live births (Butali & Mossey, 2009). This figure is likely under-reported as it excludes stillbirths, abortions and early neonatal deaths (Hlongwa, Levin, & Rispel, 2019). Cleft palate is also a feature of foetal alcohol syndrome, with rates among urban populations of Africans and South Africans of mixed ancestry being high (Mossey & Catilla, 2003). Hydrocephalus and facial defects have also been reported among the five most common birth defects in black South Africans, at an incidence of 1.3 per 1 000 and 0.3 per 1 000 births, respectively (Kromberg & Jenkins, 1982). The incidence of craniofacial conditions in South Africa, combined with the reported high incidence of hearing loss in craniofacial anomalies in developed nations, warrants inclusion of this risk factor in a registry.

Syndromes associated with hearing loss or progressive or late onset hearing loss*, such as neurofibromatosis, osteopetrosis and Usher syndrome; other frequently identified syndromes include Waardenburg, Alport, Pendred, and Jervell and Lange-Nielson
   AND

Physical findings, such as white forelock, which is associated with a syndrome known to include a sensorineural or permanent conductive hearing loss

Evidence

Hundreds of syndromes that are highly associated with hearing loss are included under the risk factor of 'syndrome associated with hearing loss'.

In addition to those listed by the JCIH and the HPCSA (listed above), the most common syndromes associated with hearing loss include Down syndrome, Muenke syndrome, DiGeorge syndrome, Crouzon/Pfeiffer syndrome, Treacher-Collins syndrome and Velocardiofacial syndrome (Beswick & Driscoll, 2013). Of particular note is Down syndrome as it continues to be the most common chromosomal disorder in many developed countries (1.4 in 1 000 births), with 38–78 percent having associated hearing loss (Shott, Joseph, & Heithaus, 2001). As with craniofacial anomalies, the type, degree and time course of hearing loss in infants and children with syndromes will vary depending on the anatomical structures involved (Beswick & Driscoll, 2013).

Contextualisation

Obtaining information regarding the prevalence of certain syndromes in South Africa is challenging given that there are no national surveys or registries on such conditions (Kromberg & Jenkins, 1982; Kromberg, Sizer, & Christianson, 2013). This is partly due to the lack of funding available for genetic services, as well as community and professional ignorance regarding the benefits of genetic testing and counselling (Kromberg et al., 2013). Despite this, Down syndrome has received some attention in the literature, with prevalence rates similar to those reported in developed nations (white 1.88/1 000; coloured 1.54/1 000; black 1.29/1 000) (Molteno, Smart, Viljoen, Sayed, & Roux, 1997). However, unlike developed nations, diagnosis frequently does not occur until 7 to 12 months of age or later, with a relatively low accuracy of clinical suspicion reported (Willoughby, Aldous, Patrick, Kavonic, & Christianson, 2016). Other syndromes, such as Waardenburg, Pendred and Usher, are reported to be uncommon in native sub-Saharan African populations (Rudman et al., 2017). If syndromes are to be included in a risk factor registry, a comprehensive list of relevant syndromes, as well as associated medical training in identification and testing, should occur to ensure appropriate referral and surveillance is undertaken.

Neurodegenerative disorders, such as Hunter syndrome, or sensory motor neuropathies, such as Friedreich's ataxia and Charcot-Marie-Tooth syndrome*

Evidence

As the initial symptoms of neurodegenerative disorders often present later in childhood, identifying children at birth with this risk factor to enable hearing monitoring is difficult. For example, Hunter syndrome is commonly diagnosed between four and eight years of age, with hearing loss frequently conductive, followed by later onset of sensorineural loss (Wraith et al., 2008). Friedreich's ataxia is typically identified between 10 and 15 years but can be detected as early as two years (Delatycki et al., 1999).

Sensorineural hearing loss has been reported in 13 percent of individuals (Dürr et al., 1996), with evidence of auditory processing disorder in 64 percent (Rance et al., 2010). As research indicates that two out of three infants born with neurodegenerative disorders will be diagnosed with congenital hearing loss (Dumanch et al., 2017), it is important to include hearing monitoring in the treatment care plan once the diagnosis of a neurodegenerative disorder occurs.

Contextualisation

There is limited prevalence data for paediatric neurodegenerative disorders in South Africa and even less is known about hearing in affected individuals. Molecular testing has identified 253 families (mainly black and coloured) with spinocerebellar ataxia and 30 families (mainly white) with Friedreich's ataxia, although this is likely an under-representation of South Africans with hereditary ataxia (Smith, Greenberg, & Bryer, 2016). Prevalence of Hunter syndrome in South Africa is unknown (Khan et al., 2017). Given the limited information available, the relevance of this risk factor in the South African context is also unknown.

Culture-positive postnatal infections associated with sensorineural hearing loss, including confirmed bacterial and viral (especially herpes viruses and varicella) meningitis*

Evidence

The presentation of hearing impairment for the infections included under the 'postnatal infection' risk factor varies given the origin of the infection and the availability of vaccinations. For example, reports globally indicate 33.9 percent of people with bacterial meningitis develop significant hearing loss (Edmond et al., 2010). Measles accounted for 5–10 percent of profound hearing losses in the United States prior to widespread vaccination (McKenna, 1997) and remains a common cause of profound bilateral sensorineural hearing loss in areas without measles vaccination (Dunmade, Segun-Busari, Olajide, & Ologe, 2006). The incidence of hearing loss from mumps infections varies and may be due to differences in national vaccination schedules (Cohen et al., 2014).

Contextualisation

Meningitis has been identified as a significant contributor to hearing loss in South Africa, with one study identifying 10 percent of children with profound hearing loss having contracted meningitis (Le Roux et al., 2015). Another study indicated that nearly one-third of children admitted with bacterial meningitis to a Cape Town tertiary hospital presented with severe to profound hearing loss (Kuschke, Goncalves, & Peer, 2018). Reports also indicate that risk of major sequelae from bacterial meningitis is twice as high in Africa than in developed nations (Edmond et al., 2010).

Despite having a vaccination schedule for measles, data indicate gaps in measles vaccination coverage. In 2017, there were three measles outbreaks in communities with low coverage, with 58 laboratory-confirmed cases in children under five years (Hong et al., 2017). Given these coverage gaps and the potentially increased risk of serious sequelae, postnatal infections may be a significant risk factor for postnatal hearing loss in South Africa.

Head trauma*, especially basal skull/temporal bone fracture requiring hospitalisation

Evidence
Head trauma can cause hearing loss in a number of ways including tympanic membrane perforation, haemotympanum, ossicular chain disruption, cochlear concussion, perilymph fistula, fracture of the bony labyrinth, eighth nerve damage and/or damage to the central auditory pathways (Basson & Van Lierop, 2009; Villarreal, Méndez, Silva, & Álamo, 2016). Depending on the nature of the injury, any degree and type of hearing loss may occur. Research indicates that up to 34 percent of children admitted to hospital with significant head injury will have hearing loss, with temporal bone fracture being the most strongly associated with hearing loss (Bowman et al., 2011).

Contextualisation
One of the obstacles in South Africa contributing to reduced insight into the occurrence of hearing impairment in children with head trauma relates to under-referral to audiologists, which may lead to unreported or unidentified hearing loss. One study indicated that only 20 percent (20/100) of children with traumatic brain injury had received formal audiological testing, of whom 70 percent had confirmed hearing loss (Penn, Watermeyer, & Schie, 2009). Given the high rate of hearing loss associated with head trauma, audiological assessment should be included in the medical review for this caseload.

Chemotherapy*

Evidence
Although there is no conclusive evidence for the ototoxic potential of prenatal exposure to anticancer drugs (Briggs & Freeman, 2017), the ototoxic effects of cisplatin and carboplatin administered postnatally are well documented. Estimates of permanent hearing loss in children following cisplatin treatment range between 10 and 85 percent, with losses varying from sloping high frequency to profound, bilateral sensorineural impairment.

Higher cumulative doses are also associated with greater ototoxic effects (Helt-Cameron & Allen, 2009). Therefore, although there is no evidence to monitor children whose mothers have received chemotherapy during pregnancy, hearing monitoring of children undergoing chemotherapy is recommended.

Contextualisation

Despite the frequency of hearing impairment in children who receive chemotherapy, reports indicate only 55 percent of paediatric oncologists from two South African hospitals counsel parents of children undergoing chemotherapy about potential ototoxic effects and refer to audiology (Moroe & Hughes, 2017). Increased knowledge sharing and collaboration between paediatric oncologists, audiologists and parents may help close this gap and improve access to hearing monitoring for infants and children undergoing chemotherapy in South Africa.

HPCSA risk factors currently published

*Maternal and/or infant HIV infection**

The HPCSA's 2007 and 2018 position statements identify HIV as a context-specific risk factor for hearing loss due to the HIV epidemic in South Africa (Rehle et al., 2007; Zuma et al., 2016). Widespread use of antiretroviral therapy by pregnant HIV-positive women reduced in-utero and perinatal mother-to-child transmission rates to 0.9 percent in 2016/17. Prevalence rates indicate 245 HIV-positive neonates per 100 000 live births (Goga et al., 2018), with an estimated 280 000 HIV-positive children aged 0 to 14 years in South Africa (UNAIDS, 2018).

Although prevalence of congenital hearing loss may not be elevated in HIV-positive infants (Fasunla et al., 2014; Manfredi, Zuanetti, Mishima, & Granzotti, 2011; Olusanya, Afe, & Onyia, 2009), a strong association between HIV and postnatal hearing loss is reported in low and middle-income countries, including South Africa. Hearing loss prevalence in HIV-infected children ranges between 22 and 39 percent, with conductive hearing loss identified as the most common type (Ensink & Kuper, 2017).

Hearing loss may occur as a direct result of the HIV exposure (that is, from infections such as meningitis, toxoplasmosis and CMV) or due to ototoxic effects of medication for co-infections. Immunocompromised children are also at higher risk of developing chronic middle ear infections and associated conductive hearing loss (Ensink & Kuper, 2017). Therefore, given the high prevalence of hearing impairment in infants and children who are HIV positive, in conjunction with the high rates of HIV in South Africa, ongoing monitoring of hearing is warranted.

Recurrent or persistent otitis media with effusion for at least three months*

Otitis media with effusion (OME) is most frequently associated with transient conductive hearing loss, but non-resolving OME can cause chronic postnatal hearing loss. HIV infection increases susceptibility to and complications of OME (Shapiro & Novelli, 1998). Despite the lack of longitudinal data, high rates of OME in children have been reported in South Africa (31.4 percent), including a higher incidence of chronic suppurative otitis media (CSOM) (4.5 percent in children aged 2 to 5 years and 9.3 percent in children aged 6 to 15 years) (Biagio, Swanepoel, Laurent, & Lundberg, 2014). CSOM can lead to serious complications including mastoiditis, cholesteatoma and meningitis, leading to sensorineural hearing loss (Papp, Rezes, Jókay, & Sziklai, 2003; Qureshi & Rehman, 2015; Smouha & Bojrab, 2011). Therefore, monitoring hearing in infants and children with persistent OME may be warranted to minimise the detrimental hearing and health sequelae.

For a screening protocol targeting bilateral hearing loss, infants with a unilateral refer result are at risk for a progressive bilateral hearing loss*

The HPCSA (2007, 2018) proposes that targeting bilateral hearing loss may be more realistic in a resource-limited context than also trying to identify unilateral hearing loss. If such an approach is adopted, infants who referred in one ear on the newborn hearing screen would still be considered to have passed the screen given that the targeted condition is bilateral hearing loss. As unilateral hearing loss may progress to bilateral hearing loss (Barreira-Nielsen et al., 2016; Brookhouser, Worthington, & Kelley, 1994), the HPCSA recommends that a unilateral refer be regarded as a risk factor for bilateral hearing loss and parents are counselled accordingly. The advantage of only targeting bilateral hearing loss through audiological assessment of bilateral refers is that fewer infants are sent for time-consuming, resource-intensive infant diagnostic audiological evaluations (De Kock, Swanepoel, & Hall, 2016).

Additional risk factors for consideration for the South African context

Malaria

In 2007, the HPCSA added malaria to the list of risk factors for PCHL in South Africa, noting that its effect on hearing in prenatally exposed infants was unknown and requires investigation (Da Silva et al., 2015; Dellicour, Hall, Chandramohan, & Greenwood, 2007). The ototoxic effect of malaria treatment was also mentioned. A few studies have reported on the relation-ship between hearing and exposure to prenatal malaria. However, these studies were inconclusive as screening, rather than diagnostic audiology outcomes, were presented (Da Silva et al., 2015) or additional risk factors were present in children diagnosed with hearing loss (Soares Aurélio et al., 2014). Given the limited evidence on the relationship between prenatal malaria exposure and hearing loss, malaria was retracted as a risk factor in the HPCSA's 2018 guidelines. Stronger evidence is required to justify inclu-sion of prenatal malaria in South Africa's risk registry.

Very low birth weight

As previously stated, VLBW does not cause congenital hearing loss (Cristobal & Oghalai, 2008) and has been removed from the JCIH risk factor registry (JCIH, 2000). However, South African research indicates that 5.5 percent of children with profound hearing loss (Le Roux et al., 2015), and 12.5 percent of children with any degree of sensorineural hearing loss or ANSD had VLBW (<1 500g) (Swanepoel et al., 2013). Therefore, for resource-limited settings such as South Africa, it may be more efficient to identify infants with VLBW as it is easily measured and has a high occurrence with other risk factors that may not be as readily detected (Kanji & Khoza-Shangase, 2012).

Consanguinity

While there is evidence that consanguinity is a risk factor for hearing loss (Bener et al., 2005), prevalence of infants born from consanguineous unions is unknown in South Africa (Bittles & Black, 2010). Whether this should be included in the HPCSA registry is unclear.

Sickle cell anaemia

Postnatal sensorineural hearing loss is common in children and adults with sickle cell anaemia (Silva, Vila Nova, & Lucena, 2012). Although sickle cell anaemia has low prevalence in South Africa, demographics are changing with immigration from other sub-Saharan countries (Wonkam et al., 2012). Relevance of this risk factor for South Africa continues to be unclear.

Identified risk factors from other developing nations

In addition to those reported by the JCIH, South Africa may benefit from reviewing risk factors identified by other developing nations. For example, a Nigerian study identified risk factors such as maternal hypertensive disorders, non-elective caesarean section, low Apgar scores, lack of skilled attendant at birth, undernutrition in the first months of life and hyperbilirubinaemia requiring phototherapy (rather than exchange transfusion) as potential risk factors for hearing loss (Olusanya, 2011b). Local research would be required to determine the relevance of these risk factors in South Africa.

Recommendations

Based on the above information, we make the following recommendations for the South African hearing screening context.

Programme recommendations

- The purpose of the programme, including the target population and hearing loss condition (congenital versus postnatal, unilateral versus bilateral, permanent versus temporary), needs to be clearly defined and communicated. This will enable risk factors to be tailored to meet the programme purpose, as well as support consistency in the collection of risk factors and provision of onward referrals.
- Increase public and professional awareness of: (i) certain risk factors (chemotherapy, head trauma) and the need for hearing assessment; (ii) the benefits of genetic testing and counselling; and (iii) culturally appropriate methods of eliciting sensitive information related to risk factors.

Risk factor recommendations

- There is good evidence to support including the following birth risk factors to identify permanent congenital and postnatal hearing loss: family history (criteria to be tightened to immediate family only and to exclude acquired hearing losses), NICU admission, in-utero infection (cCMV, toxoplasmosis, rubella), craniofacial anomalies, syndromes and neurodegenerative disorders.
- There is good evidence to include the following risk factors if the purpose of the programme is expanded to detection of all hearing losses, including conductive hearing loss, and monitoring children with postbirth causes: caregiver concern, postnatal infections, head trauma, chemotherapy, HIV, OME and unilateral screening refer outcome.
- Risk factors that require further evidence prior to inclusion in a registry are as follows: in-utero infections (HSV and syphilis), malaria, VLBW, consanguinity, sickle cell anaemia and risk factors emerging from other developing nations.

Conclusion

Risk factors can be used to identify children at risk of hearing impairment and generate onward referrals. In South Africa, to maximise the effectiveness of the registry, it is opportune to tailor the registry to meet the local context. However, the risk factor registry will not be effective in detecting hearing loss unless implemented as part of broader system change. Addressing programme-level issues, such as a clearly articulated programme purpose, as well as public and professional awareness of the importance of certain risk factors, is crucial for successful programme execution. In addition, implementation of systems to collect and report on risk factors will supply much-needed evidence on risk factor prevalence and associated hearing loss yield. In general, more research is required to inform development of a context-specific risk registry with optimal sensitivity and specificity to PCHL in South Africa.

References

Adachi, N., Ito, K., Sakata, H., & Yamasoba, T. (2010). Etiology and one-year follow-up results of hearing loss identified by screening of newborn hearing in Japan. *Otolaryngology–Head and Neck Surgery, 143*, 97–100.

Amin, S., Saluja, S., Saili, A., Orlando, M., Wang, H., Laroia, N., & Agarwal, A. (2017). Chronic auditory toxicity in late preterm and term infants with significant hyperbilirubinemia. *Pediatrics, 140*(4), e20164009.

Banatvala, J., & Peckham, C. (2007). *Rubella viruses*. Oxford, England: Elsevier.

Barkai, G., Roth, D., Barzilai, A., Tepperberg-Oikawa, M., Mendelson, E., Hildesheimer, M., & Kuint, J. (2014). Universal neonatal cytomegalovirus screening using saliva: Report of clinical experience. *Journal of Clinical Virology, 60*(4), 361–366.

Barreira-Nielsen, C., Fitzpatrick, E., Hashem, S., Whittingham, J., Barrowman, N., & Aglipay, M. (2016). Progressive hearing loss in early childhood. *Ear & Hearing, 37*, e311–e321.

Basson, O., & Van Lierop, A. (2009). Conductive hearing loss after head trauma: Review of ossicular pathology, management and outcomes. *The Journal of Laryngology & Otology, 123*(2), 177–181.

Bates, M., & Brantsaeter, A. (2016). Human cytomegalovirus (CMV) in Africa: A neglected but important pathogen. *Journal of Virus Eradication, 2*(3), 136–142.

Bener, A., Eihakeem, A. A., & Abdulhadi, K. (2005). Is there any association between consanguinity and hearing loss? *International Journal of Pediatric Otorhinolaryngology, 69*(3), 327–333.

Berg, A. L., Spitzer, J. B., Towers, H. M., Bartosiewicz, C., & Diamond, B. E. (2005). Newborn hearing screening in the NICU: Profile of failed auditory brainstem response/passed otoacoustic emission. *Pediatrics, 116*, 933–938.

Beswick, R., & Driscoll, C. (2013). Hearing loss in children with craniofacial anomalies. In S. Turner & J. Miller (Eds.), *Craniofacial disorders* (pp. 83–100). New York, NY: Nova Science Publishers.

Beswick, R., Driscoll, C., Kei, J., Khan, A., & Glennon, S. (2013). Which risk factors predict postnatal hearing loss in children? *Journal of the American Academy of Audiology, 24*(3), 205–213.

Biagio, L., Swanepoel, D., Laurent, C., & Lundberg, T. (2014). Paediatric otitis media at a primary healthcare clinic in South Africa. *South African Medical Journal, 104*(6), 431–435.

Bittles, A., & Black, M. (2010). Consanguinity, human evolution, and complex diseases. *Proceedings of the National Academy of Sciences, 107*(1), 1779–1786.

Bowman, M., Mantle, B., Accortt, N., Wang, W., Hardin, W., & Wiatrak, B. (2011). Appropriate hearing screening in the pediatric patient with head trauma. *International Journal of Pediatric Otorhinolaryngology, 75*(4), 468–471.

Briggs, G., & Freeman, R. (2017). *Drugs in pregnancy and lactation.* Philadelphia, PA: Wolters Kluwer.

Brookhouser, P. E., Worthington, D. W., & Kelley, W. J. (1994). Fluctuating and/or progressive sensorineural hearing loss in children. *The Laryngoscope, 104*, 958–964.

Brown, E., Chau, J., Atashband, S., Westerberg, B., & Kozak, F. (2009). A systematic review of neonatal toxoplasmosis exposure and sensorineural hearing loss. *International Journal of Pediatric Otorhinolaryngology, 73*(5), 707–711.

Butali, A., & Mossey, P. A. (2009). Epidemiology of orofacial clefts in Africa: Methodological challenges in ascertainment. *Pan African Medical Journal, 2*, 1–9.

Cannon, M., Schmid, D., & Hyde, T. (2010). Review of cytomegalovirus seroprevalence and demographic characteristics associated with infection. *Reviews in Medical Virology, 20*(4), 202–213.

Chau, J., Atashband, S., Chang, E., Westerberg, B., & Kozak, F. (2009). A systematic review of pediatric sensorineural hearing loss in congenital syphilis. *International Journal of Pediatric Otorhinolaryngology, 73*(6), 787–792.

Cohen, B., Durstenfeld, A., & Roehm, P. (2014). Viral causes of hearing loss: A review for hearing health professionals. *Trends in Hearing, 18*, 1–17.

Cone-Wesson, B., Vohr, B., Sininger, Y., Widen, J., Folsom, R., Gorga, M., & Norton, S. (2000). Identification of neonatal hearing impairment: Infants with hearing loss. *Ear & Hearing, 21*(5), 488–507.

Cristobal, R., & Oghalai, J. (2008). Hearing loss in children with very low birth weight: Current review of epidemiology and pathophysiology. *Archives of Disease in Childhood-Fetal and Neonatal Edition, 93*(6), F462–F468.

Da Silva, V., Sousa, M., Kuniyoshi, I., Aurelio, S., Sampaio, A., & De Oliveira, C. (2015). Risk of hearing alterations in newborns of mothers treated for malaria. *The International Tinnitus Journal, 19*(2), 20–25.

De Castro Corrêa, C., Maximino, L., & Weber, S. (2018). Hearing disorders in congenital toxoplasmosis: A literature review. *International Archives of Otorhinolaryngology, 22*(3), 330–333.

De Jong, T., Toll, M., De Gier, H., & Mathijssen, I. (2011). Audiological profile of children and young adults with syndromic and complex craniosynostosis. *Archives of Otolaryngology–Head & Neck Surgery, 137*(8), 775–778.

De Kock, T., Swanepoel, D., & Hall III, J. W. (2016). Newborn hearing screening at a community-based obstetric unit: Screening and diagnostic outcomes. *International Journal of Pediatric Otorhinolaryngology, 84*, 124–131.

Dedhia, K., Kitsko, D., Sabo, D., & Chi, D. (2013). Children with sensorineural hearing loss after passing the newborn hearing screen. *JAMA Otolaryngology–Head & Neck Surgery, 139*(2), 119–123.

Delatycki, M., Paris, D., Gardner, R., Nicholson, G., Nassif, N., Storey, E., ... Forrest, S. (1999). Clinical and genetic study of Friedreich ataxia in an Australian population. *American Journal of Medical Genetics, 87*(2), 168–174.

Dellicour, S., Hall, S., Chandramohan, D., & Greenwood, B. (2007). The safety of artemisinins during pregnancy: A pressing question. *Malaria Journal, 6*, 1–10.

Driscoll, C., Beswick, R., Doherty, E., D'Silva, R., & Cross, A. (2015). The validity of family history as a risk factor in pediatric hearing loss. *International Journal of Pediatric Otorhinolaryngology, 79*(5), 654–659.

Dumanch, K., Holte, L., O'Hollearn, T., Walker, E., Clark, J., & Oleson, J. (2017). High risk factors associated with early childhood hearing loss: A 3-year review. *American Journal of Audiology, 26*(2), 129–142.

Dunmade, A., Segun-Busari, S., Olajide, T., & Ologe, F. (2006). Profound bilateral sensorineural hearing loss in Nigerian children: Any shift in etiology? *Journal of Deaf Studies and Deaf Education, 12*(1), 112–118.

Dürr, A., Cossee, M., Agid, Y., Campuzano, V., Mignard, C., Penet, C., ... Koenig, M. (1996). Clinical and genetic abnormalities in patients with Friedreich's ataxia. *New England Journal of Medicine, 335*(16), 1169–1175.

Edmond, K., Clark, A., Korczak, V., Sanderson, C., Griffiths, U., & Rudan, I. (2010). Global and regional risk of disabling sequelae from bacterial meningitis: A systematic review and meta-analysis. *The Lancet Infectious Diseases, 10*(5), 317–328.

Ensink, R., & Kuper, H. (2017). Is hearing impairment associated with HIV? A systematic review of data from low- and middle-income countries. *Tropical Medicine & International Health, 22*(12), 1493–1504.

Fagan, J., & Jacobs, M. (2009). Survey of ENT services in Africa: Need for a comprehensive intervention. *Global Health Action, 2*(1), 1–7. doi: 10.3402/gha.v2i0.1932.

Fasunla, A., Ogunbosi, B., Odaibo, G., Nwaorgu, O., Taiwo, B., Olaleye, D., ... Akinyinka, O. (2014). Comparison of auditory brainstem response in HIV-1 exposed and unexposed newborns and their correlation with the maternal viral load and CD4 cell counts. *AIDS, 28*(15), 2223–2230.

Fowler, K., McCollister, F., Sabo, D., Shoup, A., Owen, K., Woodruff, J., ... Boppana, S. (2017). A targeted approach for congenital cytomegalovirus screening within newborn hearing screening. *Pediatrics, 139*(2), e20162128.

Goderis, J., De Leenheer, E., Smets, K., Van Hoecke, H., Keymeulen, A., & Dhooge, I. (2014). Hearing loss and congenital CMV infection: A systematic review. *Pediatrics, 134*(5), 972–982.

Goga, A., Chirinda, W., Ngandu, N., Ngoma, K., Bhardwaj, S., Feucht, U., ... Silere-Maqetseba, T. (2018). Closing the gaps to eliminate mother-to-child transmission of HIV (MTCT) in South Africa: Understanding MTCT case rates, factors that hinder the monitoring and attainment of targets, and potential game changers. *South African Medical Journal, 108*(3), 17–24.

Graham, C., Seeley, J., Gina, A., & Saman, Y. (2019). Mapping the content of mothers' knowledge, attitude and practice towards universal newborn hearing screening for development of a KAP survey tool. *PloS ONE, 14*, e0210764.

Hammond-Aryee, K., Esser, M., & Van Helden, P. (2014). Toxoplasma gondii seroprevalence studies on humans and animals in Africa. *South African Family Practice, 56*(2), 119–124.

Hayes, D. (1994). Hearing loss in infants with craniofacial anomalies. *Otolaryngology–Head and Neck Surgery, 110*(1), 39–45.

Health Professions Council of South Africa (HPCSA). (2002). *Professional board for speech, language and hearing professions: Hearing screening position statement year 2002.* Pretoria, South Africa: Health Professions Council of South Africa.

Health Professions Council of South Africa (HPCSA). (2007). *Professional board for speech, language and hearing professions: Early hearing detection and intervention programmes in South Africa position statement year 2007.* Pretoria, South Africa: Health Professions Council of South Africa.

Health Professions Council of South Africa (HPCSA). (2018). *Professional board for speech, language and hearing professions: Early hearing detection and intervention (EHDI) guidelines year 2018.* Pretoria, South Africa: Health Professions Council of South Africa.

Helt-Cameron, J., & Allen, P. J. (2009). Cisplatin ototoxicity in children: Implications for primary care providers. *Pediatric Nursing, 35*(2), 121–128.

Hlongwa, P., Levin, J., & Rispel, L. C. (2019). Epidemiology and clinical profile of individuals with cleft lip and palate utilising specialised academic treatment centres in South Africa. *PloS ONE, 15*, e0215931.

Hong, A., Makhathini, L., Mashele, M., Malfeld, S., Motsamai, T., Sikhosana, L., … Smit, S. (2017). *Annual measles and rubella surveillance review, South Africa, 2017.* Johannesburg, South Africa: National Institute for Communicable Diseases.

Hyde, M. (2005). Newborn hearing screening programs: Overview. *Journal of Otolaryngology, 34*(2), S70–S78.

Jacobs, M., & Mason, P. (1978). Prevalence of toxoplasma antibodies in southern Africa. *South African Medical Journal, 53*(16), 619–621.

Joint Committee on Infant Hearing (JCIH). (1973). Screening for infant hearing. Retrieved from www.jcih.org/JCIH1973.pdf.

Joint Committee on Infant Hearing (JCIH). (2000).Year 2000 position statement: Principles and guidelines for early hearing detection and intervention programs. *Pediatrics, 106*(4), 798–817.

Joint Committee on Infant Hearing (JCIH). (2007). Year 2007 position statement: Principles and guidelines for early hearing detection and intervention programs. *Pediatrics, 120*(4), 898–921.

Kanji, A. (2018). Early hearing detection and intervention: Reflections from the South African context. *South African Journal of Communication Disorders, 65*(1), 1–3.

Kanji, A., & Khoza-Shangase, K. (2012). The occurrence of high-risk factors for hearing loss in very low-birth-weight neonates: A retrospective exploratory study of targeted hearing screening. *South African Journal of Communication Disorders, 59*(1), 3–7.

Khan, N., Joseph, L., & Adhikari, M. (2018). The hearing screening experiences and practices of primary health care nurses: Indications for referral based on high-risk factors and community views about hearing loss. *African Journal of Primary Health Care & Family Medicine, 10*(1), 1–11.

Khan, S., Peracha, H., Ballhausen, D., Wiesbauer, A., Rohrbach, M., Gautschi, M., ... Orii, K. (2017). Epidemiology of mucopolysaccharidoses. *Molecular Genetics and Metabolism, 121*(3), 227–240.

Khan, W., & Khan, K. (2018). Congenital toxoplasmosis: An overview of the neurological and ocular manifestations. *Parasitology International, 67*, 715–721.

Khoza-Shangase, K., Kanji, A., Petrocchi-Bartal, L., & Farr, K. (2017). Infant hearing screening in a developing-country context: Status in two South African provinces. *South African Journal of Child Health, 11*(4), 159–163.

Korenromp, E., Rowley, J., Alonso, M., Mello, M., Wijesooriya, N., Mahiané, S., . . . Nagelkerke, N. (2019). Global burden of maternal and congenital syphilis and associated adverse birth outcomes: Estimates for 2016 and progress since 2012. *PloS ONE, 14*(2), e0211720.

Krishnan, L. A., & Donaldson, L. K. (2013). Newborn hearing screening in developing countries: Understanding the challenges and complexities of implementation. *Perspectives on Global Issues in Communication Sciences and Related Disorders, 3*, 54–61.

Kromberg, J., & Jenkins, T. (1982). Common birth defects in South African Blacks. *South African Medical Journal, 62*(17), 599–602.

Kromberg, J., Sizer, E., & Christianson, A. (2013). Genetic services and testing in South Africa. *Journal of Community Genetics, 4*(3), 413–423.

Kuschke, S., Goncalves, N., & Peer, S. (2018). Hearing outcomes in children with meningitis at Red Cross War Memorial Children's Hospital, Cape Town, South Africa: A silent crisis. *South African Medical Journal, 108*(11), 944–946.

Lasky, R., Wiorek, L., & Becker, T. (1998). Hearing loss in survivors of neonatal extracorporeal membrane oxygenation (ECMO) therapy and high-frequency oscillatory (HFO) therapy. *Journal of the American Academy of Audiology, 9*(1), 47–58.

Le Roux, T., Swanepoel, D., Louw, A., Vinck, B., & Tshifularo, M. (2015). Profound childhood hearing loss in a South Africa cohort: Risk profile, diagnosis and age of intervention. *International Journal of Pediatric Otorhinolaryngology, 79*(1), 8–14.

Leruez-Ville, M., Magny, J., Couderc, S., Pichon, C., Parodi, M., Bussières, L., ... Ville, Y. (2017). Risk factors for congenital cytomegalovirus infection following primary and nonprimary maternal infection: A prospective neonatal screening study using polymerase chain reaction in saliva. *Clinical Infectious Diseases, 65*(3), 398–404.

Looker, K., Magaret, A., May, M., Turner, K., Vickerman, P., Newman, L., & Gottlieb, S. (2017). First estimates of the global and regional incidence of neonatal herpes infection. *The Lancet Global Health, 5*(3), e300–e309.

Manfredi, A., Zuanetti, P., Mishima, F., & Granzotti, R. (2011). Newborn hearing screening in infants born to HIV-seropositive mothers. *Jornal da Sociedade Brasileira de Fonoaudiologia, 23*(4), 376–380.

McKenna, M. (1997). Measles, mumps, and sensorineural hearing loss. *Annals of the New York Academy of Sciences, 830*(1), 291–298.

Meyer, M., & Swanepoel, D. (2011). Newborn hearing screening in the private health care sector: A national survey. *South African Medical Journal, 101*(9), 665–667.

Molteno, C., Smart, R., Viljoen, D., Sayed, R., & Roux, A. (1997). Twenty-year birth prevalence of Down syndrome in Cape Town, South Africa. *Paediatric and Perinatal Epidemiology, 11*(4), 428–435.

Momberg, Z., & Geerts, L. (2016). An update on congenital cytomegalovirus infection. *Obstetrics and Gynaecology Forum, 26*(1), 20–24.

Montoya, J., & Liesenfeld, O. (2004). Toxoplasmosis. *The Lancet, 363*, 1965–1976.

Moroe, N., & Hughes, K. (2017). Parents are aware of the ototoxic effects of chemotherapy in paediatrics undergoing cancer treatment—Professional versus parental views: A pilot study. *South African Journal of Communication Disorders, 64*(1), 1–10.

Mossey, P., & Catilla, E. (2003). *Global registry and database on craniofacial anomalies: Report of a WHO registry meeting on craniofacial anomalies.* Geneva, Switzerland: World Health Organization.

Motaze, N., Manamela, J., Smit, S., Rabie, H., Harper, K., Duplessis, N., ... Moore, D. (2018). Congenital rubella syndrome surveillance in South Africa using a sentinel site approach: A cross-sectional study. *Clinical Infectious Diseases*, ciy758. Retrieved from https://doi.org/10.1093/cid/ciy758.

National Institutes of Health. (1993). National Institutes of Health Consensus Development Conference Statement: Early identification of hearing impairment in infants and young children. *International Journal of Pediatric Otorhinolaryngology, 27*(3), 215–227.

Olusanya, B. O. (2011a). Highlights of the new WHO report on newborn and infant hearing screening and implications for developing countries. *International Journal of Pediatric Otorhinolaryngology, 75*, 745–748.

Olusanya, B. O. (2011b). Making targeted screening for infant hearing loss an effective option in less developed countries. *International Journal of Pediatric Otorhinolaryngology, 75*, 316–321.

Olusanya, B., Afe, A., & Onyia, N. (2009). Infants with HIV-infected mothers in a universal newborn hearing screening programme in Lagos, Nigeria. *Acta Paediatrica, 98*(8), 1288–1293.

Olusanya, B., Ogunlesi, T., & Slusher, T. (2014). Why is kernicterus still a major cause of death and disability in low-income and middle-income countries? *Archives of Disease in Childhood, 99*(12), 1117–1121.

Olusanya, B., Wirz, S., & Luxon, L. (2008). Non-hospital delivery and permanent congenital and early-onset hearing loss in a developing country. *BJOG: An International Journal of Obstetrics & Gynaecology, 115*(11), 1419–1427.

Papp, Z., Rezes, S., Jókay, I., & Sziklai, I. (2003). Sensorineural hearing loss in chronic otitis media. *Otology & Neurotology, 24*(2), 141–144.

Pathirana, J., Groome, M., Dorfman, J., Kwatra, G., Boppana, S., Cutlan, C., ... Madhi, S. A. (2019). Prevalence of congenital cytomegalovirus infection and associated risk of in utero human immunodeficiency virus (HIV) acquisition in a high-HIV prevalence setting, South Africa. *Clinical Infectious Diseases,* ciz019. Retrieved from https://doi.org/10.1093/cid/ciz019.

Paz-Bailey, G., Ramaswamy, M., Hawkes, S., & Geretti, A. (2007). Herpes simplex virus type 2: Epidemiology and management options in developing countries. *Sexually Transmitted Infections, 83*(1), 16–22.

Penn, C., Watermeyer, J., & Schie, K. (2009). Auditory disorders in a South African paediatric TBI population: Some preliminary data. *International Journal of Audiology, 48*(3), 135–143.

Pourarian, S., Khademi, B., Pishva, N., & Jamali, A. (2012). Prevalence of hearing loss in newborns admitted to neonatal intensive care unit. *Iranian Journal of Otorhinolaryngology, 3,* 129–134.

Qureshi, S., & Rehman, U. (2015). Demographic influences on complicated chronic suppurative otitis media. *Indian Journal of Otology, 21*(3), 170–173.

Ramma, L., & Sebothoma, B. (2016). The prevalence of hearing impairment within the Cape Town Metropolitan area. *South African Journal of Communication Disorders, 63*(1), 1–10.

Rance, G., Corben, L., Barker, E., Carew, P., Chisari, D., Rogers, M., ... Delatycki, M. (2010). Auditory perception in individuals with Friedreich's ataxia. *Audiology and Neurotology, 15*(4), 229–240.

Rehle, T., Shisana, O., Pillay, V., Zuma, K., Puren, A., & Parker, W. (2007). National HIV incidence measures - new insights into the South African epidemic. *South African Medical Journal, 97,* 194–199.

Roizen, N. (2003). Nongenetic causes of hearing loss. *Mental Retardation and Developmental Disabilities Research Reviews, 9*(2), 120–127.

Rudman, J., Kabahuma, R., Bressler, S., Feng, Y., Blanton, S., Yan, D., & Liu, X. (2017). The genetic basis of deafness in populations of African descent. *Journal of Genetics and Genomics, 44*(6), 285–294.

Schoub, B., Harris, B., McAnerney, J., & Blumberg, L. (2009). Rubella in South Africa: An impending Greek tragedy? *South African Medical Journal, 99*(7), 515–519.

Sellars, S., & Beighton, P. (1983). Childhood deafness in southern Africa: An aetiological survey of 3,064 deaf children. *The Journal of Laryngology & Otology, 97*(10), 885–889.

Shapiro, N., & Novelli, V. (1998). Otitis media in children with vertically-acquired HIV infection: The Great Ormond Street Hospital experience. *International Journal of Pediatric Otorhinolaryngology, 45*(1), 69–75.

Shott, S., Joseph, A., & Heithaus, D. (2001). Hearing loss in children with Down syndrome. *International Journal of Pediatric Otorhinolaryngology, 61*(3), 199–205.

Silva, L., Vila Nova, C., & Lucena, R. (2012). Sickle cell anemia and hearing loss among children and youngsters: Literature review. *Brazilian Journal of Otorhinolaryngology, 78*(1), 126–131.

Smith, D., Greenberg, L., & Bryer, A. (2016). The hereditary ataxias: Where are we now? Four decades of local research: How human genetics came to SA. *South African Medical Journal, 106*(1), 38–41.

Smouha, E., & Bojrab, D. (2011). *Cholesteatoma.* New York, NY: Thieme.

Soares Aurélio, F., Pereira Dutra, Í., Braz Da Silva, V., Lopes Sampaio, A., Oliveira, C., & Augusto, C. (2014). Prevalence of hearing loss in newborns of mothers who had malaria and were treated with antimalaric drugs in pregnancy. *International Tinnitus Journal*, *19*(1), 68–76.

Störbeck, C., & Young, A. (2016). The HI HOPES data set of deaf children under the age of 6 in South Africa: Maternal suspicion, age of identification and newborn hearing screening. *BMC Pediatrics*, *16*, 45.

Swanepoel, D., & Almec, N. (2008). Maternal views on infant hearing loss and early intervention in a South African community. *International Journal of Audiology*, *47*(1), S44–S48.

Swanepoel, D., Hugo, R., & Louw, B. (2005). Implementing infant hearing screening at maternal and child health clinics: Context and interactional processes. *Health SA Gesondheid*, *10*(4), 3–15.

Swanepoel, D., Johl, L., & Pienaar, D. (2013). Childhood hearing loss and risk profile in a South African population. *International Journal of Pediatric Otorhinolaryngology*, *77*(3), 394–398.

Theunissen, M., & Swanepoel, D. (2008). Early hearing detection and intervention services in the public health sector in South Africa. *International Journal of Audiology*, *47*(1), S23–S29.

Thompson, D., McPhillips, H., Davis, R., Lieu, T., Homer, C., & Helfand, M. (2001). Universal newborn hearing screening: Summary of evidence. *Journal of the American Academy of Audiology*, *286*(16), 2000–2010.

Tshabalala, D., Newman, H., Businge, C., Mabunda, S., Kemp, W., & Beja, P. (2018). Prevalence and determinants of congenital cytomegalovirus infection at a rural South African central hospital in the Eastern Cape. *Southern African Journal of Infectious Diseases*, *33*(4), 89–92.

UNAIDS. (2018). *UNAIDS data 2018*. Geneva, Switzerland: Joint United Nations Programme on HIV/AIDS. Retrieved from https://www.unaids.org/en/resources/documents/2018/unaids-data-2018.

Villarreal, I., Méndez, D., Silva, J., & Álamo, P. (2016). Contralateral cochlear labyrinthine concussion without temporal bone fracture: Unusual posttraumatic consequence. *Case Reports in Otolaryngology*, 2016. Retrieved from https://doi.org/10.1155/2016/2123182.

Walton, J. P., & Hendricks-Munoz, K. (1991). Profile and stability of sensorineural hearing loss in persistent pulmonary hypertension of the newborn. *Journal of Speech Language and Hearing Research*, *34*(6), 1362–1370.

Wang, Z., Wang, S., Liu, H., Ma, H., Li, Z., Wei, F., ... Liu, Q. (2017). Prevalence and burden of Toxoplasma gondii infection in HIV-infected people: A systematic review and meta-analysis. *The Lancet HIV*, *4*(4), e177–e188.

Watkin, P., Baldwin, M., & Laoide, S. (1990). Parental suspicion and identification of hearing impairment. *Archives of Disease in Childhood*, *65*(8), 846–850.

Westerberg, B., Atashband, S., & Kozak, F. (2008). A systematic review of the incidence of sensorineural hearing loss in neonates exposed to Herpes simplex virus (HSV). *International Journal of Pediatric Otorhinolaryngology*, *72*(7), 931–937.

Williams, A. L., Van Drongelen, W., & Lasky, R. E. (2007). Noise in contemporary neonatal intensive care. *Journal of the Acoustical Society of America, 121,* 2681–2690.

Willoughby, M., Aldous, C., Patrick, M., Kavonic, S., & Christianson, A. (2016). Delay and poor diagnosis of Down syndrome in KwaZulu-Natal, South Africa: A retrospective review of postnatal cytogenetic testing. *South African Medical Journal, 106*(6), 626–629.

Wonkam, A., Ponde, C., Nicholson, N., Fieggen, K., Ramesar, R., & Davidson, A. (2012). The burden of sickle cell disease in Cape Town. *South African Medical Journal, 102*(9), 752–754.

Wraith, J., Scarpa, M., Beck, M., Bodamer, O., De Meirleir, L., Guffon, N., ... Zeman, J. (2008). Mucopolysaccharidosis type II (Hunter syndrome): A clinical review and recommendations for treatment in the era of enzyme replacement therapy. *European Journal of Pediatrics, 167*(3), 267–277.

Zuma, K., Shisana, O., Rehle, T. M., Simbayi, L. C., Jooste, S., Zungu, N., ... Abdullah, F. (2016). New insights into HIV epidemic in South Africa: Key findings from the National HIV Prevalence, Incidence and Behaviour Survey, 2012. *African Journal of AIDS Research, 15,* 67–75.

Section Two

Early Intervention for Hearing Impairment

7 Approaches to Early Intervention for Hearing Impairment

Amisha Kanji and Aisha Casoojee

The goal of early hearing detection and intervention (EHDI) is to provide children with hearing impairment with optimal and timely opportunities to develop linguistic, literacy and communicative competence. Early intervention (EI) for children with hearing impairment specifically focuses on timeous fitting of amplification devices followed by family-centred intervention. Prompt intervention remains a challenge in South Africa, partly due to late detection and diagnosis of hearing impairment. It is further influenced by factors related to access to EI services as well as adequately trained professionals, a high patient-to-professional ratio, and other contextual considerations such as the linguistic and cultural incongruence of trained professionals in relation to the population served. The age at amplification, approach to EI and family involvement have a significant impact on the outcomes of children with hearing impairment. The choice of communication approach used in the EI programme should be an ongoing, dynamic process between the early interventionist and the family for EI to be successful. This chapter explores EHDI within the early childhood development (ECD) framework. Various intervention approaches are discussed and factors influencing the choice of approach presented. The chapter ends by offering solutions and recommendations with respect to EI challenges in the South African context.

Developmental disabilities comprise a group of conditions resulting from a range of impairments that have an impact on a child's physical, scholastic and/or behavioural functioning (Centre for Disease Control and Prevention, 2018). These disabilities, or any developmental delay, place children at greater risk for inadequate health, educational attainment and psychosocial well-being (World Health Organization [WHO], 2012a).

Globally, there are reportedly 52.9 million children younger than five years of age with developmental disabilities, with about 95 percent of them living in low and middle-income (LAMI) countries (Olusanya et al., 2018). Of that 95 percent, three in five are at risk of suboptimal development. Findings from a global burden of disease study by Olusanya et al. (2018) highlight that the number of children in sub-Saharan Africa affected by developmental disabilities increased by more than 70 percent between 1990 and 2016. This increase may partly be attributed to the increase in survival rates of neonates, particularly premature neonates, during the period of the Millennium Development Goals (Olusanya et al., 2018).

Globally, hearing impairment is reported to be the second most prevalent developmental disability (Olusanya et al., 2018). Recent estimates indicate that 34 of the 466 million (7 percent) individuals with hearing impairment are children (Neumann, Chadha, Tavartkiladze, Bu, & White, 2019). Findings from a global burden of diseases, injuries and risk factor study (Olusanya et al., 2018) indicate that the leading causes of hearing impairment globally are otitis media and congenital abnormalities. Such identification of the causes of hearing impairment is useful as it may aid in the development of specific health-related indicators to address the special needs of affected children, particularly in resource-constrained LAMI contexts. Olusanya et al. (2018) argue that these health indicators should be linked to the 17 Sustainable Development Goals (SDGs), especially SDG 3, which focuses on promoting healthy lives and well-being across all age groups.

The SDGs are aimed at improving the broader health status of children following survival (Olusanya, 2005; United Nations, 2018). SDG 4 specifically addresses the need to monitor the proportion of children below five years of age who are achieving their developmental potential in terms of health, psychosocial well-being and education, based on age, gender, geographical location and the presence of disability and any other characteristics. Systematic monitoring of all children will assist in ensuring that optimal ECD is achieved (Olusanya et al., 2018). The South African government has ECD as one of its priorities, evidenced by the approval of the National Integrated ECD Policy in 2015 and the inclusion of ECD in the 2030 National Development Plan (Republic of South Africa, 2015). The National Integrated ECD Policy recognises that a lack of or poor-quality intervention during early childhood can be disadvantageous to children and can reduce their potential for success. It is thus aimed at transforming ECD service delivery in South Africa to ensure universally available and equitable access to these services (Republic of South Africa, 2015). Early childhood intervention (ECI) services for children with or at risk for developmental disability should be included within the broader framework of ECD service delivery.

Recognising the need for comprehensive early detection and intervention for all children with or at risk of any developmental disability from birth is essential when considering the associated negative consequences. In the South African context, it is important to consider the presence of other contextual risk factors and their influence on ECD and subsequent ECI service provision. These contextual risk factors include, but are not limited to: poverty; infectious diseases; environmental toxins; and disrupted caregiving due to absent parents, ill parents and non-parent caregivers (Republic of South Africa, 2015). Understanding these risk factors and their influence on development is essential to ensure the planning and implementation of effective and appropriately tailored EI programmes.

EI, also referred to as ECI programmes, comprises a series of comprehensive activities designed to improve and develop the cognitive, language, motor and sensory domains in young children (WHO, 2012b). ECI programmes are aimed at providing the necessary support to children who are considered to be at risk for, or who have been identified as having, a developmental delay or disability due to various factors, including hearing impairment (WHO, 2012b). These ECI programmes include specialised medical and rehabilitation services, family-centred support, social and psychological services, special education, as well as service planning and coordination for children with hearing impairment and their families.

A number of factors guide the implementation of ECI programmes, as detailed in the WHO discussion paper on ECD and disability (WHO, 2012b):

- The first three years of a child's life are considered critical and serve as the foundation for future development.
- Implementation of ECI programmes can assist in ensuring more effective developmental outcomes and educational initiatives.
- If development is fostered, and appropriate care and support provided, these children are more likely to function more optimally in adulthood, which may reduce economic expenditure.
- As stated by the Convention on the Rights of the Child and the Convention on the Rights of Persons with Disabilities, all children with disabilities have the right to develop to their maximum potential.

EHDI falls within the broader ECD framework, with a specific focus on early identification of and intervention for hearing impairment. The goal of EHDI is to timeously identify hearing impairment and to provide individuals diagnosed with hearing impairment with optimal opportunity to maximise their growth and development in linguistic, language, literacy, communicative, cognitive and social–emotional domains (Health Professions Council of South Africa [HPCSA], 2007, 2018; Joint Committee on Infant Hearing [JCIH], 2007). Aspects related to early identification of hearing impairment, such as approaches to audiological screening, are discussed in chapter 3. EHDI further encompasses appropriate diagnostic evaluation after newborn hearing screening, followed by a family-centred approach to intervention (HPCSA, 2018; JCIH, 2007). These EHDI objectives are guided by a number of principles that are paired with guidelines for implementation. Principles and guidelines related to early detection of hearing impairment are outlined in Chapters 2 and 4. With regard to EI for hearing impairment, the HPCSA's EHDI guidelines specify the need for timeous access to assistive devices and intervention services that are family centred and asset-based, with awareness of informed choice and the cultural beliefs and traditions of families of children with hearing impairment (HPCSA, 2018).

Evidence shows that the negative consequences of hearing impairment on a child and on society at large can be reduced through effective therapeutic interventions (Smith, O'Connor, Hennessy, O'Sullivan, & Gibson, 2017). However, this evidence has mostly been documented in studies from high-income countries. Findings from a study comparing early and late identified children, all enrolled in auditory–verbal EI programmes, revealed that those identified and fitted with amplification by three months of age, and enrolled into an EI programme by six months of age (regardless of the severity of hearing impairment), significantly outperformed those identified late in terms of speech and language outcomes (Fulcher, Purcell, Baker, & Munro, 2012). Similarly, early diagnosis by three months of age and earlier receipt of amplification and commencement of auditory–verbal intervention by six months of age (as per EHDI guidelines) were reported by clinicians as facilitators of speech and language outcomes in children with hearing impairment (Fulcher, Purcell, Baker, & Munro, 2015). A larger study exploring the longitudinal outcomes of children with hearing impairment (LOCHI) found that early fitting of hearing aids or cochlear implants is key to the EI process. The language, functional performance, speech perception and psychosocial skills of children with hearing impairment, fitted with amplification by three years of age, were measured at five years of age. Results from this study indicated an association between earlier amplification and higher global language scores, as well as better receptive and expressive language and, as a result, better speech perception in noise. Psychosocial skills, as rated by parents, indicated better performance that was associated with better language and functional performance skills (Ching, Dillon, Leigh, & Cupples, 2018). While these studies from high-income countries have clearly documented evidence of the positive outcomes associated with EHDI, evidence from LAMI countries is limited.

Research initiatives have primarily focused on the implementation of screening in EHDI programmes, and have explored the ages of provision of amplification, while intervention approaches and related outcomes have received limited attention in sub-Saharan Africa (Moodley & Störbeck, 2015). This limited evidence on intervention approaches from LAMI countries may be due to the lack of integrated, national EHDI programmes, resulting in the continued late diagnosis of hearing impairment in children in these contexts.

As noted, the goal of EI in EHDI is to provide children with hearing impairment with the opportunity to develop an effective communication system through timely amplification and the provision of intervention by six months of age, with the child's family being a key stakeholder in the process (HPCSA, 2018; Smith et al., 2017). A survey with parents from the LOCHI study conducted in Australia revealed that they perceived themselves as central to the EI process, assuming multiple roles not always recognised by clinicians (Ching et al., 2018), such as case manager, care provider, teacher and advocate. Clinicians in high-income countries like Australia, however, have noted challenges in working with culturally and linguistically diverse families in terms of beliefs and views regarding amplification and EI (Fulcher et al., 2015). Nevertheless, these findings highlight the importance of clinicians taking into account individual context and environment during the EI process, which is particularly vital in culturally and linguistically diverse as well as resource-constrained contexts such as sub-Saharan Africa. In chapter 11, Maluleke, Chiwutsi and Khoza-Shangase focus on family-centred EHDI, with careful deliberations around what this means in the South African context.

Evidence from South Africa that supports the efficacy of EHDI has been documented in a single pilot study comprising language assessments of 10 children diagnosed with hearing impairment (Störbeck & Pittman, 2008). Children in this study were diagnosed at an average age of 15 months and enrolled in a home-based, family-centred EI programme. All children were found to display an overall language increase of 4.66 months per quarter, with a definitive difference between children identified before seven months and those identified late (Störbeck & Pittman, 2008). A larger, retrospective review on the audiological management of children with hearing impairment (from birth to three years of age) conducted at three public sector hospitals in Gauteng, South Africa, found lack of EHDI within this context (Khoza-Shangase & Michal, 2014). In this study, enrolment into aural (re)habilitation programmes was reported to be at an average age of two years five months, which far exceeds the recommended guidelines of six to eight months in South Africa. Although early diagnosis and timeous fitting of amplification are key principles of EHDI that influence outcome, specific EI goals need to be adhered to in order to ensure strong EI systems that meet the needs of children with hearing impairment and their families.

In alignment with EHDI goals for children with hearing impairment and their families, EI programmes need to adhere to specific goals outlined in the 2013 statement of endorsement (JCIH et al., 2013) as a supplement to the 2007 JCIH position statement. The 12 goals of EI following confirmation of hearing impairment as outlined by the JCIH statement are summarised below:

- Goal 1: All children and their families have access to timely and coordinated entry into EI programmes supported by a data management system capable of tracking families and children from confirmation of hearing impairment to enrolment into EI services.
- Goal 2: All children and their families experience timely access to service coordinators who have specialised knowledge and skills related to working with individuals with hearing impairment.

- Goal 3: All children from birth to three years of age and their families have EI providers who have the professional qualifications and core knowledge and skills to optimise the child's development and child/family well-being.
- Goal 4: All children with additional disabilities and their families have access to specialists who have the professional qualifications and specialised knowledge and skills to support and promote optimal developmental outcomes.
- Goal 5: All children and their families from culturally diverse backgrounds and/or from non-English-speaking homes have access to culturally competent services with provision of the same quality and quantity of information given to families from the majority culture.
- Goal 6: All children should have their progress monitored every six months from birth to 36 months of age, through a protocol that includes the use of standardised, norm-referenced developmental evaluations for language (spoken and/or signed), the modality of communication (auditory, visual and/or augmentative), social–emotional, cognitive, and fine and gross motor skills.
- Goal 7: All children who are identified with hearing impairment of any degree, including those with unilateral or slight hearing impairment, those with auditory neural hearing impairment (auditory neuropathy), and those with progressive or fluctuating hearing impairment, receive appropriate monitoring and immediate follow-up intervention services where appropriate.
- Goal 8: Families will be active participants in the development and implementation of EHDI systems at the state/territory and local levels.
- Goal 9: All families will have access to other families who have children with hearing impairment and who are appropriately trained to provide culturally and linguistically sensitive support, mentorship and guidance.
- Goal 10: Individuals who are deaf or hard of hearing will be active participants in the development and implementation of EHDI systems at the national, state/territory and local levels; their participation will be an expected and integral component of the EHDI systems.
- Goal 11: All children with hearing impairment and their families have access to support, mentorship and guidance from hearing-impaired individuals.
- Goal 12: As best practices are increasingly identified and implemented, all children with hearing impairment and their families will be assured of fidelity in the implementation of the intervention they receive (JCIH et al., 2013).

For the purposes of the JCIH statement, the terms 'deaf' and 'hard of hearing' are intended to be inclusive of congenital and acquired hearing impairment of all types and degrees (mild to profound). Distinctions have been made in terms of audibility, with the statement specifying that severe hearing impairment results in the audition of speech sounds without a clear understanding of them. Hard of hearing children are described as those who are able to communicate through spoken language and may benefit from hearing amplification with hearing aids and cochlear implants, whereas deaf children are described as having severe or profound hearing impairment resulting in very little or no residual hearing (JCIH et al., 2013). The statement of endorsement describes that children who are deaf may benefit from hearing amplification devices such as cochlear implants as it may help them to hear and learn speech. In learning to communicate, such children may benefit from visual reinforcement, such as signs, cued speech and lip reading (JCIH et al., 2013). These distinctions highlight the need to explore the various approaches to EI for children with hearing impairment.

Approaches to early intervention for hearing-impaired children

Although not specific regarding the approaches to EI for children diagnosed with hearing impairment, the HPCSA's (2018) EHDI guidelines broadly highlight the roles and responsibilities of speech-language therapists and audiologists. These include provision and timely fitting and monitoring of amplification devices in addition to education and counselling for families, as well as provision of direct (re)habilitation services, including the assessment of cochlear implant candidacy by speech-language therapists and audiologists experienced in the area.

With regard to provision of hearing amplification, timely fitting is not yet a reality in South Africa. Earlier studies indicated an average age at amplification of between 28 and 30 months (Khoza-Shangase & Michal, 2014; Van der Spuy & Pottas, 2008). More recently, Maluleke, Khoza-Shangase, and Kanji (2019) reported age ranges between one year six months and four years four months. These delays subsequently result in the late initiation of (re)habilitation.

With regard to direct (re)habilitation services, various intervention approaches are available for a child with a hearing impairment to learn to communicate. These include auditory approaches such as auditory–verbal therapy (AVT), incorporating listening and spoken language (LSL) principles, the oral–aural approach and cued speech, as well as more visual approaches such as total communication, or sign language. The chosen mode(s) of communication extend beyond the therapy session as speech-language therapists and audiologists are often consulted regarding the educational placement of children with hearing impairment or those who are cochlear implant candidates. This decision is often intricately related to the communication strategy and whether or not to recommend an oral communication approach or total communication (Connor, Hieber, Arts, & Zwolan, 2000). The following sections explore AVT, LSL, total communication, sign language and cued speech as communication approaches for EI for children with hearing impairment.

Auditory–verbal therapy

With the global drive toward implementation of universal newborn hearing screening for early identification of hearing impairment and the availability of hearing amplification technologies such as cochlear implantation, families are now able to elect an LSL outcome for their children, regardless of the degree of hearing impairment (Rosenzweig, 2017).

AVT is a parent-coaching programme aimed at developing spoken language through listening in order to narrow the gap between the hearing-impaired child's chronological age and language ability. This is done so that they may enter a mainstream school environment with appropriate language and social skills to participate in a hearing world (Auditory Verbal UK, 2018). Sound is the primary mode for learning and parents are equipped with the skills to maximise their child's speech as well as build a foundation for language development. AVT enables children with hearing impairment who have been fitted with hearing aids or cochlear implants to make sense of the sound relayed by the assistive device (Auditory Verbal UK, 2018). This auditory–verbal or oral–aural approach makes use of minimal amounts of residual hearing to develop speech and process language through auditory pathways, thereby enabling deaf children to understand spoken language and communicate orally using this residual hearing (Auditory Verbal UK, 2016). AVT has been recommended as the mainstream approach in the (re)habilitation of children with hearing impairment in the United States, Australia and New Zealand over the past 25 years (Kaipa & Danser, 2016; Lim & Hogan, 2017; Percy-Smith et al., 2018).

Professionals certified in AVT provide services under a guiding set of 10 principles, as defined by the AG Bell Academy for Listening and Spoken Language (Estabrooks, MacIver-Lux, & Rhoades, 2016, p. 18; Goldberg, Dickson, & Flexer, 2010, p. 135):

- Principle 1: Promote early diagnosis of hearing impairment in newborns, infants, toddlers and young children, followed by immediate audiologic management and auditory–verbal therapy.
- Principle 2: Recommend immediate assessment and use of appropriate, state-of-the-art hearing technology to obtain maximum benefits of auditory stimulation.
- Principle 3: Guide and coach parents to help their child use hearing as the primary sensory modality in developing listening and spoken language.

- Principle 4: Guide and coach parents to become the primary facilitators of their child's listening and spoken language development through active, consistent participation in individualised auditory–verbal therapy.
- Principle 5: Guide and coach parents to create environments that support listening for the acquisition of spoken language throughout the child's daily activities.
- Principle 6: Guide and coach parents to help their child integrate listening and spoken language into all aspects of the child's life.
- Principle 7: Guide and coach parents to use natural developmental patterns of audition, speech, language, cognition and communication.
- Principle 8: Guide and coach parents to help their child self-monitor spoken language through listening.
- Principle 9: Administer ongoing formal and informal diagnostic assessments to develop individualised auditory–verbal treatment plans, to monitor progress and to evaluate the effectiveness of the plans for the child and family.
- Principle 10: Promote education in regular schools with peers who have typical hearing and with appropriate services from early childhood onwards.

Outcome studies related to AVT have reported various positive outcomes in children with hearing impairment. Firstly, they have been reported to develop spoken language in line with their age-matched typically hearing peers (FirstVoice, 2015; Fulcher et al., 2012). Secondly, Dornan, Hickson, Murdoch, Houston, and Constantinescu (2010) found that following AVT, hearing-impaired children demonstrate progress at the same rate as age-matched typically hearing peers in terms of listening, spoken language, self-esteem, reading and mathematics (Dornan et al., 2010). Thirdly, these children tend to benefit markedly from earlier amplification (Dettman, Wall, Constantinescu, & Dowell, 2013). Finally, Percy-Smith et al. (2018) found that the use of AVT resulted in advanced language skills in comparison to children who received standard EI.

These findings suggest that the success of AVT is the direct result of the early provision of this therapeutic approach, which incorporates family-centred care following timeous fitting of hearing amplification devices. Percy-Smith et al. (2018) report that children with hearing impairment who were enrolled in an AVT programme yielded higher odds in terms of performing at age-equivalent speech and language levels compared to children with hearing impairment who received traditional speech therapy and/or aural (re)habilitation. Although the fitting of hearing amplification devices, particularly cochlear implantation, is emphasised in AVT, the study by Percy-Smith et al. (2018) established that language outcomes were achieved regardless of the type of hearing technology. Similarly, Cupples et al. (2018) reviewed the extent to which hearing amplification improved the speech production and language outcomes in children with hearing impairment enrolled in an AVT programme. Results indicated small to moderate improvements. Outcome data from a dataset of 696 children in Queensland, Australia, indicated that with AVT, the mean language, vocabulary and speech scores of hearing-impaired children fell within the average range of typical hearing peers. Most children also obtained scores within or above the average range for language for typical hearing children (First Voice, 2015). While these studies have positively reported on outcomes following AVT, findings have been limited to the presence of hearing impairment only, and have not been inclusive of children with other, concurrent conditions.

Hitchins and Hogan (2018) explored spoken language outcomes in hearing-impaired children who received AVT. The sample comprised children with and without additional needs, such as intellectual difficulties, sensory impairments, and physical, motor or musculoskeletal difficulties and syndromes. Of the 129 children in the study, 79 percent achieved age-appropriate language. However, despite an evident enhancement in listening and spoken communication, significantly fewer children with additional needs achieved these outcomes. These authors suggest that specific access to AVT in addition to generic EI could assist these children to achieve age-appropriate language. They further assert that ensuring access to effective EI by families will increase the chances of the adoption of a suitable communication approach as early as possible and will allow a child with additional needs (acquiring LSLs) to develop at a rate proportionate to their full potential (Hitchins & Hogan, 2018).

Goal 5 of the principles and guidelines for EI emphasises that all children with hearing impairment and their families should have access to culturally competent services. Active parental engagement is at the core of AVT, thus the evolution of the role of the AV interventionist since its inception in 1973 (Akçakaya & Tavşancıl, 2016). Given South Africa's cultural diversity, AVT sessions need to reflect culturally responsive practices in order to facilitate family engagement by demonstrating and incorporating an interest, understanding and respect for family cultures, including their behaviour and interaction styles (Estabrooks et al., 2016). It is crucial that AV interventionists embrace and incorporate cultural sensitivity in its therapeutic modalities, as data indicate that insufficient cultural responsiveness creates a barrier to optimal outcomes despite the early identification of a hearing impairment (Paul & Roth, 2011). Due to the lack of contextually relevant and contextually responsive evidence, South Africa's cultural diversity has not been tapped into, which is the key to effective clinical service provision in our population. It is well established that intervention is more valid when it is relevant and culturally acceptable (Pascoe, 2011). Yet, many intervention approaches and therapy resources developed by clinicians and researchers in the developed world are still being used in South Africa due to the absence of contextually relevant resources (Pascoe, 2011).

However, South African early interventionists have made attempts to adapt the existing developed world AVT intervention approach. The application of LSL interventions and AV practice has considered current cochlear implant and acoustic technologies and models for successful treatment planning, delivery and evaluation (LSLS South Africa, 2015). The listening and spoken language specialist (LSLS) designation is a worldwide certification. It is the only voluntary certification aimed at ensuring that professionals working with hearing-impaired children have the knowledge and skills to maximise the spoken language development of these children through listening so that they can be on a par with their typically hearing peers (Goldberg et al., 2010). Adequate provision of LSLS as an intervention approach may, however, be influenced by the number of professionals trained to provide this particular approach.

Current research suggests that, overall, there is a critical shortage of professionals trained to provide EI services to infants and children with hearing impairments in high-income countries (Martin-Prudent, Lartz, Borders, & Meehan, 2016). This shortage of professionals in relation to the high prevalence of congenital or early onset permanent sensorineural hearing impairments is apparent in the South African context too. Khoza-Shangase reports in chapter 5 that in January 2020, there were 788 audiologists and 1 612 speech therapists and audiologists registered in South Africa. This situation is exacerbated by only 51 qualified AVT interventionists in the country (LSLS South Africa, 2018), and the fact that AVT training is an additional licensing course following an undergraduate qualification. Of the 51 AVT interventionists, most work in the private health care sector (LSLS South Africa, 2018). Hence, improving levels of access to EI services is crucial, with an evident need for capacity-building through certified LSLS mentoring programmes, which need to include consideration of the diversity in South Africa.

Language is one of the most challenging aspects facing AV interventionists (Estabrooks et al., 2016). South Africa has 11 official languages but most speech-language and hearing professionals in the country have English or Afrikaans as a mother tongue, with only 5 percent being black African language speakers (Khoza-Shangase & Mophosho, 2018; LSLS South Africa, 2018). These findings are particularly relevant when considering oral communication approaches to EI such as AVT, as well as the development, integration and understanding of linguistic profiles such as the Language Assessment, Remediation and Screening Procedure (LARSP) of the different languages in South Africa. The limited number of trained AV interventionists and their linguistic backgrounds make it challenging to meet the demands of parents and families who speak any of the other official languages.

Total communication

Unlike AVT, the total communication philosophy focuses on using a variety of communication methods, including sign, speech and listening, lip reading, finger spelling, facial expression and gesture, in a combination that is best suited for a particular child. This approach is based on the premise that deaf children are able to learn to communicate effectively by using any and all modes of communication. Contrary to the view that speech perception is a purely auditory phenomenon, research has shown that it is a multimodal experience and that typically hearing people routinely include a combination of auditory and visual information (Leybaert & LaSasso, 2010).

Findings from a South African study reported an evident mismatch in the modes of communication in the home environment. Family members used a variety of communication modes during interactions, including oral communication or spoken language in isiZulu and English (depending on who the communication partner was), signed communication (pointing, gestures, home signs, eye gaze, facial expressions and South African Sign Language, or SASL), a combination of all communication modes, and tactile communication (Blose & Joseph, 2017). These findings suggest the unfair burden placed on children with hearing impairment in terms of taking responsibility for establishing communication interaction with different communication partners (Blose & Joseph, 2017), as well as the possible lack of family-centred EI in these contexts. Findings thus highlight the need for and importance of family involvement and collaboration between EI service providers and caregivers or parents regarding the choice of communication approach. It is vital that the provision of EI services is responsive to the multilingual and multicultural nature of sub-Saharan Africa.

Sign language

Incorporated as one possible approach within total communication, sign language is a visual, gestural approach. Programmes supporting the bilingual approach advocate for sign language to be the first or primary language. The second language is then the learned, spoken language of the family, which facilitates literacy development (Auditory Verbal UK, 2016). The sign language approach also focuses on learning about the deaf community as a cultural group, including its history and language, in order to develop a strong positive deaf identity. The National Institute for the Deaf (NID) defines deaf culture as a shared system of accepted behaviours, with sign language being the main mode of communication. Sign language comprises five parts: handshape, orientation, location, movement and non-manual features (NID, 2018).

In South Africa, the deaf community is a minority culture, with the 2011 census indicating that 400 000 citizens use SASL as their mother tongue (NID, 2018). At least 95 percent of deaf children are born to hearing parents who are unfamiliar with SASL. These children often learn the language at school, where they are taught speech in the form of a spoken language and SASL (NID, 2018). However, access to deaf schools remains a challenge as not every town or city has one. This results in many children having to leave home and attend residential schools. Peers and staff at the school often become like family to these children, with a challenging transition as they complete school and have to adapt to a hearing culture in the workplace (NID, 2018). In 2015, SASL was introduced as a subject in all schools for the deaf. This has resulted in a shift from the use of many different signs for the same concept to a gradually more homogenised system (NID, 2018).

Cued speech

Research findings indicate that exposure to cued speech prior to implantation is beneficial for late cochlear implantees (Leybaert & LaSasso, 2010). Cued speech comprises a system of manual gestures which accompany speech production in real time, with the aim of providing deaf children with complete, unambiguous phonological messages that are based only on visual information. Hence, cued speech has two components: the visual manual component, which is the handshape, and a visual non-manual articulatory component, which is the mouth shape. Cued speech has been argued to enhance the benefits of cochlear implantation by training the brain to make better use of auditory signals to achieve oral language development (Leybaert & LaSasso, 2010).

Research investigating language outcomes and communication approaches is limited and has demonstrated mixed findings. Some studies have demonstrated that children with hearing impairment who use oral communication are more likely to achieve better language scores than those who use total communication (Yanbay, Hickson, Scarinci, Constantinescu, & Dettman, 2014). Yanbay and colleagues compared the language outcomes in children with cochlear implants enrolled in different EI programmes, namely sign and spoken language, auditory–oral and AVT. Findings were variable in terms of the scores obtained, with no significant differences in language outcomes across the three groups. The age of diagnosis and family involvement were, however, associated with positive outcomes (Yanbay et al., 2014).

While research has explored different approaches to EI and communication in high-income countries, there is a lack of research around the use and effectiveness of implementing these intervention approaches for children with hearing impairment in sub-Saharan Africa (Khoza-Shangase, 2019). The need remains to implement evidence-based EI approaches and develop appropriate cultural and linguistic resources for the African context.

Although literature from sub-Saharan Africa has not specifically explored the outcomes of particular EI approaches in hearing-impaired children, a few studies have looked at the modes of communication used by the family and educators of these children. A study conducted from the perspective of hearing-impaired children in Zimbabwe revealed that they experienced language difficulties at school and at home, as spoken language was the mode of communication at home whereas sign language was used at school (Dakwa & Musengi, 2015). The authors acknowledge that African languages are part of indigenous culture, and that children need to be exposed to their mother tongue, but emphasise the need for hearing-impaired children's families also to be proficient in sign language, as these children are able to acquire multiple languages (Dakwa & Musengi, 2015). Another study conducted in Zimbabwe sought to establish the mode of communication used by parents with their hearing-impaired children. Findings from this study revealed that most parents used total communication, while some who struggled to communicate with their child used gestures, facial expression, pointing, touching and other manual signs that are not officially recognised (Mbaluka, Kurebwa, & Wadesango, 2013). Choosing a communication approach is a complex process, with family participation potentially having a significant impact on the choice.

Choosing a communication approach

There is continuous debate and controversy regarding the choice of spoken versus visual communication approaches. However, Gravel and O'Gara (2003) suggest that less emphasis should be placed on a specific approach, method or mode of communication and more on ensuring easy and frequent language exchange between the family and child with hearing impairment. The decision around which communication approach to use should be a dynamic, ongoing family-centred exploration with the early interventionist.

A number of factors may influence families' choice of communication approach. These include the age of identification and intervention, family involvement, use of amplification, community resources, presence of co-morbid conditions and the availability of later educational options. Each factor is discussed in more detail below.

Earlier identification and intervention is advantageous in terms of language outcomes. This is an important consideration in LAMI countries like South Africa, where the identification and commencement of intervention is delayed. Furthermore, family involvement is key. A study by Moeller (2000) found that apart from age at commencement of intervention, family participation and effectiveness of communication influence language scores. In African culture, family structure and involvement may differ, and in some instances may extend to the community. Maluleke, Chiwutsi and Khoza-Shangase explore the concept of family in relation to culture in chapter 11. The chosen approach may also be influenced by the type and use of amplification (hearing aids or cochlear implants). The development of spoken language is dependent on access to the acoustic features of speech and this is also important if the goal of the family is for the child with hearing impairment to develop intelligible speech. Additionally, access to and availability of community resources, specifically access to EI programmes and early interventionists trained in any one or more approaches, are influencing factors. A study exploring caregiver experiences of EI in South Africa revealed the following factors compromising EI service delivery: limited availability of appropriate facilities for hearing-impaired children, long distances between these services, related costs, and inconsistent and conflicting professional opinions about a child's diagnosis and treatment (Khoza-Shangase, 2019). Furthermore, the presence of co-morbidities or additional sensory impairments or developmental disabilities may make the choice of communication approach more challenging. Lastly, the availability of later educational options such as special schools, residential facilities or mainstream, inclusive education may be a deciding factor (explored by Khoza-Shangase in chapter 9).

Solutions and recommendations

A number of aspects need to be actualised to facilitate prompt and adequate EI for children with hearing impairment. Firstly, due to age at amplification being a documented factor influencing outcome, early identification of hearing impairment needs to be prioritised. Earlier identification and diagnosis will allow opportunities for earlier intervention. Hence, there needs to be a greater drive toward implementing newborn hearing screening followed by timely diagnosis of hearing impairment. Secondly, EI services need to be available and accessible to children with hearing impairment. This needs to be strategically argued for using the 2030 National Development Plan, which alludes to equitable access. Lastly, there needs to be a greater focus on training speech-language therapists and audiologists as well as other professionals, such as educators and early interventionists, in communication approaches for children with hearing impairment. According to the JCIH recommendations, professionals must be educated and suitably trained to provide services to children with hearing impairment. Apart from ensuring effective service delivery, the training may assist in addressing the significant shortage of professionals qualified to work with hearing-impaired infants and toddlers in both developed and developing contexts (Martin-Prudent et al., 2016).

Currently, speech-language therapists and/or audiologists need to undergo additional training in order to be certified to provide specific intervention approaches such as AVT. There is thus a need for early interventionists to receive training that is more specialised for developing the strategies and skills necessary to provide appropriate services to children with hearing impairments, bearing in mind their diverse backgrounds (Martin-Prudent et al., 2016). More intensive training in undergraduate curricula needs to be provided so that the current shortage of professionals is not further limited by the small percentage trained in specific approaches to EI.

More concerted efforts are required to provide linguistically and culturally relevant and responsive EI services in South Africa. Khoza-Shangase and Mophosho (2018) argue that language and culture play a complex role in intervention and that these aspects of diversity should be embraced by clinicians as they influence health-seeking behaviours and decisions made by patients and their caregivers. This argument extends beyond the clinical setting to the higher educational context, where the training of linguistically and culturally skilled professionals needs to happen within the speech-language hearing professions in South Africa.

The approach to EI should be guided by the mode of communication chosen by the family, who are key stakeholders in the process. This should be an informed decision following the presentation of all available intervention options and appropriate information counselling by the audiologist. The current reality of later identification and fitting of amplification in South Africa needs to be factored in when choosing the approach to intervention. Also important to consider are other contextual factors such as family structures and support.

Although there is limited evidence to suggest that one approach is more appropriate than another, it is widely accepted that AVT has its place in the spectrum of therapeutic intervention approaches. There is, however, a need for research-based evidence on the current, adapted therapy methodologies, as is the case with Listening and Spoken Language South Africa (LSLSA), and the benefits and limitations for the South African context. Determining the outcomes associated with the use of LSLSA will contribute to literature and inform appropriate EI goal setting (Hitchins & Hogan, 2018).

Conclusion

The age at amplification, communication approach and family involvement are all key to the EI process. The chosen approach needs to be a collaborative decision to best suit the needs of the child with hearing impairment and their family. This may be a dynamic process which also considers the age at amplification. Decision-making at the commencement of EI will enable a better match in modes of communication between the home and school environments.

Unlike developed contexts, approaches to EI and their subsequent outcomes have not been well documented in LAMI countries like South Africa. There is a clear need for more evidence-based research with regard to the effectiveness of EI approaches in the South African context, which differs from that of higher-income countries. Contextual factors related to cultural and linguistic diversity, African family contexts, late identification and management of childhood hearing impairment as well as accessibility to EI services are key considerations in EI programmes.

While the AVT approach has reportedly been adapted for the South African context, the relevance and efficacy of these adaptations need to be explored. There is also a need for an increase in trained professionals, particularly in the public health care sector, which serves the majority of the population. Training needs to extend beyond the intervention approaches and ensure incorporation of linguistic and cultural diversity in order to facilitate provision of contextually responsive and relevant services.

References

Akçakaya, H., & Tavşancıl, E. (2016). Teacher opinions about auditory verbal therapy. *Journal of Qualitative Research in Education, 4*(2), 1–25.

Auditory Verbal UK. (2016). Investing in a sound future for deaf children: A cost benefit analysis of auditory verbal therapy at Audiory Verbal UK. Retrieved from https://www.avuk.org/Handlers/Download.ashx?IDMF=d3a9f385-8d03-4580-900f-41cb00562397.

Auditory Verbal UK. (2018). A sound future: Raising expectations for children with deafness position paper 2018. Retrieved from https://www.avuk.org/Handlers/Download.ashx?IDMF=55c2082e-57b1-4caa-a6a3-6f3e8de845da.

Blose, Z. M., & Joseph, L. N. (2017). The reality of every day communication for a deaf child using sign language in a developing country. *African Health Sciences, 17*(4), 1149–1159.

Centre for Disease Control and Prevention. (2018). Facts about developmental disabilities. Retrieved from https://www.cdc.gov/ncbddd/developmentaldisabilities/facts.html.

Ching, T., Dillon, H., Leigh, G., & Cupples, L. (2018). Learning from the longitudinal outcomes of children with hearing impairment (LOCHI) study: Summary of 5-year findings and implications. *International Journal of Audiology, 57*(Suppl. 2), S105–S111.

Connor, C. M., Hieber, S., Arts, H. A., & Zwolan, T. A. (2000). Speech, language and the education of children using Cochlear implants: Oral or total communication? *Journal of Speech, Language, and Hearing Research, 43*, 1185–1204.

Cupples, L., Ching, T. Y. C., Button, L., Seeto, M., Zhang, V., Whitfield, J., … Marnane, V. (2018). Spoken language and everyday functioning in 5-year old children using hearing aids or cochlear implants. *International Journal of Audiology, 57*(2), S55–S69.

Dakwa, F. E., & Musengi, M. (2015). A look at language problems experienced by children with hearing impairments: The learner's experience. *South African Journal of African Languages, 35*(2), 177–180.

Dettman, S., Wall, E., Constantinescu, G., & Dowell, R. (2013). Commuication outcomes for groups of children using cochlear implants enrolled in auditory-verbal, aural-oral, and bilingual-bicultural early intervention programs. *Otology & Neurotology, 34*(3), 451–459.

Dornan, D., Hickson, L., Murdoch, B., Houston, T., & Constantinescu, G. (2010). Is auditory-verbal therapy effective for children with hearing loss? *The Volta Review, 110*, 361–387.

Estabrooks, W., MacIver-Lux, K., & Rhoades, E. A. (2016). *Auditory verbal therapy for young children with hearing impairment and their families, and the practitioners who guide them*. San Diego, CA: Plural Publishing.

First Voice. (2015). Sound outcomes: First voice speech and language data. Retrieved from https://www.firstvoice.org.au/wp-content/uploads/2017/09/FV-Sound-Outcomes-2015-Report-Final.pdf.

Fulcher, A., Purcell, A. A., Baker, E., & Munro, N. (2012). Listen up: Children with early identified hearing loss achieve age-appropriate speech/language outcomes by 3 years-of-age. *International Journal of Pediatric Otorhinolaryngology, 76*, 1785–1794.

Fulcher, A., Purcell, A. A., Baker, E., & Munro, N. (2015). Factors influencing speech and language outcomes of children with early identified severe/profound hearing loss: Clinician-identified facilitators and barriers. *International Journal of Speech-Language Pathology, 17*(3), 325–333.

Goldberg, D. M., Dickson, C. L., & Flexer, C. (2010). AG Bell Academy certification program for listening and spoken language specialists: Meeting a world-wide need for qualified professionals. *The Volta Review, 110*(2), 129–143.

Gravel, J. S., & O'Gara, J. (2003). Communication options for children with hearing loss. *Mental Retardation & Developmental Disabilities Research Reviews, 9*, 243–251.

Health Professions Council of South Africa (HPCSA). (2007). Early hearing detection and intervention programmes in South Africa, position statement year 2007. Retrieved from http://www.hpsca.co.za/hpcsa/default.aspx?id=137.

Health Professions Council of South Africa (HPCSA). (2018). Early hearing detection and intervention (EHDI) guidelines. Retrieved from http://www.hpcsa.co.za/Uploads/editor/UserFiles/downloads/speech/Early_Hearing_Detection_and_Intervention_(EHDI)_2018.pdf.

Hitchins, A. R. C., & Hogan, S. C. (2018). Outcomes of early intervention for deaf children with additional needs following an auditory verbal approach to communication. *International Journal of Pediatric Otorhinolaryngology, 115*, 125–132.

Joint Committee on Infant Hearing (JCIH). (2007). Year 2007 position statement: Principles and guidelines for early hearing detection and intervention programs. *Pediatrics, 120*(4), 898–921.

Joint Committee on Infant Hearing (JCIH), Muse, C., Harrison, J., Yoshinaga-Itano, C., Grimes, A., Brookhouser, P. E., … Martin, B. (2013). Supplement to the JCIH 2007 position statement: Principles and guidelines for early intervention after confirmation that a child is deaf or hard of hearing. *Pediatrics, 131*(4), e1324–e1349.

Kaipa, R., & Danser, M. L. (2016). Efficacy of auditory-verbal therapy in children with hearing impairment: A systematic review from 1993–2015. *International Journal of Pediatric Otorhinolaryngology, 86*, 124–134.

Khoza-Shangase, K. (2019). Early hearing detection and intervention in South Africa: Exploring factors compromising service delivery as expressed by caregivers. *International Journal of Pediatric Otorhinolaryngology*, *118*, 73–78.

Khoza-Shangase, K., & Michal, G. (2014). Early intervention in audiology: Exploring the current status from a developing country context. *British Journal of Medicine & Medical Research*, *4*(11), 2238–2249.

Khoza-Shangase, K., & Mophosho, M. (2018). Language and culture in speech-language and hearing professions in South Africa: The dangers of a single story. *South African Journal of Communication Disorders*, *65*(1), a594.

Leybaert, J., & LaSasso, C. J. (2010). Cued speech for enhancing speech perception and first language development of children with Cochlear implants. *Trends in Amplification*, *14*(2), 96–112.

Lim, S. R., & Hogan, S. C. (2017). Research findings for AV practice. In E. A. Rhoades & J. Duncan (Eds.), *Auditory verbal practice: Family centred early intervention* (pp. 52–64). Springfield, IL: Charles Thomas.

LSLS South Africa. (2015). Listening and spoken language skills South Africa: Professional training: Introductory guidebook. Retrieved from http://www.sacig. org.za/wp-content/uploads/2014/09/LSL-SA-Information-and-Application-form-for-2015.pdf.

LSLS South Africa. (2018). LSLSA graduates 2010–2017. Official list received via email from LSLSA training coordinator/facilitator: eroberts@polka.co.za.

Maluleke, N., Khoza-Shangase, K., & Kanji, A. (2019). Communication and school readiness abilities of children with hearing impairment in South Africa: A retrospective review of early intervention preschool records. *South African Journal of Communication Disorders*, *66*(1), a604.

Martin-Prudent, A., Lartz, M., Borders, C., & Meehan, T. (2016). Early intervention practices for children with hearing impairment: Impact of professional development. *Communication Disorders Quarterly*, *38*(1), 13–23.

Mbaluka, A., Kurebwa, M., & Wadesango, N. (2013). Parents' mode of communication with their hearing impaired children in Gweru Urban. *Journal of Human Ecology*, *42*(2), 1–7.

Moeller, M. P. (2000). Early intervention and language development in children who are deaf and hard of hearing. *Pediatrics*, *106*(3), E43.

Moodley, S., & Störbeck, C. (2015). Narrative review of EHDI in South Africa. *South African Journal of Communication Disorders*, *62*(1), 1–10.

National Institute for the Deaf (NID). (2018). South African Sign Language. Retrieved from https://www.westerncape.gov.za/assets/departments/cultural-affairssport/national_institute_for_the_deaf_sa_sign_language_booklet.pdf.

Neumann, K., Chadha, S., Tavartkiladze, G., Bu, X., & White, K. R. (2019). Newborn and infant hearing screening facing globally growing numbers of people suffering from disabling hearing loss. *International Journal of Neonatal Screening*, *5*(7), 1–11.

Olusanya, B. O. (2005). State of the world's children: Life beyond survival. *Archives of Disease in Children*, *90*, 317–218.

Olusanya, B. O., Davis, A. C., Wertlieb, D., Boo, N., Nair, M. K. C., Halpern, R., ... Kassebaum, N. J. (2018). Developmental disabilities among children younger than 5 years in 195 countries and territories, 1990–2016: A systematic analysis for the global burden of disease study 2016. *Lancet Global Health, 6*(10), e1100–e1121.

Pascoe, M. (2011). Contextually-relevant resources in speech-language therapy and audiology in South Africa: Are there any? *South African Journal of Communication Disorders, 58*(1), 2–5.

Paul, D., & Roth, F. P. (2011). Guiding principles and clinical applications for speech-language pathology practice in early intervention. *Language, Speech and Hearing Services in Schools, 42*, 320–330.

Percy-Smith, L., Tonning, T. L., Josvassen, J. L., Mikkelsen, J. H., Nissen, L., Dieleman, E., & Caye-Thomasen, P. (2018). Auditory verbal habilitation is associated with improved outcome for children with cochlear implant. *Cochlear Implants International, 19*(1), 38–45.

Republic of South Africa. (2015). National integrated early childhood development policy. Retrieved from https://unicef.org/southafrica/SAF_resources_integratedecd policy.pdf.

Rosenzweig, E. A. (2017). Auditory verbal therapy: A family-centered listening and spoken language intervention for children with hearing impairment and their families. *Perspectives of the ASHA Special Interest Groups, 2*(9), 54–65.

Smith, A., O'Connor, A., Hennessy, S., O'Sullivan, P. G., & Gibson, L. (2017). Permanent childhood hearing impairment: Aetiological evaluation of infants identified through the Irish newborn hearing screening programme. *Irish Medical Journal, 110*(10), 651.

Störbeck, C., & Pittman, P. (2008). Early intervention in South Africa: Moving beyond hearing screening. *International Journal of Audiology, 47*(Suppl. 1), S36–S43.

United Nations. (2018). Sustainable development goals. Retrieved from https://www. un.org/sustainabledevelopment/%20sustainable-development-goals/.

Van der Spuy, T., & Pottas, L. (2008). Infant hearing loss in South Africa: Age of intervention and parental needs for support. *International Journal of Audiology, 47*, S30–S35. doi: 10.1080/14992020802286210.

World Health Organization (WHO). (2012a). Developmental difficulties in early childhood: Prevention, early identification, assessment and intervention in low- and middle-income countries. A review. Retrieved from http://www.who.int/maternal_ child_adolescent/documents/development_difficulties_early_childhood/en.

World Health Organization (WHO). (2012b). Early childhood development and disability: A discussion paper. Retrieved from http://apps.who.int/iris/bitstream/ 10665/75355/1/9789241504065_eng.pdf?ua=1.

Yanbay, E., Hickson, L., Scarinci, N., Constantinescu, G., & Dettman, S. J. (2014). Language outcomes for children with cochlear implants enrolled in different communication programs. *Cochlear Implants International, 15*(3), 121–135.

8 Models of Care in Early Intervention for Children with Hearing Impairment

Amisha Kanji

Early intervention (EI) is vital in ensuring children and their families are provided with the necessary support to reach their maximum potential. These services are particularly important in children who are considered at risk for developmental delay as a lack of intervention may have negative consequences on development, school readiness, educational outcomes and vocational opportunities. This chapter deliberates on models of care and their link to early childhood intervention (ECI), with a specific focus on the principles of intervention for children with hearing impairment. A discussion of the different approaches to service delivery of EI is provided, paying careful attention to contextual factors that might influence the intervention process. Considerations around educational access for children with disability in sub-Saharan Africa are highlighted. Lastly, solutions and recommendations for EI for hearing impairment in the South African context are put forward.

ECI is aimed at supporting children who are considered to be at risk for, or who have been identified as having, a developmental delay or disability (World Health Organization [WHO], 2012). ECI programmes include specialised services such as medical and rehabilitation services, family-centred support (including training and counselling), social and psychological services, special education as well as service planning and coordination (WHO, 2012). These specialised services are guided by specific reasoning and may be provided at different sites or levels of service delivery that include health care clinics, hospitals, EI centres, rehabilitation centres, community centres, homes and schools (WHO, 2012).

Exploring models of care within these levels of service delivery is important to ensure efficacious intervention that is contextually responsive and responsible. A model of care is broadly defined as the manner in which health services are delivered. It outlines best practice care and services for the patient or population concerned as they progress through the various stages of a condition or event. A model of care therefore aims to ensure provision of appropriate care by the relevant professionals at the right time and place (Agency for Clinical Innovation, 2013). The use of models of care is valuable in framing EI services as it is one stage within the multi-staged early hearing detection and intervention (EHDI) process following diagnosis of hearing impairment, and requires the implementation of appropriate and timely intervention to facilitate positive outcomes. The guiding principles of a model of care include, among others, patient-centric care, localised flexibility, and considerations for equity of access, efficient use of existing resources and quality, integrated care. These broader guiding principles align well with the specific EI principles (defined by the Joint Committee on Infant Hearing, or JCIH) that should guide the provision of EI services (JCIH et al., 2013).

As a component of ECI, EI for hearing impairment involves (re)habilitation to prevent the disability posed by restricted hearing from resulting in limited participation in society. Specific (re)habilitation is a multi-staged process that commences with the provision, fitting and adjustment of amplification devices such as hearing aids or cochlear implants, followed by early communication intervention (McPherson, 2014; Peer, 2015). Most developed countries have been able to access hearing health care through private and publicly funded aural rehabilitation systems. However, many low and middle-income (LAMI) countries, where the prevalence of child and adult hearing impairment is substantially higher, have not had these opportunities for access to amplification (McPherson, 2014; Stevens et al., 2011). A lack of access to assistive devices is further coupled with additional challenges in South Africa, such as skilled staff shortages; inequity in health access and quality of care; and health care spending that is primarily focused on improving health outcomes related to life expectancy, decreasing mortality and decreasing the burden of disease (Kerr, Tuomi, & Müller, 2012). Against the backdrop of life-threatening diseases and the prioritisation of primary health care service provision, specialised rehabilitative approaches, such as cochlear implantation, which is essentially a quaternary level of care, are not seen as a priority by the National Department of Health (Kerr et al., 2012).

The provision of affordable assistive devices in a sustainable manner is one of the key elements to successful EI programmes. Yet, in most cases, amplification devices and the related maintenance costs remain unaffordable and may still be regarded as a substantial sum to pay by many families in LAMI countries (McPherson, 2014). Obtaining a cochlear implant involves a lifetime commitment from the families of children with hearing impairment as adequate finances are required in order to access the rapidly developing technology for the rest of their lives. Related costs include assessment, implantation, rehabilitation and maintenance. In addition, families of children must be able to access a specialist facility where cochlear implantation is offered. In South Africa, accessing one of the facilities in the main cities could involve additional travel costs (Kerr et al., 2012). Kerr and colleagues (2012) explored the costs involved in using a cochlear implant in South Africa. Findings from their study revealed that in 2010, the costs for a child for the first five and ten years post implantation were R298 961 and R455 225, respectively. While cost remains a major drawback to regular cochlear implantation, there are currently 15 cochlear implantation programmes in South Africa. There is growing interest in the expansion of these programmes (Peer, 2015), which may facilitate access to specialist facilities for EI where the development of spoken language (for congenital hearing impairment) or retention of access to spoken language (for acquired hearing impairment) is the communication system of choice. These specialist facilities, as well as all other EI programmes for hearing-impaired children, should be guided by a set of key principles.

Research indicates that the provision of EI for hearing-impaired children in the first six months of life is likely to result in linguistic, speech and cognitive development that is comparable to that of their typical hearing peers (Ching et al., 2013; Fulcher, Purcell, Baker, & Munro, 2012). Factors that contribute to the outcomes include, among others, quality of intervention services and service delivery models (Ching et al., 2013; Fitzpatrick, Durieux-Smith, Eriks-Brophy, Olds, & Gaines, 2007; Pimperton & Kennedy, 2012; Wake, Poulakis, Hughes, Carey-Sargeant, & Rickards, 2005). These service delivery models may include group, individual, home-based, centre-based and/or inclusive or specialised schooling. The choice of model may vary between countries due to contextual differences, but may also differ as a child transitions through the EI process.

Individual versus group-based early intervention

The implementation of intervention approaches that provide efficient management without compromising quality of care is the focus in some developed countries (Collins, Souza, O'Neill, & Yueh, 2007) and has been provided through a programme called Advanced Clinical Access. This programme is aimed at increasing clinical capacity by offering group sessions with the rationale that more patients could be seen using the same number of resources as required by individual therapy or traditional one-on-one sessions. Collins et al. (2007) argue that sessions in audiological (re)habilitation that are focused on amplification device training and use for new patients can be accommodated in group sessions as information is standardised with common discussion themes.

A few studies have compared the effectiveness of group versus individual therapy or aural rehabilitation in the adult population (Collins, Liu, Taylor, Souza, & Yueh, 2013; Collins et al., 2007). The first study, in 2007, compared hearing aid outcomes in new hearing aid patients who received individual as opposed to group fitting and follow-up visits. Results from the Effectiveness of Auditory Rehabilitation (EAR), Hearing Handicap Inventory for the Elderly, and Satisfaction with Amplification in Daily Life questionnaires revealed that patients who attended group visits scored better, had improved hearing-related function and wore their hearing aids daily for a longer period (Collins et al., 2007). Similarly, a study in 2013 explored the effectiveness of individual versus group hearing aid fittings and follow-up in terms of hearing-related function, adherence six months post fitting as well as the costs associated with each approach. Contrary to the first study, findings indicated no significant difference in EAR scores or in the total number of hours that patients wore their hearing aids. Group sessions were thus not inferior to individual sessions. However, significantly higher costs were noted for individual fitting and follow-up visits (Collins et al., 2013).

There is a dearth of literature regarding the effectiveness of group versus one-on-one speech-language therapy for children with hearing impairment. Rehman, Khan, Malik, and Ud Din (2016) compared the effectiveness of these two models of service delivery for EI for children with hearing impairment in a developing context. Twenty children between six and seven years of age were enrolled in the study and were assessed both pre and post language intervention. Findings indicated that although both intervention models resulted in improved performance, significant differences in language development were noted between individual versus group therapy. The authors of this study concluded that language development in children with hearing impairment can be more effectively enhanced when group therapy sessions are utilised (Rehman et al., 2016). According to Roman (2018), key lessons to consider when implementing a group therapy approach with hearing-impaired individuals include:

- developing realistic, measurable goals as per any intervention approach
- recognising that group development takes time due to the diversity of backgrounds and expectations
- recognising that the group therapy approach fosters social interaction, which is beneficial in itself
- developing goals that meet the needs of the group while still addressing individual needs through home programmes or exercises.

While both group and individual models of intervention contribute to positive outcomes in children with hearing impairment, the chosen model needs to be considered in light of the long-term benefits as the child transitions through different stages of the EI process. The benefits of individual versus group therapy in terms of social integration and inclusivity when a hearing-impaired child reaches school-going age need to be considered. In this instance, group therapy may afford more opportunity for inclusivity as it fosters diversity and social interaction (Roman, 2018). The choice may also be influenced by context. Group sessions cost less than individual sessions (Rehman et al., 2016). Findings from a study by Collins et al. (2013) also indicated significantly higher costs associated with individual versus group hearing aid fittings and follow-up. These costs are important considerations for contexts such as South Africa, which have limited budgetary and human resources and, as a result, limited service delivery, which may further impact access to rehabilitation.

Access to rehabilitation in the public health care sector in South Africa is constrained, even in relatively well-resourced provinces such as the Western Cape (Maart & Jelsma, 2013). Research has demonstrated that only 26 percent of children from a peri-urban township in Gauteng accessed rehabilitation services in 2007 (Saloojee, Phohole, Saloojee, & Ijsselmuiden, 2007). Assistive devices such as hearing aids were widely unavailable or subject to long waiting lists (Saloojee et al., 2007). The lack of provision of hearing amplification results in delays with the commencement of EI, particularly for spoken language, and has serious short- and long-term implications for children with hearing impairment, including possible schooling difficulties and subsequent lack of employment opportunities (Sherry, 2015). Therapists across South Africa have cited the following reasons for the lack of provision of assistive devices: inefficient procurement processes, lack of budget allocation, lack of transport to collect and deliver devices, and lack of spare parts and repair technicians (Sherry, 2015). Additionally, the availability of adequate human resources remains a challenge to effective EI service provision, and may influence the chosen service delivery model in the public health care sector.

Human resources for rehabilitation in the public sector are subject to the same challenges as other groups of health care professionals. These include international migration, attrition, freezing of posts and relocation to the private health care sector (Sherry, 2015). While there are currently no set staffing norms for rehabilitation services (Sherry, 2015), the number of health care professionals in relation to the number of patients that need to be serviced must be considered in programme planning to ensure adequate and timely service provision. In chapter 2, Kanji discusses hearing health care services in relation to the number of trained professionals in sub-Saharan Africa.

Khoza-Shangase, in chapter 5, provides the most recent Health Professions Council of South Africa (HPCSA) statistics. These statistics indicate that in January 2020, there were 788 audiologists and 1 612 registered speech-language therapists and audiologists. The speech-language and hearing profession in South Africa has an unfavourable professional-to-patient ratio, with an incongruence with regard to capacity versus demand (Khoza-Shangase & Mophosho, 2018; Pascoe, 2011). Posts for speech-language and hearing professionals are also lacking, thus resulting in most communities not having access to these services in the public health care sector (Khoza-Shangase, Kanji, Petrocchi-Bartal, & Farr, 2017). Considering the high patient-to-professional ratio in sub-Saharan Africa, the use of group sessions may be beneficial in addressing human resource shortages. This may in turn result in reduced waiting lists, which could potentially shorten the timeframes from diagnosis to enrolment in an intervention programme.

While the number of qualified professionals in relation to the population is an important consideration for EI service delivery, the number of experienced clinicians in this field is also important to ensure quality service provision. Kanji and Casoojee highlight the shortage of trained speech-language therapists and audiologists in chapter 7. The EI principles refer to the need for hearing-impaired children and their families to have access to professionals who have the qualifications, skills and knowledge as EI providers to enhance development and well-being, as well as facilitate optimal development in children with hearing loss and any additional disability.

The linguistic and cultural competency of therapists is important considering the diversity in sub-Saharan African countries. Statistics related to the linguistic profile of South Africa indicate that isiZulu is the most commonly spoken home language (22.7 percent), followed by isiXhosa (16 percent), Afrikaans (13.5 percent) and English (9.6 percent). However, English is the most dominant language in the speech-language and hearing profession, followed by Afrikaans (Statistics South Africa, 2011). Qualified speech-language therapists and audiologists are thus not representative of the linguistic and cultural diversity of the country's population, with a further unequal distribution between public and private health care sectors (Pascoe, 2011). The linguistic incongruence also poses an ethical challenge, as an individual should not be denied intervention due to a language mismatch. However, speech-language therapists and audiologists may not be competent to offer intervention in all languages (Pascoe, 2011). A variety of linguistic profiles among children with hearing impairment may pose further challenges for the clinician in a diverse group therapy approach. This needs careful consideration when adopting such an approach to intervention. Khoza-Shangase and Mophosho (2018) argue that diversity should be embraced as a strength instead of being viewed as a complication.

Cultural awareness is considered the foundation to becoming culturally competent (Wegner & Rhoda, 2015). Campinha-Bacote (2002) proposed a model of cultural competence consisting of five constructs: cultural awareness, knowledge, skills, encounters and desire. Cultural awareness relates to reflection on one's own beliefs regarding culture. Cultural knowledge can be built by engaging with people of different cultural backgrounds. Cultural skills refer to the health care practitioners' ability to assess and manage patients while considering the differences within various cultural groups. Cultural encounters and desire refer to an individual's initiative to experience the differences among cultures.

Considering the current resource-constrained context in sub-Saharan Africa, group therapy may be a viable option. However, it needs to be weighed against other contextual aspects such as the linguistic and cultural profiles of both patients and therapists, as well as the broader African cultural context. In African culture, the philosophy of ubuntu may be a beneficial viewpoint to consider when deciding on the approach to EI. Ubuntu describes the essence of being human but also adopts a system different from western values in that it stands for 'I am because we are', which essentially suggests that there is no 'I' without the 'we'. Ubuntu thus portrays a spirit of oneness and group solidarity, with an emphasis on understanding, collaboration and partnership (Wilson & Williams, 2013).

Collaboration and partnership extend beyond the therapy context to the family context and home environment. 'Children acquire language within the family context where there is a dynamic interaction between language, culture, values and child rearing practices' (HPCSA, 2018, p. 28). Hence, families with children who are newly diagnosed with hearing impairment also require information and resources from EI professionals on how to provide an enriched language environment that supports early language learning (Yoshinaga-Itano, 2014).

Home- versus centre-based early intervention

An estimated 474 000 children live with severe disabilities in South Africa, with many more presenting with mild to moderate disabilities (Republic of South Africa, 2015). Appropriate screening and detection of these cases is hampered by the lack of services at a primary health care level as well as the shortage of appropriately skilled staff (Michelson, Adnams, & Shung-King, 2003). Intervention following identification is also hindered by services not being widely available – less than 30 percent of public health facilities offer rehabilitation/community-based rehabilitation services (Ebrahim, Seleti, & Dawes, 2013; Slemming & Saloojee, 2013). These limitations extend beyond the health care sector into early childhood development facilities that do not always provide environments conducive to learning for children with disabilities (Republic of South Africa, 2015). In addition, the current funding model does not make provision for additional funding for programmes for such children (Republic of South Africa, 2015). There is also a need to strengthen the curricula for the training of early childhood practitioners who provide services to infants and young children with disability. Other factors influencing access are adult beliefs regarding whether these children may be included in mainstream programmes, the stigma associated with disability, and that early childhood teaching strategies do not take into account children with disabilities (Republic of South Africa, 2015).

Home-based intervention is a crucial component of EI while children are not yet eligible for institution-based intervention (Couto & Carvalho, 2013; Lichtert & Van Wieringen, 2013). It is particularly beneficial in contexts such as South Africa where access to EI services remains a challenge. Perceived benefits of home-based intervention programmes include overcoming barriers to participation in EI services as a result of the lack of transportation (Collins, Jordan, & Coleman, 2010); providing intervention in the home environment, which is ideal for determining the strengths and needs of families; and increasing parental involvement in the EI process (Miedel & Reynolds, 1999).

Home-based service delivery systems for EI usually make use of a consultation model whereby the early interventionist visits the family in their home on a regular, scheduled basis (Deiner, 2013). The early interventionist has the responsibility of sharing the necessary information with the family regarding service resource availability, answering questions posed by parents about their child's impairment or disability, modelling or demonstrating appropriate activities for working with their child (Deiner, 2013) and possibly also serving as a liaison between the medical and educational sectors. Literature suggests that three aspects of home-based programmes are critical to their success (Azzi-Lessing, 2013):

- the quality of the relationship between the consultant or early interventionist, the child and the family
- the characteristics, training and support of the consultant or interventionist, as some families may be more comfortable with an individual who shares their cultural background and is able to communicate easily in their primary language (Azzi-Lessing, 2013, 2017)
- the ability to match the services delivered to the specific needs of the families and that meet their expectations (Azzi-Lessing & Schmidt, 2019).

This type of home-based intervention engages the family of the hearing-impaired child, lays a solid foundation and facilitates decision-making by families regarding mode of communication and other intervention strategies (Yang et al., 2015). A study conducted by Yang and colleagues (2015) revealed that home-based intervention facilitated understanding of common phrases and conversation in 78 percent of the children, and 98 percent were intelligible to the listener. These authors concluded that habilitation within the first 12 months after fitting of amplification is a key stage for auditory and speech development in hearing-impaired children.

In 2006, the HI HOPES (Home intervention: Hearing and language opportunities parent education services) family-centred, home-based support programme was established in South Africa's Gauteng province. This programme currently provides free EI services for children (from birth to three years of age) with mild to profound degrees of hearing impairment and their families in five of the nine provinces in South Africa. Children and their families are either self-referred to these services, or referrals are made by professionals (HI HOPES, 2019; Störbeck & Young, 2016).

The HI HOPES programme comprises family support and language development interventions that have been adapted from the SKI HI curriculum (SKI-HI Institute, 2004). The SKI HI Language Development Scale is a norm-referenced assessment performed shortly after enrolment into the programme. Language development is monitored and assessed every four months, with the Bayley Scales of Infant and Toddler Development being conducted every six months (Störbeck & Calvert-Evers, 2008). Home interventionists from a variety of vocational backgrounds, including teachers, audiologists, speech therapists and deaf mentors conduct regular home visits, and are suitably matched to the families in terms of culture. The language development intervention aspect of the programme is not biased toward any form of communication approach (sign language, spoken language or a mix). There is also no bias toward the type of amplification device – hearing aids, cochlear implants, bone-anchored devices – fitted for the hearing-impaired child (Störbeck & Young, 2016). Since the HI HOPES programme only caters for children up to three years of age, there is a need for integration and transition to a preschool or other educational setting (Störbeck & Calvert-Evers, 2008). While home-based intervention may be beneficial in terms of providing cost-effective access to families in LAMI countries, this type of service delivery model is highly reliant on follow-through by families. Due to consultants or early interventionists typically working according to a daytime schedule, the caregiver that is at home has the responsibility of carrying out the intervention and interpreting the information from the consultant for the other family members (Deiner, 2013). In instances where families are headed by single parents or caregivers, very young parents, elderly grandparents, chronically ill parents or caregivers, more support is required from the early interventionist. Although a primary-caregiver-centred approach is often considered, extended family members, grandparents and daytime caregivers may also be trained to achieve intervention goals in the African context (SASLHA Ethics and Standards Committee, 2017). The role and definition of family in Africa is discussed in chapter 11.

Centre-based EI service delivery systems may be based in a variety of contexts and usually comprise a team of specialists. Staff at these EI centres are usually well trained in special education and therapists conduct assessments, provide therapy in the setting and contribute to the child's educational programme (Deiner, 2013). According to the National Integrated Early Childhood Development Policy in South Africa, centre-based programmes are partial care facilities that focus on early learning and development of children from birth until the year before entering grade R or formal schooling (Republic of South Africa, 2015). While access to these early childhood development programmes is increasing, access to early learning and care remains inequitable, especially for vulnerable children (Republic of South Africa, 2015). This is primarily due to the cost, which is unaffordable for many parents or caregivers of affected children (Republic of South Africa, 2015).

Centre-based EI programmes in South Africa are often located in pre-primary or preschool settings, and include but are not limited to the Children's Communication Centre in Johannesburg, Whispers Speech and Hearing Centre in Pretoria and the Carel du Toit Centre in Cape Town. Some of these centres collaborate closely with audiologists in both the public and private sectors, offer EI outreach programmes, and act as resource centres for parent and teacher training. Two studies exploring the enrolment and outcomes of children with hearing impairment in centre-based EI programmes revealed suboptimal initiation of these services due to late identification of hearing loss (Maluleke, Khoza-Shangase, & Kanji, 2019b). As a result, these children presented with below average communication skills and school readiness abilities (Maluleke, Khoza-Shangase, & Kanji, 2019a)

Special schooling versus mainstream inclusion

Childhood development is embedded in education, which impacts on the progression through life (United Nations Children's Fund [UNICEF], 2016). All children, including those with disabilities, should thus have access to quality education to ensure literacy and participation in society as well as assist in enhancing both the social and economic security of individuals (UNICEF, 2016). However, in sub-Saharan Africa (UNICEF, 2016), children with disability are disproportionately affected by a lack of access to education and are far less likely than their peers to access quality education (UNICEF, 2016). There are more than 40 schools for the deaf in South Africa. In addition, the Institute for the Deaf in Worcester operates a deaf college which trains deaf people for jobs, and the University of the Witwatersrand in Johannesburg has a Centre for Deaf Studies that offers programmes in deaf education (Government Communications, 2016).

A number of policies and programmes support education for children with disabilities in many countries in eastern and southern Africa. One is the UN Convention on the Rights of Persons with Disabilities (CRPD), which states in regard to education that children with disabilities must (UNICEF, 2016):

• not be excluded from the general education system
• be afforded access to an inclusive, quality education
• be provided with support and reasonable accommodations to facilitate learning
• be able to access alternative means of learning or communication such as sign language

- be able to receive education in their respective mode or means of communication
- be taught by teachers who are qualified in the respective means or modes of communication (including teachers with disabilities), and who are trained in disability
- be made aware of the use of appropriate augmentative and alternative modes, means and formats of communication.

Countries in sub-Saharan Africa that have signed and ratified the CRPD protocol include Angola, Burundi, Mozambique, Namibia, Rwanda, South Africa, Swaziland, Uganda, Tanzania and Zimbabwe. Botswana, Eritrea, Somalia and South Sudan have not done so. Hearing impairment is one of the most commonly identified and recognised disabilities, and appears to have been formally recognised in Angola, Botswana, Eritrea, Ethiopia, Kenya, Malawi, Namibia, Rwanda, South Sudan, Swaziland, Uganda, United Republic of Tanzania and Zimbabwe (UNICEF, 2016).

'Special educational needs', 'disability' and 'inclusive education' are common terms utilised in studies from various country contexts. 'Special educational needs' is sometimes used interchangeably with the term 'children with disabilities'. In some instances, children with disabilities are viewed as a subgroup of children with special educational needs. Inclusive education has commonly been viewed in terms of the educational placement of the child to avoid segregation, for which special needs schooling is often critiqued (Haug, 2017; Mitchell, 2017). However, it has been suggested that this may be a narrow approach to defining inclusive education, and that an alternative may be to define inclusive education not as complete membership in a mainstream classroom, but rather as the best place for learning (Haug, 2017).

The definitions of these terms have been disputed as disability is also interpreted as an interaction between impairment, the environment and personal factors (WHO, 2002). For example, a child with a hearing impairment may not be able to effectively participate in a mainstream school due to a variety of factors that act as barriers or enablers at individual and environmental levels (Figure 8.1).

A child's participation in a mainstream environment may be influenced by personal factors or barriers such as the severity of the hearing impairment, and how much spoken language has been acquired if it is a postlingual hearing loss. Participation will also be influenced by how these factors interact with other enabling factors, such as the availability of hearing amplification, and teacher training and involvement. Other demand-side factors also play a role, such as parental views, an appropriate curriculum, learning materials or resources, and teachers' adequate understanding of the hearing impairment (UNICEF, 2016).

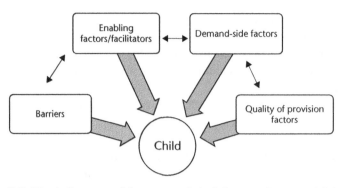

Figure 8.1 The influence of factors and their interaction on children with hearing impairment

Source: WHO, 2002

Inclusive education remains in a pilot phase in much of sub-Saharan Africa (Mariga, McConley, & Myezwa, 2014; Srivastava, De Boer, & Pijl, 2015). This is due to various barriers that hinder participation of children with disabilities, and obstruct the realisation of inclusive education (Mitchell, 2017). These barriers include lack of infrastructure and resource constraints which result in inadequate provision of education and disproportionately disadvantage children with sensory or motor impairments (Abdo & Semela, 2010; Mariga et al., 2014; Tassew, Jones, & Bekele, 2005).

Solutions and recommendations

A model of care for EI for children with hearing impairment needs to be developed for the South African context to ensure that change is effected through consistent improvements in service delivery that is contextually responsive and responsible. These models of care need to be evidence-based and linked to national strategic plans and initiatives by government in both the health and educational sectors. Due to the involvement of various stakeholders in the EHDI process, these models of care need to be developed in collaboration with clinicians, educators and families of children with hearing impairment. This is particularly important as the journey of the child with hearing impairment extends across different service providers (Agency for Clinical Innovation, 2013).

Since EI commences following fitting of amplification, there is a need for effective provision of hearing amplification devices. Hlayisi and Ramma (2018) propose a multi-pronged approach to ensure that supply meets the need for the provision of hearing aids. These authors suggest that audiologists in developing countries advocate for increased budget allocation and explore low-cost hearing amplification devices and rehabilitation intervention. One such low-cost intervention approach is group therapy, especially when considering the shortage of skilled human resources in South Africa.

EI should commence with home-based intervention services delivered by professionals trained specifically in managing hearing impairment. This will allow for early language learning and provide support for families with children with hearing impairment. South Africa could provide support for the development of these services to other countries in the sub-Saharan region given the establishment of home-based intervention programmes nationally. Due to the shortage of skilled professionals, alternative methods should be explored to increase access to services in South Africa and across sub-Saharan Africa. One such alternative method is the use of remote service delivery or tele-intervention, with innovative use of task shifting as a delivery model. A task-shifting model should include training the caregivers of children with hearing impairment, who are then able to provide services to other families. This will assist in expanding human resources to deal with patient demand in homes, centres and schools, with the added advantages of capacity-building, community engagement, caregiver empowerment and creation of local jobs and new opportunities for caregivers of hearing-impaired children (WHO, 2007).

Tele-intervention is a viable option in contexts where it is difficult or too costly for the health care practitioner to consult with the patient in person (Havenga, Swanepoel, Le Roux, & Schmid, 2017). Implementation of these services has resulted in practitioners saving time and resources, and increasing their reach. In addition to practitioner benefits, parent benefits include satisfaction as a result of reduced cost, reduced waiting lists and fewer travel arrangements for appointments. A study conducted in South Africa revealed no significant differences between tele-intervention and conventional face-to-face intervention in terms of the communication performance of children with hearing impairment (Havenga et al., 2017). Despite both methods being effective, the choice of preferred intervention needs to be made in consultation with the family and needs to take into account contextual factors such as access to technology (Havenga et al., 2017). Khoza-Shangase explores the use of tele-audiology in an educational setting in chapter 9, and Naudé and Bornman highlight the core ethical aspects around implementing tele-audiology for EHDI in chapter 13.

Home-based intervention programmes need to act as a referral source for centre-based intervention once children reach the age of three to ensure continuity of care. Referral pathways are often the focus in the early detection of hearing impairment in order to ensure timely diagnosis. An equal focus needs to be placed on the EI stage to facilitate transition through the EHDI process.

Irrespective of the service delivery model or approach to EI, effective service provision should be cognisant of the principles related to the models of care, and should include the contextual diversity in South Africa. Provision of appropriate service delivery should commence during student clinical training and should ensure that cultural awareness forms part of the undergraduate curriculum, particularly as it is the cornerstone of cultural sensitivity.

The government's promulgation and ratification of relevant policies specifically geared towards managing hearing impairment is the first step to actualising ECI at an effective level. Intrinsic to this is EI service access for those with hearing impairment. Health care professionals and teachers need to collaboratively advocate for access to these services in less developed contexts, particularly those where a high percentage of childhood disability exists. All educators and teachers should have some training in childhood disabilities, which should be initiated in the university curriculum, as this will assist in reducing communication barriers with respect to inclusive education.

Conclusion

The importance and benefits of EI are well known. While there are defined principles for EI in children with hearing impairment, they are not always implemented in developing world contexts, specifically countries in sub-Saharan Africa. Home-based EI may be more accessible for parents and families in these contexts, and group therapy a more cost-effective and resource-savvy approach to EI. However, linguistic and cultural diversity need to be considered when implementing a specific approach to EI. At present, inclusive education and special education needs remain a challenge in sub-Saharan Africa due to resource limitations and a lack of trained educators. This must be considered in proposed EI strategies.

References

Abdo, M., & Semela, T. (2010). Teachers of poor communities: The tale of instructional media use in primary schools of Gedeo Zone, southern Ethiopia. *Australian Journal of Teacher Education, 35*(7), 78–92.

Agency for Clinical Innovation. (2013). Understanding the process to develop a model of care: An ACI framework. Retrieved from https://www.aci.health.nsw.gov.au/__data/assets/pdf_file/0009/181935/HS13-034_Framework-DevelopMoC_D7.pdf.

Azzi-Lessing, L. (2013). Serving highly vulnerable families in home-visitation programs. *Infant Mental Health Journal, 34*(5), 376–390.

Azzi-Lessing, L. (2017). *Behind from the start: How America's war on the poor is harming our most vulnerable children.* New York, NY: Oxford University Press.

Azzi-Lessing, L., & Schmidt, K. (2019). The experiences of early childhood development home visitors in the Eastern Cape province of South Africa. *South African Journal of Childhood Education, 9*(1), a748.

Campinha-Bacote, J. (2002). The process of cultural competence in the delivery of healthcare services: A model of care. *Journal of Transcultural Nursing, 13*(3), 181–184.

Ching, T. Y. C., Dillon, H., Marnane, V., Hou, S., Day, J., Seeto, M., ... Yeh, A. (2013). Outcomes of early- and late-identified children at 3 years of age: Findings from a prospective population-based study. *Ear and Hearing, 34*(5), 535–552.

Collins, D., Jordan, C., & Coleman, H. (2010). *An introduction to family social work (3rd ed.)*. Pacific Grove, CA: Brooks.

Collins, M. P., Liu, C., Taylor, L., Souza, P. E., & Yueh, B. (2013). Hearing aid effectiveness after aural rehabilitation: Individual versus group trial results. *Journal of Rehabilitation Research & Development, 50*(4), 585–598.

Collins, M. P., Souza, P. E., O'Neill, S., & Yueh, B. (2007). Effectiveness of group versus individual hearing aid visits. *Journal of Rehabilitation Research & Development, 44*(5), 739–750.

Couto, M. I., & Carvalho, A. C. (2013). Factors that influence the participation of parents in the oral rehabilitation process of children with cochlear implants: A systematic review. *Codas, 25*, 84–91.

Deiner, P. L. (2013). *Inclusive early childhood education: Development, resources and practice (6th ed.)*. Belmont, Australia: Wadsworth Cengage Learning.

Ebrahim, H., Seleti, J., & Dawes, A. (2013). Learning begins at birth: Improving access to early learning. In L. Berry, L. Biersteker, A. Dawes, L. Lake, & C. Smith (Eds.), *South African child gauge 2013* (pp. 66–71). Cape Town, South Africa: Children's Institute, UCT.

Fitzpatrick, E., Durieux-Smith, A., Eriks-Brophy, A., Olds, J., & Gaines, R. (2007). The impact of newborn hearing screening on communication development. *Journal of Medical Screening, 14*, 123–131.

Fulcher, A., Purcell, A. A., Baker, E., & Munro, N. (2012). Listen up: Children with early identified hearing loss achieve age-appropriate speech/language outcomes by 3 years-of-age. *International Journal of Pediatric Otorhinolaryngology, 76*, 1785–1794.

Government Communications. (2016). South Africa yearbook 2015/16: Social development. Retrieved from https://www.southafrica-newyork.net/consulate/Yearbook_2016/SocialDevelopment-SAYB1516.pdf.

Haug, P. (2017). Understanding inclusive education: Ideals and reality. *Scandinavian Journal of Disability Research, 19*(3), 206–217.

Havenga, E., Swanepoel, D., Le Roux, T., & Schmid, B. (2017). Tele-intervention for children with hearing loss: A comparative pilot study. *Journal of Telemedicine and Telecare, 23*(1), 116–125.

Health Professions Council of South Africa (HPCSA). (2018). Early hearing detection and intervention (EHDI) guidelines. Retrieved from http://www.hpcsa.co.za/Uploads/editor/UserFiles/downloads/speech/Early_Hearing_Detection_and_Intervention_(EHDI)_2018.pdf.

HI HOPES. (2019). Our vision. Retrieved from https://www.hihopes.co.za/.

Hlayisi, V., & Ramma, L. (2018). Rehabilitation for disabling hearing loss: Evaluating the need relative to provision of hearing aids in the public health care system. *Disability and Rehabilitation, 63*(1), a105.

Joint Committee on Infant Hearing (JCIH), Muse, C., Harrison, J., Yoshinaga-Itano, C., Grimes, A., Brookhouser, P. E., ... Martin, B. (2013). Supplement to the JCIH 2007 position statement: Principles and guidelines for early intervention after confirmation that a child is deaf or hard of hearing. *Pediatrics, 131*(4), e1324–e1349.

Kerr, G., Tuomi, S., & Müller, A. (2012). Costs involved in using a cochlear implant in South Africa. *South African Journal of Child Health, 59*(1), 16–26.

Khoza-Shangase, K., Kanji, A., Petrocchi-Bartal, B., & Farr, K. (2017). Infant hearing screening from a developing country context: Status from two South African provinces. *South African Journal of Child Health, 11*(4), 159–163.

Khoza-Shangase, K., & Mophosho, M. (2018). Language and culture in speech-language and hearing professions in South Africa: The dangers of a single story. *South African Journal of Communication Disorders, 65*(1), a594.

Lichtert, G., & Van Wieringen, A. (2013). The importance of early home-based guidance (EHBG) for hearing-impaired children and their families in Flanders. *B-ENT, 9*(Suppl. 21), 27–36.

Maart, S., & Jelsma, J. (2013). Disability and access to health care: A community-based descriptive study. *Disability and Rehabilitation, 36*(18), 1489–1493.

Maluleke, N., Khoza-Shangase, K., & Kanji, A. (2019a). Communication and school readiness abilities of children with hearing impairment in South Africa: A retrospective review of early intervention preschool records. *South African Journal of Communication Disorders, 66*(1), a604.

Maluleke, N., Khoza-Shangase, K., & Kanji, A. (2019b). Hearing impairment detection and intervention in children from centre-based earlyintervention programmes. *Journal of Child Health Care, 23*(2), 232–241.

Mariga, L., McConley, R., & Myezwa, H. (2014). *Inclusive education in low-income countries: A resource book for teacher educators, parent trainers and community development workers.* Rondebosch, South Africa: Disability Innovations Africa.

McPherson, B. (2014). Hearing assistive technologies in developing countries: Background,achievements and challenges. *Disability and Rehabilitation Assistive Technology, 9*(5), 360–364.

Michelson, L., Adnams, C., & Shung-King, M. (2003). The Western Cape screening programme for developmental disabilities in pre-school children: Results of an evaluation. *MCH News, 21*, 2–3.

Miedel, W. T., & Reynolds, A. J. (1999). Parental involvement in early development for disadvantaged children: Does it matter? *Journal of School Psychology, 37*(4), 379–402.

Mitchell, R. (2017). Inclusive education in sub-Saharan Africa. In E. Sarton, M. Smith, R. Mitchell, & D. Were (Eds.), *Inclusive education in Uganda: Examples of best practice* (pp. 17–34). Enable-Ed and USDC. Retrieved from https://afri-can.org/wpcontent/uploads/2017/11/Inclusive-Education-in-Uganda-examples-of-best-practice-March-2017..pdf.

Pascoe, M. (2011). Contextually relevant resources in speech-language therapy and audiology in South Africa: Are there any? *South African Journal of Communication Disorders, 58*(1), 2–5.

Peer, S. (2015). Turning up the volume on hearing loss in South Africa. *South African Medical Journal, 105*(1), 31–32.

Pimperton, H., & Kennedy, C. R. (2012). The impact of early identification of permanent childhood hearing impairment on speech and language outcomes. *Archives of Disease in Childhood, 97*, 648–653.

Rehman, A., Khan, M. S. G., Malik, M. A., & Ud Din, N. (2016). Comparative effects of group and one to one speech and language therapy on language development of hearing impaired children. *Journal of Riphah College of Rehabilitation Sciences, 4*(2), 65–68.

Republic of South Africa. (2015). National integrated early childhood development policy. Retrieved from https://unicef.org/southafrica/SAF_resources_integratedecd policy.pdf.

Roman, A. M. (2018). It takes a village: Lessons in group aural rehabilitation therapy. *Audiology Today, 30*(2), 12–14.

Saloojee, G., Phohole, M., Saloojee, H., & Ijsselmuiden, C. (2007). Unmet health, welfare and educational needs of disabled children in an impoverished South African peri-urban township. *Child Health Care and Development, 33*(3), 230–235.

SASLHA Ethics and Standards Committee. (2017). Practice guidelines for audiologists and speech-language therapists in early communication intervention. Retrieved from https://www.saslha.co.za/Content/Documents/Guidelines_for_Early_Communi cation_Intervention_2017.pdf.

Sherry, K. (2015). Disability and rehabilitation: Essential considerations for equitable, accessible and poverty-reducing health care in South Africa. In A. Padarath, J. King, & R. English (Eds.), *South African Health Review 2014/15* (pp. 89–100). Durban, South Africa: Health Systems Trust.

SKI-HI Institute. (2004). *Ski Hi curriculum.* Logan, Utah: Hope Inc.

Slemming, W., & Saloojee, H. (2013). Beyond survival: The role of health care in promoting ECD. In L. Berry, L. Biersteker, A. Dawes, L. Lake, & C. Smith (Eds.), *South African child gauge 2013* (pp. 50–55). Cape Town, South Africa: Children's Institute, UCT.

Srivastava, M., De Boer, A., & Pijl, S. J. (2015). Inclusive education in developing countries: A closer look at its implementation in the last 10 years. *Educational Review, 67*(2), 179–195.

Statistics South Africa. (2011). Census in brief. Retrieved from http://www.statssa.goc. za/census/census_2011/census_products/Censusinbrief.pdf.

Stevens, G., Flaxman, S., Brunskil, E., Mascarenhas, M., Mathers, C. D., & Finucane, M. (2011). Global and regional hearing impairment prevalence: An analysis of 42 studies in 29 countries. *The European Journal of Public Health, 23*(11), 146–152.

Störbeck, C., & Calvert-Evers, J. (2008). Towards integrated practices in early detection of and intervention for deaf and hard of hearing children. *American Annals of the Deaf, 153*(3), 314–321.

Störbeck, C., & Young, A. (2016). The HI HOPES data set of deaf children under the age of 6 in South Africa: Maternal suspicion, age of identification and newborn hearing screening. *BMC Pediatrics, 16*(45), 1–10.

Tassew, W., Jones, N., & Bekele, T. T. O. Y. L. (2005). *Children's educational comple-tion rates and achievement: Implications for Ethiopia's second poverty reduction strategy (2006–10)*. Oxford, England: Young Lives.

United Nations Children's Fund (UNICEF). (2016). Eastern and southern Africa regional study on the fulfilment of the right to education of children with dis-abilities. Retrieved from https://www.unicef.org/esaro/Regional-children-with-disabilities-UNICEF-EDT-2016.pdf.

Wake, M., Poulakis, Z., Hughes, E. K., Carey-Sargeant, C., & Rickards, F. W. (2005). Hearing impairment: A population study of age at diagnosis, severity, and language outcomes at 7–8 years. *Archives of Disease in Childhood, 90*, 238–244.

Wegner, L., & Rhoda, A. (2015). The influence of cultural beliefs on the utilisation of rehabilitation services in a rural South African context: Therapists' persepective. *African Journal of Disability, 4*(1), 128–135.

Wilson, D., & Williams, V. (2013). Ubuntu: Development and framework of a specific model of positive mental health. *Psychology Journal, 10*(2), 80–100.

World Health Organization (WHO). (2002). The world health report 2002: Reducing risks, promoting healthy life. Retrieved from https://www.who.int/whr/2002/en/whr02_en.pdf?ua=1.

World Health Organization (WHO). (2007). Task shifting to tackle health worker short-ages. Retrieved from https://www.who.int/healthsystems/task_shifting_booklet.pdf.

World Health Organization (WHO). (2012). Early childhood development and disabil-ity: A discussion paper. Retrieved from http://apps.who.int/iris/bitstream/10665/75355/1/9789241504065_eng.pdf?ua=1.

Yang, Y., Liu, Y., Fu, M., Li, C., Wang, L., Wang, Q., & Sun, X. (2015). Home-based early intervention on auditory and speech development in Mandarin-speaking deaf infants and toddlers with chronological aged 7–24 months. *Chinese Medical Journal, 128*(16), 2202–2207.

Yoshinaga-Itano, C. (2014). Principles and guidelines for early intervention after con-firmation that a child is deaf or hard of hearing. *The Journal of Deaf Studies and Deaf Education, 19*(2), 143–175.

9 Continuity of Care at School for the Hearing-Impaired Child

Katijah Khoza-Shangase

The National Development Plan 2030 has a clear vision about an inclusive education system in South Africa, where every child has access to as well as success within the South African education system. All initiatives aimed at ensuring successful inclusive education for learners with disabilities are important. Early hearing detection and intervention (EHDI), one of these initiatives, has well-established and documented benefits for the development of children with hearing impairment. Achieving these benefits is not easy, even in high-income countries which do not face the resource constraints that low and middle-income (LAMI) countries like South Africa do, where social determinants of health are significantly poor. Political will, health care spending, intersectoral collaboration between health and education departments, the burden of life-threatening diseases such as tuberculosis and HIV/AIDS, and resource constraints are some of the contextual realities that initiatives such as EHDI have to contend with in South Africa. Despite these challenges, access to basic education has been an important goal of the South African government.

Evidence of the increased efforts towards attaining educational goals can be seen in initiatives such as the early childhood development (ECD) programmes that the South African government has adopted. Access, however, without a similar emphasis on success, is problematic and translates into unproductive expenditure for all stakeholders, especially for learners with barriers to learning, such as the hearing impaired. Efforts to facilitate success include continuity of care for hearing-impaired children, from the health sector to the education sector, through access to therapeutic services that remediate barriers to learning, as well as exploration of other models of service delivery, such as the use of telehealth to increase access where limited therapeutic services are available, as is the case in South Africa. This chapter explores early intervention with the goal of inclusive education for the hearing impaired in the South African educational setting. Telehealth in the form of tele-audiology is proposed as one way to increase and improve access.

Evidence points to the link between early identification of communication and hearing impairment, and resulting intervention, and speech and language development, social and emotional development, as well as scholastic outcomes in children with hearing impairment (Maluleke, Khoza-Shangase, & Kanji, 2019b; Sininger, Grimes, & Christensen, 2010; Van Dyk, Swanepoel, & Hall, 2015). The positive outcomes of early intervention programmes are dependent on a number of factors.

Firstly, evidence indicates that children with communication disorders are at risk of not achieving the necessary skills to prepare them for school. This has a negative influence on their education and academic success, which ultimately impacts their ability to find employment later in life (Maluleke et al., 2019a; Marschark, 2007). Secondly, health challenges and the social determinants of health in the South African context play a significant role in the success or failure of these early intervention programmes. The social determinants of health are defined as 'the circumstances in which people are born, grow up, live, work and age, and the systems put in place to deal with illness' (World Health Organization [WHO], 2008). For example, a report from a 2013 meeting between the departments of Basic Education (DBE) and Public Service and Administration and the deputy minister of Women, Children and Persons with Disability revealed that a majority of children with communication disorders (in this case, deaf and hearing-impaired children) did not have access to ECD programmes for stimulation and development of sign language (Parliamentary Monitoring Group, 2013). They thus entered school without the necessary language development that facilitates learning. The report also noted that most (80 percent) teachers in schools for the deaf were poorly prepared to teach deaf children as they were unable to use sign language. As a consequence, few deaf learners were reported to have progressed beyond grade 12 (Parliamentary Monitoring Group, 2013). This reality underlines the importance of early intervention for children with hearing impairment in the South African educational setting.

The prevalence of disabling hearing impairment is rising globally. However, I believe the figures to be underestimated, particularly in LAMI countries, thus my call for strategies to be put in place in ECD centres to overcome barriers to learning.

Hearing impairment has been described as an overlooked epidemic in LAMI countries due to its silent and non-life-threatening nature (Swanepoel, Delport, & Swart, 2007). It is reported as the most prevalent of all congenital sensory disorders, affecting more than twice the number of neonates than all other screened newborn disorders combined (Olusanya, 2005). Early identification of hearing impairment is not only the first but also the most important step for obtaining successful outcomes in children who are deaf or hard of hearing (Arehart, Yoshinaga-Itano, Thomson, Gabbard, & Stredler, 1998). Early diagnosis and treatment of hearing impairment is also critical to the educational and social development of children with such an impairment (Olusanya, Luxon, & Wirz, 2004). Early identification of hearing impairment creates the opportunity for developing normal language skills (Prendergast, Lartz, & Fiedler, 2002), which are critical to educational outcomes.

Early intervention refers broadly to intervention practices with children from birth to three years of age, especially aspects which provide services for hearing-impaired and deaf children and their families for the purpose of lessening the effects of the condition (Bowe, 2004; Guralnick, 2005). In audiology, early audiological intervention involves ensuring that all infants and toddlers with hearing impairment are identified as early as possible and provided with timely and appropriate audiological, educational and medical intervention, where necessary (Moeller, 2000). This is the definition adopted in this chapter and throughout the book. Early hearing detection and intervention effects include improved academic performance, social and communicative functioning, and achievement of developmental milestones, including motor, cognitive, speech, language and hearing development (Guralnick, 2005). Additionally, long-term financial benefits are evident, parent–child interactions are strengthened, a supportive family environment is provided and an overall improvement in the quality of life is achieved (Olusanya & Newton, 2007; Rossetti, 2004).

There is considerable evidence that undetected hearing impairment has profound consequences on the language abilities and skills of infants, which may result in language delays of at least two to four years (Yoshinaga-Itano, 2004). Negative social and economic outcomes are also evident, posing a threat to quality of life in areas such as education, employment and integration in society (Moeller, 2000; Olusanya, 2005; Yoshinaga-Itano, 2004). The positive effects of intervention justify considerable attention being directed towards early identification and intervention with respect to hearing-impaired children. This includes ensuring maintained continuity of care and intervention in the educational setting.

Early intervention for children with hearing impairment in South Africa faces many challenges (Khoza-Shangase, 2019). There is a paucity of published South African research into epidemiological trends and the use and effectiveness of different interventions for hearing impairment. The Joint Committee on Infant Hearing (JCIH) set international standards stating that all infants with hearing impairment be identified and intervention implemented by six months of age (JCIH, 2000, 2007). Khoza-Shangase (2019) argues that, in LAMI countries such as South Africa, evidence indicates that there are still significant delays in the age of diagnosis as well as between the age at which hearing impairment is first identified and the initiation of early intervention services. This means that a majority of South African children might only have access to early intervention when they are of school-going age. Therefore, in order to achieve the positive outcomes of effective early intervention, a system that ensures continuity of care for the hearing-impaired child, and that includes intervention at school, must be put in place (Guralnick, 2005).

It is generally accepted that infants and young children in LAMI contexts such as South Africa are not receiving adequate intervention services (Franz et al., 2018; Khoza-Shangase, 2019; Samuels, Wiedaad, & Balton, 2012). Very little state subsidy is allocated, for example for cochlear implants. This service is primarily available in private implantation centres, which are accessed by less than 20 percent of the South African population. However, the South African health care system does provide hearing aids to individuals with hearing impairment at minimal cost, and for free for children under the age of six years, although availability is inconsistent and often limited to one hearing aid per client regardless of whether they have a unilateral or bilateral hearing impairment. Due to a shortage of qualified staff, audiologists' use of traditional institution-based models of service delivery is the standard practice, despite evidence indicating this to be ineffective in reaching the majority of vulnerable and disadvantaged communities in South Africa (Khan, Joseph, & Adhikari, 2018).

Educational intervention for infants and young children with hearing impairment in South Africa has not been conducive to including these individuals in broader society (Khoza-Shangase, 2019). Children with hearing impairment are primarily placed in the country's limited number of special schools for the deaf. There are not enough of these schools to meet the needs of the number of children with hearing impairment, and they are known to be poorly resourced, with overcrowded classrooms and large teacher–child ratios (Human Sciences Research Council, 2018). These schools also contradict the South African ethos of inclusive education.

The impact of hearing impairment is far-reaching, with direct consequences for inclusive education possibilities and outcomes. Studies have documented that children with hearing impairment may have delayed speech and language development, delayed and/or impaired literacy development, psycho-emotional problems and cognitive developmental problems (Ching, 2015; DesJardin, Ambrose, Martinez, & Eisenberg, 2009; Maluleke et al., 2019b; Olusanya, 2005; WHO, 2018). All of these lead to vocational challenges later in life, thus impacting on the quality of life of the affected family and individual. In the classroom, some studies have found that children with hearing impairment easily become fatigued when compared to their hearing peers, and are therefore unable to concentrate (Gustafson, Key, Hornsby, & Bess, 2018; Hornsby et al., 2017). Similarly, patterns of delayed development are also observed in children with recurrent and persistent middle ear disorders (Roberts & Hunter, 2002). This has significant implications for hearing-impaired children's educational access and prospects.

South African educational setting and access

According to Statistics South Africa (2016), more South African children are attending school than pre-1994, with increased access for all children, including those in rural areas. The General Household Survey (Statistics South Africa, 2018) reported that while two-thirds of learners attend no-fee schools, financial constraints remain the main reason for dropping out. The percentage of learners in no-fee schools increased from 21.4 percent in 2007 to 67.2 percent by 2018. More than three-quarters (77.1 percent) of learners who attended public schools were part of the school feeding schemes in 2018, compared to 63.1 percent in 2009. The National Development Plan states that by 2024 South Africa will have introduced two years of compulsory ECD for all children before they enter grade 1, with 75 percent of four to five year olds participating in formal early childhood education, in pre grade R or grade RR.

As part of the DBE's *Action Plan* (2015), the minister of basic education, Angie Motshekga, reported on the department's plan to work towards achieving the Millennium Development Goals for access, participation and gender equity in basic education. To this end, the department developed three streams of curricula: academic, vocational and technical. These streams take into account the diversity in the developmental and learning needs of learners, which has implications for children with hearing impairment. Twenty-seven Schooling 2030 goals were crafted. Goals 1 to 13 deal with outputs the department wants to achieve in relation to learning and enrolments; goals 14 to 27 deal with how the outputs are to be achieved.

Since the advent of South Africa's democracy in 1994, the democratically elected government has adopted policies that aim at equitable and fair provision of services to all South Africans. This includes social development and educational service provision for learners with special needs, as well as the development of an inclusive education system in line with the Constitution (Act No. 108 of 1996) (Dalton, Mckenzie, & Kahonde, 2012).

Specifically, the Bill of Rights (Section 29 of the Constitution) states that everyone has the right to a basic education which the state, through reasonable measures, must make progressively available and accessible to all. Section 29 emphasises that the state may not discriminate directly or indirectly against anyone on one or more grounds, including disability. It is within this framework that efforts at supporting the process of early detection and intervention of hearing impairment are seen as a fundamental human right, as they facilitate inclusive education. The principle of inclusivity is a social model, as opposed to the special needs principle which is based on a medical model. The social model is not about learners with disabilities, but rather about the needs of all learners.

The benefits of EHDI allow for children with hearing impairment to have access to the same resources as their hearing peers, hence the importance of ensuring that such resources allow for a successful inclusive education process. Donohue and Bornman (2014) outline three benefits of inclusive education. These benefits comprehensively cover all relevant stakeholders: learners, teachers and parents. For learners, inclusive education fosters a celebration of diversity. Children gain a greater acceptance of themselves because of their exposure to peers from different backgrounds or who are differently abled. For teachers, inclusivity encourages and calls for the acquisition of a larger skill set comprising different teaching methods. This is required in order to cope with the diverse learning needs of the children. For parents, inclusive education offers opportunities and inspiration for their children with disabilities to prove their capabilities without being disadvantaged. A fourth benefit of inclusive education is the benefit to the country as a whole. In *MEC for Education: KwaZulu-Natal v Pillay*, Judge Langa stated that the Constitution 'does not tolerate diversity as a necessary evil; but affirms it as one of the primary treasures of our nation'. Inclusive education ensures that diversity is seen as a contextual strength which provides South Africa with unique opportunities for development, innovation and growth in all spheres of life (Khoza-Shangase & Mophosho, 2018).

EHDI in a South African educational setting is supported by a number of policies. These policies guide inclusive education, over and above what is enshrined in the Constitution (Bill of Rights, Chapter 2), and include the following: United Nations Convention on the Rights of Persons with Disabilities; the National Education Policy Act (No. 27 of 1996); the South African Schools Act (No. 84 of 1996); White Paper 6: Special Needs Education (Department of Education [DoE], 2001); and the revised Screening, Identification, Assessment and Support policy (DBE, 2014). These policies are supported by guideline documents, including Guidelines for Inclusive Teaching and Learning (DoE, 2010a); Guidelines for Responding to Learner Diversity in the Classroom through Curriculum and Assessment Policy Statements (DoE, 2011); Guidelines for Full-Service/Inclusive Schools (DoE, 2010b); Guidelines to Ensure Quality Education and Support in Special Schools and Special School Resource Centres (DoE, 2014); the Integrated School Health Policy (Health Basic Education, 2012); the Policy Framework on Care and Support for Teaching and Learning (Southern African Development Community, 2016); as well as the Children's Act (No. 38 of 2005) and the Children's Amendment Act (No. 41 of 2007). Most recently, the Health Professions Council of South Africa (HPCSA) released guidelines for minimum standards for hearing screening in schools. These guidelines aim to regulate hearing screening in schools to ensure that it occurs timeously to detect, identify and refer school-age children for management of hearing impairment and ear pathology (HPCSA, 2018). These policies and guideline documents are targeted at addressing the diverse needs of all learners who experience barriers to learning, including hearing impairment.

White Paper 6 (DoE, 2001) asserts that in order to make inclusive education a reality, there needs to be a conceptual shift regarding the provision of support for learners who experience barriers to learning. Barriers to learning are described as challenges that prevent access to learning and development.

These barriers can occur singly or in combination and include internal learner barriers such as neurological, physiological and genetic challenges; school barriers, which are systemic challenges; and environmental barriers such as socio-economic difficulties (DBE, 2014). Specific to internal learner barriers, deafness or being hard of hearing has been listed as a physiological barrier to learning.

Despite existing policies and guidelines, the implementation of inclusive education in South Africa has been slow and incomplete (Wildeman & Nomdo, 2007). The reasons for this are numerous and relate to problems that affect the education system as a whole, the role of special schools, and other support structures and conditions of poverty, among others (Stofile, 2008; Stofile & Green, 2007). I argue that failure to implement early identification of and intervention for disabilities such as hearing impairment worsens the situation for hearing-impaired learners.

Of the numerous challenges that have been reported in the basic education sector in South Africa, inadequacies in education for children with special needs, including the deaf and hard of hearing, are well documented (Tandwa, 2017). In their review of the challenges in realising inclusive education in South Africa, Donohue and Bornman (2014) report that up to 70 percent of children of school-going age with disabilities are out of school, which is contrary to the Statistics South Africa (2018) report, which notes that in 2018 approximately 4 percent of the total population of learners attending school were learners with disabilities. This trend has been constant since 2016. The percentage of enrolments of learners with disabilities in the country is generally lower than the percentage of other learners attending educational institutions. For example, around 72 percent of 16 to 18 year olds with disabilities attended educational institutions in 2018, which is significantly lower than the 86 percent of all 16 to 18 year olds attending educational institutions (Statistics South Africa, 2018, p. 3). This is despite White Paper 6, which was designed to transform the South African educational system by building an integrated system for all learners; utilising a flexible and suitable curriculum that takes into consideration the diversity in the needs and abilities of learners; developing district-based support teams to provide systemic support for any and all teachers who need it; and strengthening the skills of teachers to cope with more diverse classes (Muthukrishna & Schoeman, 2000). Even the existing specialised schooling system is largely inadequate and inaccessible to the majority of learners with hearing impairment. For example, there are just over 40 schools across the country catering to the needs of deaf South African learners (Berke, 2018). A majority of these schools are located in urban areas, with limited access for children who do not reside in such areas. Additionally, a number of teachers of the deaf are not proficient in South African Sign Language (SASL) (DeafSA, n.d.; Parliamentary Monitoring Group, 2013). SASL has been recognised by the South African Constitution of 1996 and the South African Schools Act (No. 84 of 1996), as well as by the Pan South African Language Board (2009), as an appropriate and necessary medium of education for deaf learners.

In chapter 5, Khoza-Shangase discusses how the global shortage of health care workers influences intervention strategies, and calls for innovative ways of confronting this challenge. Globally, there is predicted to be a net shortage of 15 million health care workers by 2030, with middle-income countries unable to meet their own demand. Wilford et al. (2018) suggest that in order to maximise efficiency, all health systems will need to look to task shifting and upskilling, making maximal use of community health workers. In the case of early intervention for the hearing impaired in the educational setting, I recommend trained volunteers as teacher assistants. Clear minimum standards for training non-professionals need to be established to ensure quality. This is necessary over and above the upskilling of teachers in early intervention.

Chapter 5 presents health care staffing profiles in the South African context, with specific data for the speech-language and hearing (SLH) professions. Reasons for the employment profiles shown in Figure 5.1 and Table 5.1 may include the lack of posts in the government sector, in addition to practitioners' preferences for working in private practice. No figures are available for these health care professionals in the educational setting. However, from the available data one can deduce that the figures are negligible. These numbers do not reflect all who are allowed to function within EHDI, but are an illustration of the contextual realities of SLH professions in South Africa, clearly showing the demand–capacity challenge. This is further complicated by the fact that the demographic profile of most SLH professionals is not congruent with the population they serve, with the majority being white and English or Afrikaans speaking.

Given these resource disparities in the South African educational setting, I argue for the adoption of tele-audiology in this context for children with hearing impairment. This innovation could be of significant benefit in ensuring successful implementation and maximum benefits from early intervention for hearing impairment at all levels of the child's development, regardless of whether the child is in a special schooling or inclusive education system.

Tele-audiology possibilities

Tele-audiology is an audiology service delivery model that forms part of telehealth, aimed at increasing access to hearing care, primarily in areas with limited access to health care due to a shortage of human resources.

This model of care utilises telecommunication technologies to extend services to patients, reduce hurdles to best care in underserved areas, enhance user satisfaction and accessibility to specialists, lessen professional isolation in rural areas, aid medical practitioners to expand their practice reach, and save patients time and money from having to travel or be transported to receive high-quality care (Krupinski, 2015). In contexts like South Africa, where obvious demand–capacity challenges exist, this mode of service delivery may serve the very basic function of access. This includes an increased ability to overcome common barriers to services like obtaining hearing aids, such as cost and distance from service providers (Schweitzer, Moritz, & Vaughan, 1999). Furthermore, in South Africa, tele-audiology can also facilitate continuity of care. Children identified in the health care sector can continue to receive intervention in the education sector when they enter schooling. There are currently no therapeutic services, except for very limited access to special schools, that cater for children who have special educational needs due to learning difficulties, physical disabilities or behavioural problems.

As a LAMI country, South Africa continues to experience challenges to health care service delivery. While there are numerous contributory factors (Khoza-Shangase & Mophosho, 2018), demand–capacity challenges inspired the establishment of tele-audiology, which was aimed at addressing the extreme shortages of audiologists, speech-language pathologists and ear, nose and throat specialists (Fagan & Jacobs, 2009; Mulwafu, Ensink, Kuper, & Fagan, 2017). These professionals are located mainly in health centres in large cities and private practices, with a large percentage of the South African population not being able to access their services. This limited professional resource availability is even worse in the education sector. There are limited posts available, and they are only in special schools such as schools for the deaf. There is a need to advocate for community service post placements, as done in the health care sector. Tele-audiology is slowly becoming an alternative model of service delivery to reach those that cannot travel long distances to health centres. I believe that tele-audiology can also be explored as a strategy in the education sector to improve access and success of children with hearing impairment. Swanepoel et al. (2010) consider the scope of application for telehealth in audiology. This can be applied in the education context for continuity of care of hearing-impaired children. Swanepoel and colleagues (2010) suggest synchronous and asynchronous possibilities for the various fields of application, such as education and training, screening, diagnosis and intervention.

Through the use of computer-based technology and internet connectivity, tele-audiology in the education sector can be used to reach children with barriers to learning in various communities. However, in South Africa, this would require connectivity challenges being addressed. Tele-audiology delivery can be done in a variety of ways: synchronous, asynchronous or hybrid. Synchronous delivery requires the presence of the service provider (audiologist), albeit in a different location to the learner, during the session, for example through video-conferencing or remote programming of hearing aids. Evidence shows that this method is useful for programming hearing technologies such as cochlear implants (Hughes, Sevier, & Choi, 2018). This is important in the South African context, where there is no seamless transition or relationship between health sector services and the basic education sector. However, despite its value, implementation of synchronous tele-audiology may not yet be feasible in South Africa. Steuerward, Windmill, Scott, Evans, and Kramer (2018) emphasise that synchronous telehealth techniques require the audiologist to be present during remote testing, and also require computer network connectivity. As challenging as this type of telehealth might be, if network connectivity difficulties can be overcome, it might be the next best option for intervention with a professional who is located far from the school in question, with teacher assistants as aids.

Asynchronous telehealth delivery can be done without an audiologist present. Paraprofessionals can be trained, as part of task shifting, to conduct certain audiological tests, save the results, and forward them to the audiologists at a later stage for review and analysis. This is one reason why tele-audiology would be ideal for the South African basic education set-up, where the services of audiologists are not readily available. Studies in South Africa have demonstrated the accuracy of asynchronous tele-audiology when compared to traditional face-to-face diagnosis performed by qualified professionals (Biagio, Adeyemo, Hall, & Vinck, 2013; Biagio, Swanepoel, Laurent, & Lundberg, 2014). Such findings instil confidence around the use of asynchronous delivery, particularly in the context of connectivity challenges that impact negatively on synchronous tele-audiology.

A strong argument exists for adopting hybrid tele-audiology – the combined use of synchronous and asynchronous methods – in the South African education sector. This is particularly important when one considers the challenges around network connectivity, particularly in rural and peri-urban areas, as well as the shortages of audiologists available for synchronous testing and intervention.

The potential applications and possible impacts of tele-audiology in the South African education sector are substantial. The sector could integrate tele-audiology into school health programmes to increase access to services. This would include access not only to South African audiologists, but also to volunteer audiologists from around the world who perform humanitarian audiology through a tele-audiology network (see www.teleaudiology.org).

Tele-audiology in the South African educational setting

Evidence supports the use of telehealth to improve health care access and reach (Dansky, Joseph, & Bowles, 2008; Jin, Ishikawa, Sengoku, & Ohyanagi, 2000; Swanepoel, Olusanya, & Mars, 2010; Tousignant, Moffet, Cabana, & Simard, 2011). Nevertheless, certain concerns need careful deliberation, particularly in the South African context. Firstly, a key concern is the training and education of health care students in the use and implementation of telehealth (Edirippulige, Armfield, & Smith, 2013; Govender & Mars, 2018). In a systematic review, Edirippulige et al. (2013) report on a lack of evidence in African education and training programme records. A strategy recommended to promote telehealth at a national level in LAMI countries such as South Africa, including in the education sector, is to introduce telehealth into the education and training programmes of health care professionals. This should occur at both undergraduate and postgraduate levels so that students are aware of and can use telehealth methods to provide health care to their patients (Edirippulige et al., 2013). Introducing short courses for continued professional development is an additional strategy to reach those who are not in formal education and training programmes. This will have direct benefits for the education sector as professionals who are competently trained in the methodology will be able to deliver efficient services (Rena, 2000; Rice, 2003) that are grounded in research (Shulman, 1986).

A second concern, noted in the *South African Health Review*, is that no specific provision is made for health technology assessment (HTA) in the National Health Act, and that HTA is narrowly and incompletely defined (Siegfried, Wilkinson, & Hofman, 2017). The *Review* highlights the need to improve telehealth capacity-building, acknowledges that educational opportunities in telehealth are limited, but notes that government aims to promote capacity development in telehealth through education and research. Universities have been identified as key stakeholders to facilitate this capacity development process by:

- developing education and training courses that are well structured
- adhering to minimum standards to provide the theoretical and practical competencies required for administering clinical and educational services via a telehealth model
- developing appropriate ICT infrastructure support specific to telehealth.

This will ensure that where tele-audiology is implemented in an educational setting, it is done efficaciously and ethically, with a contextually relevant and responsive evidence base within well-resourced telehealth models of care.

Thirdly, while identification of middle ear pathology and hearing loss as well as auditory processing problems through asynchronous tele-audiology has an evidence base from resource-constrained contexts, including school settings (Olusanya, Okolo, & Adeosun, 2004; Potgieter, Swanepoel, & Smits, 2018; Swanepoel, Myburgh, Howe, Mahomed, & Eikelboom, 2014), intervention through tele-audiology is beginning to gain attention too. However, very little contextually relevant evidence has considered the linguistic and cultural diversity of the South African context, as well as the professional-to-patient incongruency in terms of this diversity.

Fourthly, identifying auditory pathologies such as hearing impairment and middle ear disorders and implementing appropriate management such as hearing aid fitting, are important in alleviating barriers to the success of learners. However, tele-audiology can also be used as a preventive and promotive tool to educate learners, teachers, parents and caregivers about ear and hearing care, as well as about other barriers to learning such as auditory processing, language disorders and specific learning disorders. The challenge is how to include this in school programmes and schedules without interfering with the academic imperative. Nonetheless, awareness programmes around some of the causes of auditory pathologies in children that are self-induced and preventable, such as excessive exposure to noise through the use of iPods and mp3 players (WHO, 2017), remain a key benefit of telehealth in primary prevention. While audiologists are expected to educate people about the risk of excessive exposure to noise, the use of earbuds and so on, their scarcity in the country makes it challenging to provide these preventive services in schools. Therefore, using others through telehealth to provide this service could be beneficial.

Fifthly, there appears to be limited synergy between the South African departments of Health and Basic Education in managing children with special needs and providing continuity of care. Although various Acts and policies increasingly recognise the value of ICT in health, particularly in the context of the fourth industrial revolution, and support the use of telehealth applications and technology in the health care service delivery model (Govender & Mars, 2018), this has not been extended to the school health programmes currently in place. The recognition of ICT in health led to the development of the National eHealth Strategy (DoH, 2012). These efforts from the health ministry need to be extended to the education sector.

Lastly, a number of challenges are envisaged in the implementation of tele-audiology in the South African education system: the computer competency and literacy of potential users (Carter, Horrigan, & Hudyma, 2010; Lamb & Shea, 2006; Picot, 2000); the availability of network connectivity; understanding and adhering to ethical and legal prescripts around the use of tele-audiology (Grogan-Johnson, Meehan, McCormick, & Miller, 2015; Lamb & Shea, 2006; Picot, 2000); understanding the protocols and standards that guide good practice by practitioners and para-practitioners (Grol & Grimshaw, 2003); data management relating to online transmission, retrieval and storage (Grogan-Johnson et al., 2015); and the possible influences of linguistic and cultural diversity (Khoza-Shangase & Mophosho, 2018). Careful deliberation and planning around these challenges is key to the successful implementation of telehealth to facilitate early intervention in the educational setting.

Conclusion

Evidence suggests that most children with disabilities in South Africa are still not taught in classrooms together with their typically developing peers, despite education White Paper 6 advocating for this (DoE, 2001). There is also evidence that EHDI has not been successfully implemented in South Africa, for various reasons. This has a direct impact on inclusive education possibilities, despite various policies and guidelines. Translation of policy into practice is heavily influenced by resource constraints, among other factors. As far as inclusive education is concerned, numerous barriers and challenges exist to achieving quality and inclusive education for learners with disabilities. These include the inability to address barriers to learning because of a lack of (human) resources, specifically access to rehabilitation professionals such as audiologists, as well as a significant mismatch between capacity and demand, especially in the basic education sector. This chapter proposed telehealth in the form of tele-audiology as a strategy to overcome access barriers in order to enhance the success of early intervention initiatives. It is believed that the use of telehealth will allow for transfer and carry-over of early intervention benefits from the health sector to enhance outcomes in the educational sector. This will lead to children with hearing impairment becoming productive and contributing members of society.

The positive impact of telehealth is increasingly evident in several areas of health care and its scope is continually broadening with advances in technology and internet connectivity. In South Africa, the planned upscaling of e-health and e-education make this an opportune time to include telehealth in the educational setting. Applying telehealth to hearing health care has a broad scope of application possibilities, including training and education, screening, diagnosis and intervention. These services are not bound by distance or location and can facilitate access to patients isolated from the audiological services they require.

Like any new intervention strategy, contextually relevant research needs to be conducted to ensure a contextually relevant evidence base that will allow for best practice. Issues such as linguistic and cultural diversity also need to be considered. There is an urgent need for the DBE to understand and address the range of diverse learning needs in South African classrooms, if the country is to address the exclusion of learners from the education system due to various barriers to learning. In order to achieve this, the DBE needs to embrace ICT innovations such as telehealth. Furthermore, teachers, teacher assistants, therapists, audiologists and parents need to find ways to plan and work collaboratively for the greatest benefit to their learners. This includes embracing ICT in the form of tele-practice as a way of bridging the existing gap.

References

Arehart, K. H., Yoshinaga-Itano, C., Thomson, V., Gabbard, S. A., & Stredler, B. (1998). State of the states: The status of universal new-born hearing screening, assessment, and intervention systems in 16 states. *American Journal of Audiology, 7*(2), 101–114.

Berke, J. (2018). Deaf community and culture in South Africa. Retrieved from https://www.verywellhealth.com/deaf-community-south-africa-1048924.

Biagio, L., Adeyemo, A., Hall, J. W., & Vinck, B. (2013). Asynchronous video-otoscopy with a telehealth facilitator. *Telemedicine and e-Health, 19*(4), 252–258.

Biagio, L., Swanepoel, D. W., Laurent, C., & Lundberg, T. (2014). Paediatric otitis media at a primary healthcare clinic in South Africa. *South African Medical Journal, 104*(6), 431–435.

Bowe, F. W. (2004). *Early childhood special education: Birth to eight.* New York, NY: Delmar Learning.

Carter, L., Horrigan, J., & Hudyma, S. (2010). Investigating the educational needs of nurses in telepractice: A descriptive exploratory study. *Canadian Journal of University Continuing Education, 36*(1), 1–20.

Ching, T. (2015). Is early intervention effective in improving spoken language outcomes of children with congenital hearing loss? *American Journal of Audiology, 24,* 345–348.

Dalton, E. M., Mckenzie, J. A., & Kahonde, C. (2012). The implementation of inclusive education in South Africa: Reflections arising from a workshop for teachers and therapists to introduce Universal Design for Learning. *African Journal of Disability, 1*(1), a13. doi: 10.4102/ajod.v1i1.13.

Dansky, K. H., Joseph, V., & Bowles, K. (2008). Use of telehealth by older adults to manage heart failure. *Research in Gerontological Nursing, 1*(1), 25–32.

DeafSA (n.d.). Portfolio committee on basic education: Deaf education. Retrieved from http://pmg-assets.s3-website-eu-west-1.amazonaws.com/180912DeafSA.pdf.

Department of Basic Education (DBE). (2014). Screening, identification, assessment and support policy. Retrieved from https://www.naptosa.org.za/doc-manager/90-provinces/94-kwazuly-natal/kwz-archived/367-sias-final-19-december-2014/file.

Department of Basic Education (DBE). (2015). Action plan to 2019 towards the realisation of schooling 2030: Taking forward South Africa's national development plan 2030. Retrieved from https://www.education.gov.za/Portals/0/Documents/Publications/Action%20Plan%202019.pdf.

Department of Education (DoE). (2001). *Education white paper 6: Special needs education: Building an inclusive education and training system*. Pretoria, South Africa: Government Printer.

Department of Education (DoE). (2010a). *Guidelines for inclusive teaching and learning 2010*. Pretoria, South Africa: Government Printer.

Department of Education (DoE). (2010b). *Guidelines for full-service/inclusive schools 2010*. Pretoria, South Africa: Government Printer.

Department of Education (DoE). (2011). *Guidelines for responding to learner diversity in the classroom through curriculum and assessment policy statements*. Pretoria, South Africa: Government Printer.

Department of Education (DoE). (2014). *Guidelines to ensure quality education and support in special schools and special school resource centres*. Pretoria, South Africa: Government Printer.

Department of Health (DoH). (2012). *South Africa. eHealth strategy for SA (2012–2016)*. Pretoria, South Africa: Department of Health.

DesJardin, J., Ambrose, S., Martinez, A., & Eisenberg, L. (2009). Relationships between speech perception abilities and spoken language skills in young children with hearing loss. *International Journal of Audiology, 48*, 248–259.

Donohue, D., & Bornman, J. (2014). The challenges of realising inclusive education in South Africa. *South African Journal of Education, 34*(2), 1–14.

Edirippulige, S., Armfield, N. R., & Smith, A. (2013). A qualitative study of the careers and professional practices of graduates from an e-health postgraduate programme. *Journal of Telemedicine and Telecare, 18*(8), 455–459.

Fagan, J. J., & Jacobs, M. (2009). Survey of ENT services in Africa: Need for a comprehensive intervention. *Global Health Action, 2*(1). doi: 10.3402/gha.v2i0.1932.

Franz, L., Adewumi, K., Chambers, N., Viljoen, M., Baumgartner, J. N., & De Vries, P. J. (2018). Providing early detection and early intervention for autism spectrum disorder in South Africa: Stakeholder perspectives from the Western Cape province. *Journal of Child and Adolescent Mental Health, 30*(3), 149–165.

Govender, S. M., & Mars, M. (2018). The perspectives of South African academics within the disciplines of health sciences regarding telehealth and its potential inclusion in student training. *African Journal of Health Professions Education, 10*(1), 38–43.

Grogan-Johnson, S., Meehan, R., McCormick, K., & Miller, N. (2015). Results of a national survey of preservice telepractice training in graduate speech-language pathology and audiology programs. *Journal of Contemporary Issues in Communication Science and Disorders, 42*, 122–137.

Grol, R., & Grimshaw, J. (2003). From best evidence to best practice: Effective implementation of change in patient care. *The Lancet, 362*(9391), 1225–1230.

Guralnick, M. (2005). *The developmental systems approach to early intervention*. Baltimore, MD: Paul H. Brookes Publishing.

Gustafson, S. M., Key, A. P., Hornsby, B. W. Y., & Bess, F. H. (2018). Fatigue related to speech processing in children with hearing loss: Behavioral, subjective, and electrophysiologyical measures. *Journal of Speech, Language, Hearing Research, 61,* 1000–1011.

Health Basic Education. (2012). *Integrated school health policy 2012.* Pretoria, South Africa: Government Printer.

Health Professions Council of South Africa (HPCSA). (2018). Minimum standards for the hearing screening in schools. Retrieved from https://www.hpcsa.co.za/Uploads/ SLH/Minimum%20Standards%20for%20the%20Hearing%20Screening%20in%20 Schools.pdf.

Hornsby, B. W. Y., Gustafson, S. M., Lancaster, H., Cho, S. J., Camarata, S., & Bess, F. H. (2017). Subjective fatigue in children with hearing loss assessed using self-and parent-proxy report. *American Journal of Audiology, 26*(35), 393–407.

Hughes, M. L., Sevier, J. D., & Choi, S. (2018). Techniques for remotely programming children with Cochlear implants using pediatric audiological methods via teleprac- tice. *American Journal of Audiology, 27,* 385–390.

Human Sciences Research Council. (2018). SA is failing deaf and hard-of-hearing learners: Can a bilingual model of education be the solution to acquiring liter- acy? Retrieved from http://www.hsrc.ac.za/en/review/hsrc-review-oct-dec-2018/ sa-is-failing-deaf-and-hard-of-hearing-learners.

Jin, C., Ishikawa, A., Sengoku, Y., & Ohyanagi, T. (2000). A telehealth project for sup- porting an isolated physiotherapist in a rural community of Hokkaido. *Journal of Telemedicine and Telecare, 6*(Suppl. 2), S35–S37.

Joint Committee on Infant Hearing (JCIH). (2000). Year 2000 position statement: Principles and guidelines for early hearing detection and intervention programs. *Pediatrics, 106*(4), 798–817.

Joint Committee on Infant Hearing (JCIH). (2007). Year 2007 position statement: Principles and guidelines for early hearing detection and intervention programs. *Pediatrics, 120,* 898–921.

Khan, N., Joseph, L., & Adhikari, M. (2018). The hearing screening experiences and practices of primary health care nurses: Indications for referral based on high-risk factors and community views about hearing loss. *African Journal of Primary Health Care & Family Medicine, 10*(1), a1848. https://doi.org/10.4102/ phcfm.v10i1.1848.

Khoza-Shangase, K. (2019). Early hearing detection and intervention: Exploring factors compromising service delivery as expressed by caregivers. *International Journal of Pediatric Otorhinolaryngology, 118,* 73–78. https://doi.org/10.1016/j. ijporl.2018.12.021.

Khoza-Shangase, K., & Mophosho, M. (2018). Language and culture in speech-lan- guage and hearing professions in South Africa: The dangers of a single story. *South African Journal of Communication Disorders, 65*(1), 594.

Krupinski, E. (2015). Innovations and possibilities in connected health. *Journal of American Academy of Audiology, 26,* 761–767.

Lamb, G. S., & Shea, K. (2006). Nursing education in telehealth. *Journal of Telemedicine and Telecare*, *12*(2), 55–56.

Maluleke, N. P., Khoza-Shangase, K., & Kanji, A. (2019a). Hearing impairment detection and intervention in children from centre-based early intervention programmes. *Journal of Child Health Care*, *23*(2), 232–241. doi: 10.1177/1367493518788477.

Maluleke, N. P., Khoza-Shangase, K., & Kanji, A. (2019b). Communication and school readiness abilities of children with hearing impairment in South Africa: A retrospective review of early intervention preschool records. *South African Journal of Communication Disorders*, *66*(1), a604. https://doi.org/10.4102/ sajcd.v66i1.604.

Marschark, M. (2007). *Raising and educating a deaf child (2nd ed.)*. New York, NY: Oxford University Press.

Moeller, M. (2000). Early intervention and language development in children who are deaf and hard of hearing. *Pediatrics*, *106*, e43.

Mulwafu, W., Ensink, R., Kuper, H., & Fagan, J. (2017). Survey of ENT services in sub-Saharan Africa: Little progress between 2009 and 2015. *Global Health Action*, *10*(1). doi: 10.1080/16549716.2017.1289736.

Muthukrishna, N., & Schoeman, M. (2000). From 'special needs' to 'quality education for all': A participatory approach to policy development in South Africa. *International Journal of Inclusive Education*, *4*(4), 315–335.

Olusanya, B. (2005). Can the world's infants with hearing loss wait? *International Journal of Pediatric Otorhinolaryngology*, *69*, 735–738.

Olusanya, B., Luxon, L., & Wirz, S. (2004). Benefits and challenges of newborn hearing screening for developing countries. *International Journal Pediatric Otorhinolaryngology*, *68*(3), 287–305.

Olusanya, B., & Newton, V. (2007). Global burden of childhood hearing impairment and disease control priorities for developing countries. *The Lancet*, *369*, 1314–1317.

Olusanya, B., Okolo, A., & Adeosun, A. (2004). Predictors of hearing loss in school entrants in a developing country. *Journal of Postgraduate Medicine*, *50*(3), 173–179.

Pan South African Language Board. (2009). Linguistic human rights and advocacy. Retrieved from http://www.southafrica.info/about/democracy/pansalb.htm.

Parliamentary Monitoring Group. (2013). *Disabled people's employment & learning challenges: Deputy minister women, children & people with disabilities, departments of public service and basic education briefings*. Pretoria, South Africa. Retrieved from https:// pmg.org.za/committee-meeting/15545/.

Picot, J. (2000). Meeting the need for educational standards in the practice of telemedicine and telehealth. *Journal of Telemedicine and Telecare*, *6*(2), 59–62.

Potgieter, J., Swanepoel, D. W., & Smits, C. (2018). Evaluating a smartphone digits-in-noise test as part of the audiometric test battery. *South African Journal of Communication Disorders*, *65*(1), a574. doi: 10.4102/sajcd.v65i1.574.

Prendergast, S. G., Lartz, M. N., & Fiedler, B. C. (2002). Ages of diagnosis, amplification, and early intervention of infants and young children with hearing loss: Findings from parent interviews. *American Annals of the Deaf*, *147*(1), 24–29.

Rena, U. (2000). *Who will teach: A case study of teacher education reform*. San Francisco, CA: Caddo Gap Press.

Rice, J. K. (2003). *Teacher quality: Understanding the effectiveness of teacher attributes*. Washington, DC: Economic Policy Institute.

Roberts, J., & Hunter, L. (2002). Otitis media and children's language and learning. *ASHA Leader, 7*(18). https://doi.org/10.1044/leader.FTR2.07182002.6.

Rossetti, L. (2004). *Communication intervention: Birth to three* (2nd ed.). New York: Delmar Cengage Learning.

Samuels, A., Wiedaad, S., & Balton, S. (2012). Early childhood intervention in South Africa in relation to the developmental systems model. *Infants and Young Children, 25*(4), 334–345.

Schweitzer, C., Moritz, M. S., & Vaughan, N. (1999). Perhaps not by prescription – but by perception. In S. Kochkin & K. E. Strom (Eds.), *High performance hearing solutions, Vol. 3. Hearing Review, 6*(1) [suppl], 58–62.

Shulman, L. S. (1986). Those who understand: Knowledge growth in teaching. *Educational Researcher, 15*(2), 4–14.

Siegfried, N., Wilkinson, T., & Hofman, K. (2017). Where from and where to for health technology assessment in South Africa? A legal and policy landscape analysis. In A. Padarath & P. Barron (Eds.), *South African Health Review 2017* (pp. 41–48). Durban, South Africa: Health Systems Trust. Retrieved from http://www.hst.org.za/publications/south-african-health-review-2017.

Sininger, Y. S., Grimes, A., & Christensen, E. (2010). Auditory development in early amplified children: Factors influencing auditory-based communication outcomes in children with hearing loss. *Ear Hear, 31*(2), 166–185. doi: 10.1097/AUD.0b013e3181c8e7b6.

Southern African Development Community. (2016). Policy framework on care and support for teaching and learning. Retrieved from http://www.cstlsadc.com/wp-content/uploads/2016/10/SADC_CSTL_Policy_Framework_Final_English.pdf.

Statistics South Africa. (2016). Education series volume III: Educational enrolment and achievement, 2016. Retrieved from http://www.statssa.gov.za/publications/Report%2092-01-03/Report%2092-01-032016.pdf.

Statistics South Africa. (2018). General Household Survey 2018. Retrieved from http://www.statssa.gov.za/?p=12180.

Steuerward, W., Windmill, I., Scott, M., Evans, T., & Kramer, K. (2018). Stories from the webcams: Cincinnati Children's Hospital Medical Center audiology telehealth and pediatric auditory device services. *American Journal of Audiology, 27*, 391–402.

Stofile, S. Y. (2008). Factors affecting the implementation of inclusive education policy: A case study in one province in South Africa. PhD thesis, Cape Town, University of the Western Cape. Retrieved from http://etd.uwc.ac.za/usrfiles/modules/etd/docs/etd_gen8Srv25Nme4_7965_1269472515.pdf.

Stofile, S. Y., & Green, L. (2007). Inclusive education in South Africa. In P. Engelbrecht & L. Green (Eds.), *Responding to the challenges of inclusive education in southern Africa* (pp. 52–65). Pretoria: Van Schaik.

Swanepoel, D. W., Clark, J. L., Koekemoer, D., Hall, J. W., Krumm, M., & Ferrari, D. V. (2010). Telehealth in audiology: The need and potential to reach underserved communities. *International Journal of Audiology, 49*, 195–202.

Swanepoel, D. W., Delport, S., & Swart, J. (2007). Equal opportunities for children with hearing loss by means of early identification. *South African Family Practice, 49*, 3.

Swanepoel, D. W., Myburgh, H. C., Howe, D. M., Mahomed, F., & Eikelboom, R. H. (2014). Smartphone hearing screening with integrated quality control and data management. *International Journal of Audiology, 53*, 841–849.

Swanepoel, D. W., Olusanya, B. O., & Mars, M. (2010). Hearing healthcare delivery in sub-Saharan Africa: A role for teleaudiology. *Journal of Telemedicine and Telecare, 16*(10), 53–56.

Tandwa, L. (2017). *Education gets largest chunk of Gauteng budget.* Retrieved from https://www.news24.com/SouthAfrica/News/education-gets-largest-chunk-of-gauteng-budget-20170307.

Tousignant, M., Moffet, H., Cabana, F., & Simard, J. (2011). Patients' satisfaction of healthcare services and perception with in-home telerehabilitation and physiotherapists' satisfaction toward technology for post-knee arthroplasty: An embedded study in a randomized trial. *Telemedicine Journal and E-Health, 17*(5), 376–382.

Van Dyk, M., Swanepoel, D., & Hall, J. W. (2015). Outcomes with OAE and AABR screening in the first 48h - implications for newborn hearing screening in developing countries. *International Journal of Pediatric Otorhinolaryngology, 79*(7), 1034–1040. http://dx.doi.org/10.1016/j.ijporl.2015.04.021.

Wildeman, R. A., & Nomdo, C. (2007). *Implementation of inclusive education: How far are we?* Occasional Paper, Idasa Budget Information Service.

Wilford, A., Phakathi, S., Haskins, L., Jama, N. A., Mntambo, N., & Horwood, C. (2018). Exploring the care provided to mothers and children by community health workers in South Africa: Missed opportunities to provide comprehensive care. *BMC Public Health, 18*(1), 171.

World Health Organization (WHO). (2008). Social determinants of health: Key concepts. Retrieved from https://www.who.int/social_determinants/thecommission/finalreport/key_concepts/en/.

World Health Organization (WHO). (2017). Current practices in the assessment of recreational noise-induced hearing loss: A review. Retrieved from https://www.who.int/pbd/deafness/Monograph_on_current_Practices_in_the_assessment_of_NIHL_in_recreational_settings.pdf?ua=1.

World Health Organization (WHO). (2018). Deafness and hearing loss. Retrieved from https://www.who.int/news-room/fact-sheets/detail/deafness-and-hearing-loss.

Yoshinaga-Itano, C. (2004). Levels of evidence: Universal new-born hearing screening (UNHS) and early hearing detection and intervention systems (EHDI). *Journal of Communication Disorders, 37*, 451–465.

Section Three

Complexities of Early Hearing Detection and Intervention

10 Sensory Impairments in Early Hearing Detection and Intervention

Nomfundo F. Moroe

Blindness separates us from things. Deafness separates us from people
 – Helen Keller
Deafblindness separates us from things and people.
 (Psychological Musings, 2013)

A plethora of studies exist on congenital hearing impairment and its lifelong impact on speech, language, cognitive and psychological development in children with hearing impairment (Kanji, Khoza-Shangase, & Moroe, 2018; Maluleke, Khoza-Shangase, & Kanji, 2019; Moroe & Kathrada, 2016). In the last few decades, the focus of these studies shifted to early hearing detection and intervention (EHDI). While they provide notable and impressive evidence-based benefits of EHDI, they have tended to neglect the co-morbid visual impairment that occurs in 1 percent of the population with hearing impairments. The impact of a concomitant visual impairment should not be underestimated. Therefore, if the goal of EHDI is to be optimally realised, audiologists and other health care professionals should be cognisant of other sensory impairments, such as blindness, that may potentially foil the optimal delivery of EHDI programmes. This chapter deliberates on deafblindness in EHDI efforts.

The goal of early EHDI is to provide children with hearing impairment with optimal and timely opportunities to develop linguistic, literacy and communicative competence in keeping with their full potential (Health Professions Council of South Africa [HPCSA], 2018). According to Olusanya et al. (2007), of all congenital or early onset sensory disabilities, a permanent hearing impairment is the most devastating. I argue that this is because a hearing impairment has a pronounced impact on speech, language, cognitive and psychological development (Olusanya et al., 2007).

Congenital hearing impairment can occur in isolation or in conjunction with another sensory impairment, the most common being a visual impairment. According to Aitken (2000), globally, it is generally accepted that approximately 10 percent of the population has a hearing impairment, of whom approximately 1 percent is also blind or has a serious visual impairment. A visual impairment in developing children is devastating, as most learning occurs through vision (Barnhardt, Borsting, Deland, Pham, & Vu, 2005). Consequently, a visual impairment affects play, motor, cognitive, social and communication skills of developing children (Chen, 2001; Owens, 2012). Authors such as Berg et al. (2009), House and Davidson (2000), and Mosca, Kritzinger, and Van der Linde (2015) believe that the impact of visual impairment on the communication development of visually impaired children is underestimated and undertreated.

It is thus clear that the combined sensory impairment of hearing and visual, referred to as deafblindness, is most catastrophic, particularly in developing children. 'Deafblindness' is the umbrella term used to refer to any degree of combined vision and hearing impairment (Ask Larsen & Damen, 2014; Wittich, Jarry, Groulx, Southall, & Gagné, 2016; Wittich, Southall, Sikora, Watanabe, & Gagné, 2013). It is a lifelong condition that significantly affects communication, socialisation, orientation and mobility, as well as access to information and daily living (Aitken, 2000; Jaiswal, Aldersey, Wittich, Mirza, & Finlayson, 2018; Janssen, Riksen-Walraven, & Van Dijk, 2003). In developing children in particular, deafblindness creates learning/educational needs that cannot be accommodated by interventions and programmes designed solely for individuals who are deaf or blind (Wiley, Parnell, & Belhorn, 2016). Thus, without appropriate early detection and intervention, children who are deafblind may not achieve optimal and timely opportunities to develop communication, socialisation, orientation and mobility as well as access to information – the ultimate goal of early detection and intervention.

Before discussing EHDI in the context of deafblindness, I differentiate between sensory impairment and sensory processing impairment. This differentiation is critical for the current discussion as it justifies the focus on deafblindness rather than on autism spectrum disorder (ASD), another condition often classified as a multisensory impairment in the paediatric population.

Sensory impairments versus sensory processing disorders

Sensory impairment refers to when one of the senses – sight, hearing, smell, touch, taste or spatial awareness – is not working as it should (Dunlop, 2019). Where more than one sense is involved, this is known as multisensory impairment. Multisensory impairment is rare (Early Support, 2012), with the most common condition being deafblindness. Sensory integration or processing, on the other hand, can be defined as 'the neurological process that organizes sensation from one's own body and from the environment and makes it possible to use the body effectively within the environment' (Ayres, 1972, p. 11). Therefore, a sensory processing disorder is a diagnosis given when the neurological process or the brain's ability to integrate and convert sensory information into effective and meaningful responses is compromised.

Numerous studies indicate that more than 80 percent of children with ASD exhibit co-occurring sensory processing problems (Ben-Sasson et al., 2007; Case-Smith, Weaver, & Fristad, 2015). But there are authors who classify ASD as a multisensory impairment (Dammeyer, 2014a ; Probst & Borders, 2017). Autism is a

> pervasive neurodevelopmental disorder, or difference, that is commonly recognized by the individual's diminished or unusual communication style, difficulty socially interacting successfully with others, desire to be alone, obsessive insistence on sameness and routine, heightened or diminished sensory responses, and in some instances unexpected and unexplainable abilities and skills that do not match skills in other developmental areas. (Belote & Maier, 2014, p. 1)

While it is plausible that both these conditions are classified as multisensory impairments, the manifestation and processing of sensory information differs in deafblindness and autism. Arguably, both conditions are lifelong, and they both affect communication and social interactions and future educational and vocational attainment. Furthermore, they both impact on how an individual accesses and processes sensory information (Belote & Maier, 2014). With children who are deafblind, vision and hearing may be:

- totally impaired, meaning that the individual may not be able to perceive light and may present with a profound hearing impairment
- decreased, that is, an individual may present with legal blindness or low vision and is hard of hearing
- distorted due to cerebral or cortical visual impairment and central auditory processing disorder or auditory neuropathy
- deafblindness can be related to specific conditions linked to the complex structure of the ear/eye, but can also be related to the way the information travels along the auditory/optic nerves and/or the way the brain processes this sensory information (Belote & Maier, 2014).

Individuals who are deafblind may experience both eye and ear issues combined with visual and auditory processing problems.

Individuals with ASD, among other developmental, cognitive and physical difficulties, also present with difficulty processing visual and auditory stimulations. This is largely attributed to sensory processing differences rather than sensory loss or impairment (Belote & Maier, 2014). Sensory processing is concerned with how well an individual perceives and responds to sensory stimulation, and the sensory processing patterns that develop determine how an individual responds in a particular situation (Belote & Maier, 2014;

Dunn, 2008). In individuals with ASD, the differences in processing incoming sensory information and the subsequent unique or unusual behavioural responses are related to how the brain processes this information (Belote & Maier, 2014). In essence, individuals with ASD experience difficulty in effectively gathering and filtering incoming information and then accurately perceiving all of the sensory information present in an environment or an interaction with another person (Dunn, 2008). There is evidence that individuals with ASD are highly adept at recognising patterns and details, but have difficulty 'seeing the entire picture'. As such, attention to detail, component parts and/or one sensory aspect over another is neurologically based and not due to sensory impairment (Belote & Maier, 2014).

Since this chapter's focus is on EHDI in the context of other sensory impairments and not sensory processing impairments, it is therefore deemed appropriate that the focus be specifically on deafblindness. Furthermore, this chapter focuses solely on deafblindness because it is a unique disability with its own concepts and terminology, its own methods of assessment and means of education and its own modes of communication (Rehabilitation Council of India, n.d.). This distinction separates deafblindness from deafness and blindness. According to the Rehabilitation Council of India (n.d.), deafblindness is not a medical concept but a developmental one, which aids with understanding the nature and scope of a disability consequent to deafblindness. Additionally, inherent in the deafblindness definition are the following assumptions:

- simultaneous presence of impaired vision and hearing which may vary in degree
- does not imply total loss of either vision or hearing
- communication is most severely affected
- highly individualised training is needed to cope with the condition
- the world is much narrower as the distance senses (vision and hearing) are affected, restricting experience to what is within arm's reach
- affects person in totality
- associated medical conditions with hearing and visual loss may be present (Rehabilitation Council of India, n.d.).

Deafblindness is not afforded the prominence it deserves as a unique disability as it is often misdiagnosed or confused with sensory processing disorders or classified under deafness or blindness. To minimise confusion and assist health care professionals in differentiating between ASD and deafblindness, Belote and Maier (2014) describe key features associated with ASD. They explain how each feature might be reflected in children with ASD, and provide clarity on why children with deafblindness might appear similar. Features include: delays in verbal and nonverbal communication; delays in social interaction; restricted areas of interest; repetitive activities and/or speech; stereotyped movements; resistance to environmental change; resistance to change in daily routines; unusual responses to sensory experiences; and difficulties with executive function skills such as self-regulation of behaviour, controlling inhibition, planning and organising, working memory and problem-solving.

Various authors classify deafblindness into four distinct groups (Aitken, 2000; Dammeyer, 2014b, Simcock, 2017; Wittich, Watanabe, & Gagné, 2012):

- Group 1: Congenital/prelingual deafblindness – from birth or early onset before developing language.
- Group 2: Acquired/postlingual deafblindness – those who simultaneously acquire both types of impairment during their lives.
- Group 3: Congenital single sensory impairment (vision or hearing) and then subsequently acquire another (vision or hearing) impairment.
- Group 4: Age-related dual sensory impairment of vision and hearing loss in varying degrees and order and time of onset.

These classifications have an impact on assessment and management in this population, and must be taken cognisance of in all research, teaching and clinical management plans.

Deafblindness is a progressive condition and in some cases may not be apparent at birth. This influences the reported incidence of deafblindness, in that acquired deafblindness may not be classified as deafblindness at birth. Furthermore, this condition is caused by a number of factors such as viral infections, premature birth and genetic conditions.

Causes of deafblindness

Prenatal viral infections

The most common prenatal viral disease to cause deafblindness is rubella, also known as German measles. Rubella is a rare but potentially devastating infectious viral disease with lifelong consequences (Boshoff & Tooke, 2012). It can be passed to the unborn child if a pregnant woman contracts it during her pregnancy, causing damage to the eyes, ears and heart of the unborn baby (Boshoff & Tooke, 2012). Literature indicates that rubella is the most common cause of deafblindness in low and middle-income (LAMI) countries. Since South Africa is a LAMI country and not much is known about deafblindness in this context, it can therefore be deduced that the incidence of rubella can be used to infer numbers of possible deafblindness in South Africa. The exact incidence of congenital rubella in South Africa is not known; however, on average, 660 cases are reported annually (Boshoff & Tooke, 2012). Rubella is completely preventable through effective immunisation programmes but, according to Boshoff and Tooke (2012), routine rubella vaccination does not form part of the expanded programme for immunisation in South Africa. This may explain why rubella is the leading cause of deafblindness in LAMI countries. Boshoff and Tooke (2012) highlight the need for a multidisciplinary team approach involving medical, surgical, educational and rehabilitative professionals in managing rubella. For the purpose of this chapter, rehabilitative management speaks to the services offered by audiologists, speech therapists, occupational therapists and physiotherapists in this population.

Premature birth

Premature birth contributes to the causes of deafblindness. Historically, it was thought that too much oxygen from excessive oxygen therapy administered to premature babies caused deafblindness. However, current research shows that oxygen levels (either too low or too high) play only a contributing factor (Batshaw, Pellegrino, & Roizen, 2007). According to Batshaw et al. (2007), infants born prematurely are exposed to increased levels of medications such as antibiotics and diuretics, which can be harmful to the auditory system. Depending on the intensity of the medication, the underdeveloped blood vessels in the inner ear may rupture and thereby interrupt the flow of blood to the inner ear, which may result in the destruction of hair cells. Subsequently, this destruction can lead to a sensorineural hearing impairment in the premature infant. With regard to vision, the eyes of premature infants are fragile and vulnerable to injury after birth, resulting in a condition known as retinopathy of prematurity, or ROP (Higuera, 2016). ROP is abnormal growth of blood vessels in an infant's eye, characterised by retarded growth of blood vessels which results in the development of scar tissue and retinal detachment, increasing the risks of vision loss or blindness (Higuera, 2016).

Genetic conditions

A number of genetic conditions are known to cause congenital and acquired deafblindness. A common condition is CHARGE syndrome – an acronym for several of the features common in the disorder: coloboma, heart defects, atresia choanae (also known as choanal atresia), growth retardation, genital abnormalities and ear abnormalities. CHARGE syndrome reportedly causes a pattern of related birth defects known to affect the eyes, heart, nose, genitals and ears, as well as stunting the child's growth (Ask Larsen & Damen, 2014). These birth defects are usually observed at birth and the child may be classified as presenting with congenital deafblindness. Usher syndrome is one of the causes in acquired cases of deafblindness. Individuals with Usher syndrome are born deaf and then develop a condition referred to as retinitis pigmentosa as they get older. Retinitis pigmentosa causes the retina to slowly deteriorate. Consequently, the retina loses the ability to transmit information to the brain, resulting in blindness (Dammeyer, 2012).

Other

Deafblindness, particularly acquired deafblindness, can also occur as a result of unrelated conditions that cause loss of vision and loss of hearing, or it can occur as a result of ageing.

Deafblindness in South Africa

Maguvhe (2014) describes deafblindness as a minority within a minority. This may be attributed to the fact that, in general, people with disabilities are viewed by the broader population as a minority and, as such, they experience difficulties in exercising their fundamental social, political and economic rights (Marumoagae, 2012). Consequently, their rights and interests are downtrodden (Maguvhe, 2014). The World Federation of the Deafblind (WFDB, 2018) stresses that persons with disabilities are not homogeneous, and some people with certain disabilities such as deafblindness are marginalised and invisible.

In South Africa, there are at least 920 000 people with various degrees of deafblindness (DispatchLIVE, 2019; Thisability, 2017). However, almost a decade later, statistics on the exact incidence of deafblindness remain unknown. Arguably, the incidence of deafblindness globally is generally low and the South African figure is thus not unique (Dammeyer, 2014a; Maguvhe, 2014). The WFDB (2018) states that persons with deafblindness represent between 0.2 and 2.0 percent of the global population and are more likely to live in poverty and be unemployed, with lower educational outcomes than other persons with disabilities. This is a reality for most children with disabilities in South Africa. According to Tswanya (2019), approximately 600 000 children with disabilities are not in school in South Africa. Nearly 121 500 learners with disabilities are in mainstream schools, with only 119 500 enrolled in special schools (Tswanya, 2019). In 2017, approximately 11 500 children with disabilities were on waiting lists to enrol in schools for learners with special educational needs (Tswana, 2019). As of February 2020, this situation seemed not to have improved, as there were still long waiting lists for special school placements (Tswanya, 2019). These figures attest to the marginalisation of children with disabilities in South Africa. Children who are deafblind, as a minority within this minority, are potentially not accounted for in these figures, which speaks to their further marginalisation and invisibilisation.

Failure to account for the educational needs of children who are deafblind has implications for the roll-out of early detection and intervention in this population. These children's marginalisation and invisibilisation is also highlighted by the dearth of literature on deafblindness in South Africa. There are many studies on children with single sensory impairments (Kanji et al., 2018; Maluleke et al., 2019; Thompson & Merino, 2018), cognitive impairment (Stadskleiv, 2020), physical impairment (Spinazola, Cia, Azevedo, & Gualda, 2018) and sensory integration/processing impairment (Dammeyer, 2015), but limited evidence exists on children with deafblindness. Apart from a brief mention of deafblindness on the website of DeafBlind South Africa – an organisation established in 1996 for individuals who are deafblind – and the information available from the University of the Witwatersrand's Library Guides Deafblind Resources (see https://libguides.wits.ac.za/deaf_and_hardofhearing/deafblind), not much is known or documented on deafblindness in the South African context. A scoping review on deafblindness in South Africa yielded very few studies with a focus on the curriculum and educational outcomes of children with deafblindness, with only one study conducted by health care professionals working in the field of deafblindness (Mosca et al., 2015). The few studies conducted on the learning outcomes of children who are deafblind are encouraging and show that generally children who are deafblind are first diagnosed at a school facility (Aitken, 2000; Hersh, 2013; Knoors & Vervloed, 2003). The absence of studies conducted by health care professionals is concerning, however, as these are often the people to first work with children who are deafblind (House & Davidson, 2000). This indicates a need for increased focus and attention on this condition by policymakers, researchers, academics, health professionals and educators.

Impact of congenital deafblindness on children

Vision and hearing are referred to as the distance senses (Marschark & Spencer, 2012), meaning that they connect an individual to the world that extends beyond their personal body space and reach (Gleason, 2017). These distance senses are the main avenues for communication, learning and socialisation (Christoffel-Blindenmission [CBM], 2016). They collect and organise information from the environment into meaningful concepts for children's learning and social development (Gleason, 2017). Moreover, vision and hearing facilitate 'accidental' learning of language and other important concepts without overtly planned instruction (Marschark & Hauser, 2012).

Congenital deafblindness places severe limitations on a child's access to communication and language. Most children who are deafblind are unable to observe the use of language shared between others or to use others as models to imitate (Gleason, 2017). A child with a visual impairment typically relies on their hearing to compensate for the visual impairment. Similarly, a child with a hearing impairment relies on their vision to compensate for the hearing impairment (Cappagli, Finocchietti, Cocchi, & Gori, 2017; Newton & Moss, 2001). For a child who is deafblind, neither sense can adequately compensate for the lack of the other. Consequently, access to the clear and consistent flow of visual and auditory information necessary for learning, interaction and overall development is negatively affected. Impairment in these senses thus potentially results in serious consequences for a developing child, unless early detection and intervention are provided timeously.

The impact of hearing and vision impairment extends far beyond early development and early childhood communication and learning. Without early detection and intervention, deafblindness restricts experience to the here and now – what is happening at this moment, within arm's reach. Therefore, children who are deafblind may not realise that the wider world exists, or they may find it so confusing and chaotic that they retreat internally (Gleason, 2017; Newton & Moss, 2001).

The impact of deafblindness extends beyond communication, mobility and educational outcomes. According to the WFDB (2018), to facilitate participation and inclusion in education, children with deafblindness require the removal of environmental barriers as well as those that prevent access to quality support services. Accessibility for children with deafblindness extends into the built, information and communication environments, as devices such as braille and loop systems may not be sufficient for them (WFDB, 2018). The WFDB (2018) notes that society assumes that services for children who are deaf or blind are also sufficient for children who are deafblind, which is not the case.

Early deafblindness detection and intervention

The goal of early detection and intervention for children who are deafblind is threefold. Firstly, it is to open up a new channel of communication and exploring the environment (Anthony, 2016). Secondly, it facilitates and reinforces appropriate social–emotional bonding and early communication, language, emergent literacy, and access to learning materials and educational experiences (Anthony, 2016). Thirdly, it mitigates the multiplicative effects of this condition in developing babies, particularly in early onset cases, where children may not have developed language (Anthony, 2016). The benefits of early detection and intervention in this group include:

- Providing health care professionals with information regarding the unique accessibility, communication and learning needs of the developing child, so minimising the potential for fragmented learning and creating optimal reciprocal relationships between the child and caregivers (Rowland, 2011).
- Spurring prompt and timeous referrals to appropriate early intervention services and support that may include specialised materials and

equipment, as screening and diagnostic programmes are counterproductive if the goal is not to provide appropriate, individualised, targeted and high-quality intervention (American Academy of Pediatrics, 2013).

- Improving prognosis for subsequent development of speech and language, which paves the way for more positive educational and vocational outcomes (Anthony, Wiggin, Yoshinaga-Itano, & Raver, 2015).
- Using medical and clinical information about the diagnosis, prognosis and degree of deafblindness specific to each child to determine communication approaches and customised educational intervention (Chen, 2004).
- Using referral to early intervention services to facilitate opportunities for education professionals to help identify and address other disabilities (Anthony et al., 2015).

Therefore, delayed or absent early detection programmes can result in missing the critical period of early neurodevelopment, thereby reducing the opportunities to learn language and negatively impacting the health and quality of life of the affected child (Anthony, 2016). This is likely to result in children with deafblindness falling behind in their communication, cognition, reading and social–emotional development (Joint Committee on Infant Hearing, 2007).

Evidence suggests that there are no active early detection and intervention programmes in South Africa specifically geared towards children who are deafblind. This lack is the consequence of various factors, discussed next.

The incidence of deafblindness is low and, in most cases, deafblind individuals are 'invisible' to society. According to Maguvhe (2014, p. 1486), deafblindness 'is rarely discussed in public circles. Minor coverage in public talk goes with low societal preparedness to accommodate people who are deafblind. Literally, society has forgotten that it is made up of members who include the deafblind'. This exclusion of deafblind individuals is exemplified in the lack of services designed exclusively for this population. In 2007, the South African government ratified the Convention on the Rights of Persons with Disabilities (South African Human Rights Commission, 2017). Subsequently, in 2015, the White Paper on the Rights of Persons with Disabilities was approved (Palime, 2016). The White Paper makes explicit mention of deafblindness. Yet, despite this, individuals who are deafblind, particularly children, continue to face discrimination, marginalisation and a lack of services. Maguvhe (2014) notes that decisions and plans concerning the education of deafblind children are influenced by society's misconception of and negative attitudes towards deafblind people. This results in compromised or inappropriate delivery of comprehensive services to this population. Despite the active and deliberate effort of the Joint Committee on Infant Hearing (JCIH, 2007) and the HPCSA's (2018) EHDI guidelines to provide neonatal hearing screening programmes in order to detect and offer intervention services for children diagnosed with a hearing impairment, deafblindness is silent in these initiatives.

In most cases, deafblindness results from the same conditions causing hearing impairments. It can therefore be argued that the deafblind population is not entirely neglected, as screening, identification and intervention can be conducted through already existing programmes and projects. However, evidence suggests that health care professionals such as audiologists, speech therapists, occupational therapists, physiotherapists and ophthalmologists are not trained to provide detection and intervention services to individuals with multisensory impairments. According to Mosca et al. (2015), the JCIH endorses the ophthalmological assessment of all infants in South Africa with confirmed hearing impairment, but there is no evidence to confirm if this is routinely done. Arguably, in cases where the need to refer to other professionals is clear, as mandated by the scope of practice of health care professionals, referrals are indeed made. However, in cases where latent symptoms or accompanying impairments are not routinely investigated, those children may not be referred to other professionals, or referred early enough. A reason could be that although health care professionals may be aware of the impact of visual and hearing impairments on the developing child, there is a lack of training for professionals who deal with deafblind individuals (House & Davidson, 2000). Internationally, a number of training institutions train practitioners in speech pathology, audiology and aural (re)habilitation. Nevertheless, for many preservice programmes, academic units and practicum, hours specific to hearing impairments remain limited to the minimum competencies as required by the American Speech-Language-Hearing Association. Very few, if any, provide training in visual impairments and deafblindness (House & Davidson, 2000). The lack of adequately trained health care professionals impacts on the timely provision of early detection and intervention programmes for these children.

Under ideal conditions, early detection and intervention should take place within the first year of life. Global trends indicate early detection programmes for children who are deafblind typically take place in special schools for the blind, in schools for the deaf, or in schools for learners with special educational needs (Aitken, 2000; Hersh, 2013; Knoors & Vervloed, 2003). This is attributable to misdiagnosis, resulting in children being sent to these special schools. In South Africa, there are no schools exclusively for children who are deafblind. These children therefore probably end up in schools for learners with special educational needs. Given that up to 70 percent of South African children of school-going age with disabilities are out of school (Donohue & Bornman, 2014), the percentage is likely higher for deafblind children. In a study conducted by Maguvhe (2014) on curriculum design for children who are deafblind, findings reveal that curricula for the deafblind are not streamlined to the national curriculum and 'their unique needs are not considered and advocated for' (Maguvhe, 2014, p. 1487). This schooling context is thus not ideal for early detection and intervention to take place for children who are deafblind. Furthermore, while some schools for learners with special educational needs employ health care professionals or teachers to work with the children, there is a dearth of knowledge on the competence of these individuals, and whether they can provide adequate services to deafblind learners.

The shortage of health care professionals and teachers specialising in deafblindness education influences active programmes for the deafblind. In South Africa, there is a paucity of evidence on the availability of therapists and teachers with expertise in the management of children who are deafblind. In ideal conditions, where health care professionals are deployed at schools for learners with special educational needs, learners with deafblindness should be referred timeously for screening, evaluation and treatment of communication and learning difficulties (House & Davidson, 2000). According to House and Davidson (2000), experts such as teachers, physiotherapists, audiologists and speech therapists should facilitate this referral process. Therefore, in order to best serve this population, it is imperative that these professionals be available and understand how the visual system works, how the auditory system works, the implications for development and intervention planning, as well as the importance of consistent access to professional colleagues and other specialists for critical information sharing and ongoing support. This highlights the need for schools designed specifically for children who are deafblind, as deafblindness creates learning/educational needs that cannot be accommodated by schools, interventions and programmes designed solely for individuals who are deaf or blind (CBM, 2015) or who present with a disability other than deafblindness.

Finally, the concept of family-centred early intervention (FCEI) is relatively new in South Africa. As discussed in chapter 11, FCEI is integral to early detection and intervention. The recommendations and principles around FCEI are applicable to children who are deafblind, and should be adopted for their comprehensive and effective management. Adopting this approach will go a long way towards optimising the deafblind child's developmental outcomes, while also taking into account the quality of life of the whole family. Health care professionals should work collaboratively with families to identify suitable communication strategies, and environmental accommodation to enhance visual and hearing sensory input. Ideally, communication interventions should be individualised to each family's needs and context of daily interactions, while taking into account activities to target concepts and skills that the child may be lacking due to being deafblind (Aitken, 2000; Anthony, 2016; Ferrell, Bruce, & Luckner, 2014).

Solutions and recommendations

There are no clear-cut solutions for the identification and management of children who present with deafblindness, as this condition is unique and complex and cannot be accommodated in contexts designed for single sensory impairment such as a hearing or visual impairment. Also, there are few professionals adequately trained to serve children who are deafblind and their families. With this is mind, the following recommendations are made:

- Prevention is better than cure and timely preventive interventions can be less costly and more effective than providing services later in life (Gardner et al., 2019). For example, if rubella is a leading cause of deafblindness, it is imperative that routine rubella vaccinations form part of the expanded programme for immunisation in South Africa. Rubella vaccinations will go a long way towards reducing the burden of disease already experienced by the South African health care sector, by significantly reducing the incidence of this condition in children.

- There is a need to ensure that early intervention programmes are provided by health care practitioners with expertise in hearing and vision impairments as well as educators of children who are deafblind (American Academy of Pediatrics, 2013). This calls for collaborative partnership among health care professionals and other relevant stakeholders who work with deafblind children. Furthermore, for effective collaborations, dedicated training of competent health care practitioners who are well equipped to serve deafblind children is required (House & Davidson, 2000). I acknowledge that the low incidence of deafblindness may not necessarily warrant dedicated training, especially in countries like South Africa where there are limited resources. However, it is recommended that health care professionals working with children with unisensory impairments, such as hearing impairment or visual impairment, consider the possibility of including other sensory impairments in their training, as most conditions causing sensory impairment are the same conditions that cause deafblindness. It is prudent for these practitioners to consider potential co-morbidities as the combination of hearing and visual impairment impacts various domains of development in children.

- Programmes for early detection should be selected carefully and systematically while taking into account the potential to lessen the long-term impact of deafblindness and counteract any negative effects through intervention. Careful deliberations are required around expanding existing programmes, such as EHDI. An emphasis on screening for possible multisensory impairments should be considered by health care professionals who engage with this population, such as paediatricians and audiologists. This will facilitate mandatory and routine screening for multisensory impairments.

- Parents of children who are deafblind are a critical link in the identification and intervention processes. Intervention programmes should be family-centred and individualised to each child's needs. Intervention programmes will be successful only with the active engagement and involvement of families. Family-centred interventions will also ensure contextually relevant and responsive care for the child.
- Most children are diagnosed with deafblindness in school settings. This highlights the need to have school-based health care practitioners; educators who are knowledgeable about the impact of deafblindness on developing children; the involvement of family members; and supportive environments for continuity of care for deafblind children, from the health care sector to the education sector.
- Every health care professional working with children who are deafblind needs to familiarise themselves with the White Paper on the Rights of Persons with Disabilities, and other regulations and policies relating to deafblindness. The White Paper outlines the rights of deafblind individuals in South Africa. If health care practitioners are cognisant of the needs and rights of children who are deafblind, they can play a critical role in not only advocating for but also upholding those rights. This would ensure that health care professionals provide services with dignity to children who are deafblind and keep their families well informed.

Specific recommendations for national governments as articulated in the WFDB (2018) include the need to:
- recognise deafblindness as a unique disability in law and practice
- raise awareness of the specific requirements of persons with deafblindness
- collect and analyse data about the experiences, barriers and support requirements of persons with deafblindness
- recognise the specificity of communication systems used by persons with deafblindness
- include deafblindness as a specific disability group and facilitate eligibility determination procedures
- carry out outreach, awareness raising and advocacy.

Conclusion

There is a paucity of knowledge globally on the impact and experiences of deafblindness in children. However, it can be argued that the outcomes for deafblind children in a LAMI context are worse than for deafblind children in high-income countries, for various reasons: limited resources in terms of availability of schools for learners who are deafblind; lack of health care professionals adequately trained to serve children who are deafblind, impacting on both early detection and intervention; and the stigma associated with disability. Therefore, to ensure that sensory development in these children is not neglected or undermined, it is important to implement carefully conceived and well-executed early detection and intervention programmes that either take into account or are specific to deafblindness.

Professionals have an important role to play in making sure that children who are deafblind get access to all the resources they require in order to improve their quality of life as well as their future prospects. Early detection and intervention programmes should be family-centred, as success in managing children who are deafblind relies on the active and informed involvement of their families.

Assessment and management programmes that involve all relevant members of the team, with the family in the centre, are key to ensure the child is managed holistically and each family has access to the resources, assistance and support they need. Adequate intervention programmes will maximise and enhance learning, particularly in the early critical years of the child's development. Consequently, this will lead to the improved physical, communication, cognitive, social and emotional development of the deafblind child (Malloy et al., 2009).

References

Aitken, S. (2000). *Understanding deafblindness*. London, England: David Fulton.

American Academy of Pediatrics. (2013). Statement of endorsement: Supplement to the JCIH 2007 position statement: Principles and guidelines for early intervention after confirmation that a child is deaf or hard of hearing. *Pediatrics, 13*(14), 1324–1349.

Anthony, T. L. (2016). Early identification of infants and toddlers with deafblindness. *American Annals of the Deaf, 161*(4), 412–423.

Anthony, T. L., Wiggin, M. P., Yoshinaga-Itano, C., & Raver, A. (2015). *Strategies for infants and toddlers with sensory disabilities*. Baltimore, MD: Brookes.

Ask Larsen, F., & Damen, S. (2014). Definitions of deafblindness and congenital deafblindness. *Research in Developmental Disabilities, 35*(10), 2568–2576.

Ayres, A. J. (1972). Types of sensory integrative dysfunction among disabled learners. *American Journal of Occupational Therapy, 26*(1), 13–18.

Barnhardt, C., Borsting, E., Deland, P., Pham, N., & Vu, T. (2005). Relationship between visual-motor integration and spatial organization of written language and math. *Optometry Visual Science, 82*, 138–143.

Batshaw, M., Pellegrino, L., & Roizen, N. (2007). *Children with disabilities (6th ed.)*. Baltimore, MD: Paul H. Brookes Publishing.

Belote, M., & Maier, J. (2014). Why deaf-blindness and autism can look so much alike. *Resources, 19*(2), 1–16.

Ben-Sasson, A., Cermak, S. A., Orsmond, G. I., Tager-Flusberg, H., Carter, A. S., Kadlec, M. B., & Dunn, W. (2007). Extreme sensory modulation behaviors in toddlers with autism spectrum disorders. *American Journal of Occupational Therapy, 61*, 584–592.

Berg, R. L., Pickett, W., Fitz-Randolph, M., Broste, S. K., Knobloch, M. J., Wood, D. J., … Marlenga, B. (2009). Hearing conservation program for agricultural students: Short-term outcomes from a cluster-randomized trial with planned long-term follow-up. *Preventive Medicine, 49*(6), 546–552. doi: 10.1016/j.ypmed.2009.09.020.

Boshoff, L., & Tooke, L. (2012). Congenital rubella: Is it nearly time to take action? *South African Journal of Child Health, 6*(4), 106–108.

Cappagli, G., Finocchietti, S., Cocchi, E., & Gori, M. (2017). The impact of early visual deprivation on spatial hearing: A comparison between totally and partially visually deprived children. *Frontiers in Psychology, 8*, 467.

Case-Smith, J., Weaver, L. L., & Fristad, M. A. (2015). A systematic review of sensory processing interventions for children with autism spectrum disorders. *Autism, 19*(2), 133–148.

Chen, D. (2001). *Visual impairment in young children: A review of the literature with implications for working with families of diverse cultural and linguistic backgrounds.* University of Illinois at Urbana Champaign.

Chen, D. (2004). Young children who are deaf-blind: Implications for professionals in deaf and hard of hearing services. *Volta Review, 104*(4), 273–284.

Christoffel-Blindenmission CBM. (2015). International day of deafblindness. Retrieved from https://www.cbm.org/news/news/news-2015/international-day-of-deafblindness/.

Christoffel-Blindenmission (CBM). (2016). Deafblind awareness week 2016. Retrieved from https://www.cbm.org/news/news/news-2016/deafblind-awareness-week-2016/.

Dammeyer, J. (2012). Children with Usher syndrome: Mental and behavioral disorders. *Behavioral and Brain Functions, 8*(1), 1–5.

Dammeyer, J. (2014a). Symptoms of autism among children with congenital deafblindness. *Journal of Autism and Developmental Disorders, 44*, 1095–1102.

Dammeyer, J. (2014b). Deafblindness: A review of the literature. *Scandinavian Journal of Public Health, 42*(7), 554–562.

Dammeyer, J. (2015). Deafblindness and dual sensory loss research: Current status and future directions. *World Journal of Otorhinolaryngology, 5*(2), 37–40.

DispatchLIVE. (2019). Big push to start deafblind branch. Retrieved from https://www.dispatchlive.co.za/news/2019-09-30-big-push-to-start-deafblind-branch/.

Donohue, D., & Bornman, J. (2014). The challenges of realising inclusive education in South Africa. *South African Journal of Education, 34*(2), 1–14.

Dunlop, J. (2019). Understanding sensory impairment. *Teach Early Years, 53*–55. https://www.teachearlyyears.com/images/uploads/article/sen-understanding-sensory-impairment.pdf.

Dunn, W. (2008). *Sensory processing: Identifying patterns and support strategies.* Shawnee Mission, KS: Autism Asperger Publishing Company.

Early Support. (2012). Information about multi-sensory impairment. Retrieved from https://councilfordisabledchildren.org.uk/sites/default/files/field/attachemnt/earlysupportmulti-sensoryimpairmentsfinal2.pdf.

Ferrell, K. A., Bruce, S., & Luckner, J. L. (2014). Evidence-based practices for students with sensory impairments. Document No. IC-4. University of Florida, Collaboration for Effective Educator, Development, Accountability, and Reform Center.

Gardner, F., Leijten, P., Melendez-Torres, G. J., Landau, S., Harris, V., Mann, J., … Scott, S. (2019). The earlier the better? Individual participant data and traditional meta-analysis of age effects of parenting interventions. *Child Development, 90*(1), 7–19.

Gleason, D. (2017). *Early interactions with children who are deaf-blind (Revised ed.).* Monmouth, OR: National Center on Deaf-Blindness.

Health Professions Council of South Africa (HPCSA). (2018). Early hearing detection and intervention (EHDI) guidelines. Retrieved from http://www.hpcsa.co.za/Uploads/editor/UserFiles/downloads/speech/Early_Hearing_Detection_and_Intervention_(EHDI)_2018.pdf.

Hersh, M. (2013). Deafblind people, communication, independence, and isolation. *The Journal of Deaf Studies and Deaf Education, 18*(4), 446–463.

Higuera, V. (2016). Premature birth complications. *Healthline.* Retrieved from https://www.healthline.com/health/pregnancy/premature-baby-complications.

House, S. S., & Davidson, R. C. (2000). Speech-language pathologists and children with sensory impairments: Personnel preparation and service delivery survey. *Communication Disorders Quarterly, 21*(4), 224–236.

Jaiswal, A., Aldersey, H., Wittich, W., Mirza, M., & Finlayson, M. (2018). Participation experiences of people with deafblindness or dual sensory loss: A scoping review of global deafblind literature. *PLoS ONE, 13*(9), e0203772. https://doi.org/10.1371/journal.pone.0203772.

Janssen, M. J., Riksen-Walraven, J. M., & Van Dijk, J. P. M. (2003). Toward a diagnostic intervention model for fostering harmonious interactions between deafblind children and their educators. *Journal of Visual Impairment & Blindness, 97*(4), 197–214.

Joint Committee on Infant Hearing (JCIH). (2007). Position statement: Principles and guidelines for early hearing detection and intervention programs. *Pediatrics, 120*(4), 898–921.

Kanji, A., Khoza-Shangase, K., & Moroe, N. (2018). Newborn hearing screening protocols and their outcomes: A systematic review. *International Journal of Pediatric Otorhinolaryngology, 115*, 104–109. https://doi.org/10.1016/j.ijporl.2018.09.026.

Knoors, H., & Vervloed, M. (2003). *Educational programming for deaf children with multiple disabilities: Accommodating special needs (Vol. 1).* Oxford Handbooks Online.

Maguvhe, M. O. (2014). Curriculum design, implementation and parental involvement in the education of the deafblind: South African teachers' perspectives. *Mediterranean Journal of Social Sciences, 5*(20), 1186–1492.

Malloy, P., Stremel Thomas, K., Schalock, M., Davies, S., Purvis, B., & Udell, T. (2009). *Early identification of infants who are deaf-blind.* National Consortium on Deaf-Blindness. Retrieved from https://files.eric.ed.gov/fulltext/ED548231.pdf.

Maluleke, N. P., Khoza-Shangase, K., & Kanji, A. (2019). Hearing impairment detection and intervention in children from centre-based early intervention programmes. *Journal of Child Health Care, 23*(2): 232–241. doi: 10.1177/1367493518788477.

Marschark, M., & Hauser, P. C. (2012). *How deaf children learn: What parents and teachers need to know (1st ed.)*. New York, NY: Oxford University Press.

Marschark, M., & Spencer, P. E. (2012). *Oxford handbook of deaf studies, language, and education (Vol. 2)*. Oxford, England: Oxford Library of Psychology.

Marumoagae, M. C. (2012). Disability discrimination and the right of disabled persons to access the labour market. *PER: Potchefstroomse Elektroniese Regsblad, 15*(1), 344–365. Retrieved from http://www.scielo.org.za/scielo.php?script=sci_arttext&pid=S1727-37812012000100010&lng=en&tlng=en.

Moroe, N., & Kathrada, N. (2016). The long-term concerns post cochlear implantation as experienced by parents/caregivers of prelingually deaf children between the ages of 3 and 5 years in Gauteng province, South Africa. *South African Journal of Child Health, 10*(2), 126. doi: 10.7196/SAJCH.2016.v10i2.1049.

Mosca, R., Kritzinger, A., & Van der Linde, J. (2015). Language and communication development in preschool children with visual impairment: A systematic review. *South African Journal of Communication Disorders, 62*, 1–10.

Newton, G., & Moss, K. (2001). Early identification of hearing and vision loss is critical to a child's development. *SEE/HEAR, 6*(3), 27–30.

Olusanya, B. O., Swanepoel, D. W., Chapchap, M. J., Castillo, S., Habib, H., Mukari, S. Z., … McPherson, B. (2007). Progress towards early detection services for infants with hearing loss in developing countries. *BMC Health Services Research, 7*(1), 1–15.

Owens, R. (2012). *Language development: An introduction (8th ed.)*. Boston, MA: Pearson.

Palime, B. (2016). White paper on the rights of persons with disabilities. Presentation to the Expanded Public Works Programme Summit, 15 November. Retrieved from http://www.epwp.gov.za/documents/Summit/2016/Day_One/Mr%20B%20Palime.Expanded%20Public%20Works%20Programme%20Summit%20Disability%20presentation.pdf

Probst, K. M., & Borders, C. M. (2017). Comorbid deafblindness and autism spectrum disorder: Characteristics, differential diagnosis, and possible interventions. *Review Journal of Autism and Developmental Disorders, 4*(2), 95–117.

Psychological Musings. (2013). Blindness and deafness. Retrieved from http://psychological-musings.blogspot.com/2013/08/blindness-and-deafness.html.

Rehabilitation Council of India. (n.d.). Deafblindness. Retrieved from http://www.rehabcouncil.nic.in/writereaddata/deafblind.pdf.

Rowland, C. (2011). Using the communication matrix to assess expressive skills in early communicators. *Communication Disorders Quarterly, 32*, 190–201.

Simcock, P. (2017). Ageing with a unique impairment: A systematically conducted review of older deafblind people's experiences. *Ageing & Society, 37*(8), 1703–1742.

South African Human Rights Commission. (2017). Research brief on disability and equality in South Africa 2013–2017. Retrieved from https://www.sahrc.org.za/home/21/files/RESEARCH%20BRIEF%20ON%20DISABILITY%20AND%20EQUALITY%20IN%20SOUTH%20AFRICA%202013%20to%202017.pdf.

Spinazola, C. D. C., Cia, F., Azevedo, T. L. D., & Gualda, D. S. (2018). Children with physical disability, Down syndrome and autism: Comparison of family characteristics in the maternal perspective in Brazilian reality. *Revista Brasileira de Educação Especial, 24*(2), 199–216. Retrieved from http://www.scielo.br/scielo. php?script=sci_arttext&pid=S1413-65382018000200199&nrm=iso.

Stadskleiv, K. (2020). Cognitive functioning in children with cerebral palsy. *Developmental Medicine and Child Neurology, 62*(3), 283–289. doi: 10.1111/ dmcn.14463.

Thisability. (2017). Tracking the footprint of deafblind persons in SA. Retrieved from https://www.thisability.co.za/2017/07/12/tracking-the-footprint-of-deafblind-persons-in-sa/.

Thompson, S. D., & Merino, S. (2018). Visual impairments in young children: Fundamentals of and strategies for enhancing development. *Young Exceptional Children, 21*(3), 157–169.

Tswanya, Y. (2019). About 600 000 children with disabilities have never been to school. *African News Agency (ANA) Archives.* Retrieved from https://www.iol.co.za/ capetimes/news/about-600-000-children-with-disabilities-have-never-been-to-school-24870542.

Wiley, S., Parnell, L., & Belhorn, T. (2016). Promoting early identification and intervention for children who are deaf/hard of hearing, children with vision impairment, and children with deaf-blind conditions. *Journal of Early Hearing Detection and Intervention, 1*(1), 26–33.

Wittich, W., Jarry, J., Groulx, G., Southall, K., & Gagné, J-P. (2016). Rehabilitation and research priorities in deafblindness for the next decade. *Journal of Visual Impairment and Blindness, 110*(4), 219–231.

Wittich, W., Southall, K., Sikora, L., Watanabe, D., & Gagné, J. (2013). What's in a name: Dual sensory impairment or deafblindness? *British Journal of Visual Impairment, 31*(3), 198–207.

Wittich, W., Watanabe, D. H., & Gagné, J-P. (2012). Sensory and demographic characteristics of deafblindness rehabilitation clients in Montréal, Canada. *Ophthalmic and Physiological Optics, 32*(3), 242–251.

World Federation of the Deafblind (WFDB). (2018). At risk of exclusion from CRPD and SDGs implementation: Inequality and persons with deafblindness. Retrieved from http://www.internationaldisabilityalliance.org/sites/default/files/wfdb_complete_ initial_global_report_september_2018.pdf.

11 Family-Centred Early Hearing Detection and Intervention

Ntsako Precious Maluleke, Rudo Chiwutsi and Katijah Khoza-Shangase

According to the Health Professions Council of South Africa (HPCSA, 2018), early intervention services following diagnosis of a hearing impairment must be family-centred and within a community-based model of service delivery that is culturally congruent. This chapter discusses family-centred early hearing detection and intervention (EHDI) in South Africa, with due recognition of the unique concept of what constitutes a family in this context; the multilingual and multicultural nature of society; as well as power and decision-making dynamics. The chapter also outlines the principles of family-centred early intervention (FCEI) and provides a discussion of current evidence and practice in the field with recommendations for the implementation of family-centred EHDI programmes in the African context.

The concept of family-centred practice made an appearance in discussions about early intervention in the early 1980s and has become an integral principle guiding the design and delivery of service models since then (Kuo et al., 2012). Consequently, over the past few decades, there has been an increasing shift towards emphasising the importance of the child's family taking an active role in the habilitation process, through FCEI programmes. In the case of early intervention services for children with hearing impairment identified through early hearing detection initiatives, the term 'family-centred EHDI' is used (Moeller, Carr, Seaver, Stredler-Brown, & Holzinger, 2013).

Deliberations around family-centred EHDI are crucial because, according to the World Health Organization (WHO, 2018), around 466 million people worldwide have disabling hearing impairment. Thirty-four million (7 percent) of these individuals are children; in 60 percent of cases, their hearing impairment is due to preventable causes. It is estimated that the number of people with disabling hearing impairment will increase to over 900 million by 2050 (WHO, 2019). This has significant implications for low and middle-income (LAMI) countries such as South Africa, where resource constraints are a challenge. The WHO (2018) states that unaddressed hearing impairment costs an annual global amount of 750 billion international dollars. Thus, initiatives to prevent, identify and provide early intervention for hearing impairment in a family-centred context are cost-effective and can bring great benefits to individuals, families and societies. Children with hearing impairment benefit from early identification and intervention; amplification through the use of hearing aids, cochlear implants and other assistive devices; speech-language therapy, captioning and sign language; and other forms of educational and social support, including that of their families (WHO, 2018; Yoshinaga-Itano, 2014).

Epidemiological data pertaining to hearing impairment, particularly early onset hearing impairment, is largely unknown in the developing world. However, incidence figures for hearing impairment in resource-poor countries are estimated at six per 1 000 live births (Olusanya, 2008). According to Swanepoel, Ebrahim, Joseph, and Friedland (2007), true prevalence data on infant hearing impairment in South Africa is unavailable because newborn hearing screening programmes are limited, often inefficiently managed and poorly supported. The hearing screening services available in the public health care sector, where over 80 percent of the South African population access health care services, are reported to be rare and mostly unsystematic (Kanji & Khoza-Shangase, 2016; Khoza-Shangase, Kanji, Petrocchi-Bartal, & Farr, 2017; Petrocchi-Bartal & Khoza-Shangase, 2016; Theunissen & Swanepoel, 2008). In South Africa, the incidence of congenital and early onset hearing impairment is considered to be three in 1 000 live births in the private sector and between four and six in 1 000 in the public sector (Swanepoel, Störbeck, & Friedland, 2009). This high prevalence of hearing impairment in a context facing demand–capacity challenges (see chapter 5) highlights the importance of collaborative work with all stakeholders, including the family.

With approximately 20 babies born with hearing impairment daily in South Africa, appropriate EHDI for these children to curb hearing and communication disability has become an important goal for the audiology community (Petrocchi-Bartal & Khoza-Shangase, 2016). However, this goal faces many challenges and is far from being realised. Early Hearing Detection Intervention in the South African context is significantly different to that in the United States, and Khoza-Shangase (2019) argues that there is a paucity of published South African research into the use and effectiveness of different interventions in early childhood hearing impairment. She notes that EHDI services in South Africa are not systematic, centralised or comprehensive, with limited resources being a significant contributing factor. There is thus an urgent need for the development and implementation of early holistic multidisciplinary services and resources, taking into account the unique South African context and the needs of the caregivers and families of children with hearing impairment. Before further exploring the concept of family-centred EHDI, we establish what a family is in the African context.

The African family defined

Family is an essential factor without which no society can function. It is through the family that children are born, socialised and cared for until they attain independence (Department of Social Development [DSD], 2013). The child's development of personality and independence is facilitated through the family's provision of physical and emotional care, security, appreciation and affection, positive communication, time spent together and spiritual well-being. The family also acts as a protective buffer against risk behaviours in order to promote resilience and coping during difficult times (Aldersey, 2012).

Despite being a foundational social institution, the concept of family is difficult to define, especially in the South African context (DSD, 2013). This is primarily because family structures and functions are in a constant state of flux due to:

- population migration as a result of high unemployment rates and limited economic opportunities, especially in rural contexts, with many African women working as domestic workers and raising their employers' children
- the high prevalence of HIV/AIDS, which has resulted in many women having to take on the roles of both breadwinner and caregiver in challenging circumstances of high unemployment
- the absence of parents due to the HIV/AIDS epidemic, resulting in grandparents and older children caring for their grandchildren or younger siblings, respectively, with child-headed households being common.

The South African population is made up of various cultures, ethnic groups and 12 official languages: isiZulu, isiXhosa, isiSwati, isiNdebele, seSotho, seTswana, sePedi, Xitsonga, Tshivenda, English and Afrikaans. The 12th official language is South African Sign Language (SASL), the acknowledged official language of teaching for the deaf. In his 2020 State of the Nation address, President Cyril Ramaphosa noted that SASL is now recognised in the Constitution and other bodies of law as one of the country's official languages.

The concept of family may differ from culture to culture and is based on the social context. Given the multilingual and multicultural nature of South Africa, no standard definition of family is comprehensive enough to cover the various kinds of families that exist. However, for the purpose of legislative frameworks, the DSD (2013, p. 11) defines the family as 'a societal group that is related by blood (kinship), adoption, foster care or the ties of marriage (civil, customary or religious), civil union or cohabitation, and goes beyond a particular physical residence'. Thus, in the African context, family constitutes a wider circle of relatives than just the nuclear family with its biological or adopted children. Instead, members of the extended family automatically become part of the immediate family: paternal and maternal grandparents, uncles, aunts, nephews, nieces, cousins, sons- and daughters-in-law (Chataika & McKenzie, 2013).

In patriarchal contexts, the roles of various family members are often hierarchical and gendered. In the case of Africa, males are generally considered the heads of the family, and females play the most significant role in day-to-day child rearing and caregiving (Masuku & Khoza-Shangase, 2018). However, as a collective, family members can take responsibility for caring for relatives when it comes to provision of shelter, clothing, food, tuition fees and health care. Similarly, hospitality and mutual aid towards one's relatives are important cultural values (Chataika & McKenzie, 2013).

Despite differences in family structures in the African context versus western contexts, children are an important factor in any family. Their care and upbringing are of concern not only for the biological parents, but also for relatives and extensive networks such as the community. Based on the adage 'your child is mine and my child is yours', communities in Africa assist in raising children to ensure they follow community values, norms and religious beliefs. This brings a sense of unity in the community. Children belong to the whole community and community members are there to ensure that they become significant members of the community. This communal child-rearing practice is underpinned by the philosophy of ubuntu – an African value system that means humanness or being human and is characterised by values such as caring, sharing, compassion and communalism. This child-rearing practice by people in the community with similar lifestyles and views about good parenting and good child development is complementary to the community's larger cultural system. It is often successful in promoting children's health and well-being in light of cultural considerations as well as possibilities and limitations within their environment (Morelli et al., 2018). Thus, in this context, the concept of family-centred may be viewed as community-centred or village-centred, particularly in rural areas. Khoza-Shangase (2019) argues that the philosophy of ubuntu and the cultural belief that a child is raised by the whole village should thus form part of any conceptualisation of intervention plans or initiatives to ensure that they are culturally congruent.

Family-centred EHDI

Family-centred early intervention is a family–professional partnership that places the needs of the child in the context of their family in order to optimise the child's developmental outcomes (Iversen, Shimmel, Ciacera, & Prabhakar, 2003; MacKean, Thurston, & Scott, 2005). This type of intervention is the preferred approach in paediatric care, where families are most involved with their children. Its purpose is to educate and support family members and the family system of the child with hearing impairment (Moeller et al., 2013). Recognising the centrality of family–child interactions represents a paradigm shift from viewing the family as a peripheral player in child-focused interventions, to a service delivery model where professionals focus on strengthening family interactions (Woods, Wilcox, Friedman, & Murch, 2011). This family–professional partnership fundamentally challenges the care paradigm of unilateral responsibility for decision-making by the professional, and also empowers the family, who are the ones the child spends the majority of their time with (Woods et al., 2011).

To summarise, FCEI is a philosophy, belief and value system where professionals support the development and capacities of families in order to promote the progress of the child with disabilities (Dalmau et al., 2017; Epley, Summers, & Turnbull, 2010). It is based on the following principles:

- The client is the child and their family, rather than just the child. Therefore, the best way to meet the needs of the child with hearing impairment is to acknowledge the needs of the family members as well (Epley et al., 2010; Kuo et al., 2012).
- Caregivers are invited to become involved in their child's care and have the opportunity to share their opinions, needs and preferences with professionals (Moeller et al., 2013; Yoshinaga-Itano, 2014).
- Information sharing between the professional and the caregiver is open, objective and unbiased in order to ensure that families can make appropriate decisions that best fit the needs, strengths and values of the child and family (Kuo et al., 2012; Moeller et al., 2013).
- Caregivers are encouraged to collaborate with professionals to acquire knowledge and competencies that allow them to mediate or extend the intervention for their child with hearing impairment. Conversely, professionals acknowledge the family as the expert of their child's development (Turan, 2012; Moeller et al., 2013).
- Social opportunities through parent-to-parent support are encouraged, which affords families of children with hearing impairment an opportunity to network and meet other families of children with hearing impairment (Henderson, Johnson, & Moodie, 2014; Yoshinaga-Itano, 2014).

The concept of FCEI is broad, and different stakeholders have emphasised different aspects of this philosophy. Consequently, an international consensus statement became available in 2013 to articulate tenets of the philosophy and promote wider implementation of validated, evidence-based principles of FCEI for children with hearing impairment and their families. A better understanding of which components of FCEI lead to positive outcomes will allow for more targeted development of effective interventions. The consensus statement highlights 10 principles guiding FCEI (Moeller et al., 2013, pp. 430–443):

- Principle 1: Early, timely, and equitable access to services – screening and confirmation of the hearing impairment is effective when linked to immediate, timely and equitable access to appropriate interventions.
- Principle 2: Family/provider partnerships – the goal is to develop a balanced partnership between families and health care professionals, characterised by reciprocity, mutual trust, respect, honesty, shared tasks and open communication.
- Principle 3: Informed choice and decision-making – families gain the necessary knowledge, information and experiences to make fully informed decisions.
- Principle 4: Family social and emotional support – families are connected to support systems so they can accrue the knowledge and experiences that can enable them to function effectively on behalf of their child with hearing impairment.
- Principle 5: Family–infant interaction – families and health care professionals work together to create optimal environments for language learning.
- Principle 6: Use of assistive technologies and supporting means of communication – providers must be skilled in the tools, assistive devices and mechanisms necessary to optimally support the child's language and communication development.
- Principle 7: Qualified providers – health care professionals must possess the core competencies to support families in optimising the child's development and child–family well-being.
- Principle 8: Collaborative teamwork – an optimal FCEI team focuses on the family and includes professionals with experience in promoting early development of children with hearing impairment.
- Principle 9: Progress monitoring – FCEI must be guided by regular monitoring/assessment of child and family outcomes.
- Principle 10: Programme monitoring – FCEI programmes must evaluate health care professional's adherence to best practice and include quality assurance monitors of all programme elements.

Incorporation of these principles in any intervention plan will enhance the outcomes of that plan, and improve the chances of achieving maximum benefits from early intervention for the child with hearing impairment.

Evidence-based practice and family-centred EHDI

Various authors have reported the positive effects on child outcomes through strengthening the family's role and responsibility, and allowing caregivers their rightful position as advocates, decision makers and partners with early intervention professionals (Epley et al., 2010; Kuo et al., 2012; Sass-Lehrer, Porter, & Wu, 2015). Outcomes of interest in this approach focus on more than just the child; they also consider key outcomes of satisfaction with services, reduced stress and worry, as well as follow-through with intervention programmes. Careful consideration of the family where early intervention is being implemented, including their views, is critical to efficacious clinical service provision in this population (Moodie, 2018). This is particularly key in contexts like South Africa, where there is significant economic, linguistic, cultural and literacy diversity. South Africa is one of the most unequal societies in the world, with poverty, HIV/AIDS and other infectious diseases, such as tuberculosis, dominating the country's attention and resources. The sharp increase in the prevalence of hearing impairment and its pervasive impact on the individual and their family call for increased attention to family-centred EHDI in order to minimise or eliminate the negative ramifications of poor intervention outcomes. Including the service users (families) in the development and implementation of intervention plans is crucial to ensuring that minimal wasteful expenditure occurs and maximum benefits of EHDI are derived from national programmes (Khoza-Shangase, 2019). The poor professional-to-patient ratio as well as the cultural and linguistic mismatch between the majority of professionals and children with hearing impairment also stress the need to involve families in intervention programmes.

The next sections present a literature review of published evidence on family-centred EHDI.

Caregiver involvement

A caregiver is defined as the person responsible for providing care to the child on a daily basis. This includes biological caregivers, legal guardians or family members. It is widely accepted that caregivers make the greatest difference to children's achievements (American Psychological Association, 2009; Magnuson & Schindler, 2019; Niklas, Cohressen, & Teyler, 2018). Thus, they are crucial to the success of EHDI initiatives.

We discuss two studies that sought to explore the influence of emotional and motivational characteristics on caregiver involvement, as well as the behaviours and practices associated with their involvement. Ingber, Al-Yagon, and Dromi (2010) investigated the contribution of maternal characteristics in explaining Israeli Hebrew-speaking mothers' involvement in early intervention for their children with hearing impairment. They found that increased curiosity, motivation and perceived social support, as well as decreased pessimism about a child's potential, resulted in increased caregiver involvement in early intervention. However, increased anger resulted in decreased caregiver involvement.

However, given the power dynamic created by South Africa's sociopolitical history of apartheid, professionals may perceive curiosity, motivation and anger incorrectly. Caregivers may experience discomfort and reluctance in seeking information from a health care professional from a different linguistic and cultural background. Moreover, different cultural groups have vastly different perceptions of the causes of disability and disease, which influences their health-seeking behaviour. Thus, it is imperative for professionals to be cognisant of caregivers' health-seeking behaviour, which may include consulting a traditional healer with the same linguistic and cultural background in conjunction with biomedical options.

According to Ingber et al. (2010), pessimism about a child's potential and perceived social support also influences caregiver involvement. Similar results may be expected in the South African context. The current state of the departments of Health, Social Development and Basic Education does not raise optimism about the potential for children with hearing impairment or the availability of social and educational support. Khoza-Shangase delves into these challenges in chapter 9, with a specific focus on educational support for the child with hearing impairment.

Through linguistically and culturally appropriate FCEI, caregivers and families in South Africa can be empowered with knowledge to optimise their children's developmental outcomes and be guided to resolve challenges associated with anger, motivation, pessimism and perceived support services. Thus, implications for this context include incorporating the effects of language and culture in clinical decision-making in audiology curricula. Such FCEI programmes may mitigate the effects of the reported barrier of poor access to health care due to a shortage of health care professionals.

In Erbasi, Scarinci, Hickson, and Ching's (2018) study, conducted in Queensland, Australia, findings revealed that caregiver involvement is multifaceted, incorporating a broad range of behaviours and practices. These include caregivers:

- creating an optimal environment for habilitation and learning at home and helping the child adapt to hearing technology as well as managing the use and maintenance of the devices
- working as case managers, including arranging and attending appointments and meetings, communicating with various professionals, educating others and advocating on behalf of their child
- supporting their child's language development by giving up work or reducing their workload to help their child achieve successful communication outcomes, incorporating interactive activities into daily routines, and encouraging their child to use communication strategies
- advocating for all children with hearing impairment through contributing to education and support for other families of children with hearing impairment, and participating in research to improve products and services
- showing affection and being responsive to their child's needs, involving their child in daily and weekly routines, encouraging and supporting their child to explore new things, as well as participating in school activities and helping with school work.

Erbasi et al.'s (2018) study sought to understand caregiver involvement from their own perspective. Their findings highlight that caregiver involvement is more extensive than previously reported and provide a more comprehensive understanding of the various roles that caregivers of children with hearing impairment fulfil in their children's daily lives. However, caution needs to be exercised when using these findings in order to ensure that epistemic knowledge from developed contexts is not used as the norm, without incorporating knowledge obtained from the South African context. Thus, the constructs of caregiver involvement need to be explored in this context in order to ensure that caregivers are adequately capacitated to carry out their role and participate in their child's development. That said, however, we believe that Erbasi and colleagues' (2018) findings are applicable to children and families everywhere, including in the South African context.

Caregiver coaching and information sharing

Information sharing refers to the exchange of information in an open, objective and unbiased manner. Caregivers should be guided and coached through information that supports their ability and confidence to care for their child and provide learning opportunities that have a positive impact on their development without threatening self-confidence, and cultural, religious or family traditions (Bruder, 2000; Dalmau et al., 2017; Turan, 2012). We looked at 11 studies addressing caregiver coaching and/or information sharing, discussed next.

Caregiver coaching

Ekberg, Scarinci, Hickson, and Meyer's (2018) Australian study describes how caregiver-directed commentaries during assessment or intervention tasks can be used to enhance caregivers' knowledge of habilitation procedures and facilitate FCEI. Similarly, Sacks et al.'s (2014) study, conducted in Chicago in the United States, describes how providing linguistic feedback for caregiver–child interactions resulted in increased adult word count, conversation turn count and child vocalisation count.

Caregiver coaching has been shown to empower and prepare caregivers to function effectively in their social contexts and daily lives, and as a result promote their quality of life. Caregiver coaching through modelling and provision of linguistic feedback is essential in order to ensure that caregivers are adequately equipped to extend the therapy environment into the home environment, where the child with hearing impairment spends most of their time. However, this is only effective if contextual factors are taken into account. For example, studies by Watermeyer, Kanji, and Cohen (2012) as well as Watermeyer, Kanji, and Sarvan (2017), conducted in South Africa, have demonstrated poor caregiver recall and understanding of information provided by professionals during information counselling sessions. This is partly a result of the information not being tailored to the communicative needs of the individual caregiver. It has also been shown that the use of an interpreter does not necessarily address the challenges associated with multi-lingualism and multiculturalism in South Africa (Mophosho, 2018). A multi-pronged approach is thus required to address this challenge:

- The Department of Health should invest in recruiting trained interpreters to assist health care professionals.
- The induction of all newly appointed health care professionals should include introductory knowledge on the language and culture of the community in which they serve.
- Additional opportunities for clarification through initiating community support group structures should be put in place.
- Transformation of the admission criteria to the speech-language and hearing programme should be effected to increase accessibility for students who speak African languages, and a curriculum implemented that incorporates cultural awareness and cultural competence.

Khoza-Shangase and Mophosho (2018) argue that as part of the transformation, speech-language and hearing professions in the country need to respond to the national calls to Africanise institutions and service delivery. This includes curriculum changes to incorporate more African-centred courses and courses that are based on evidence that is contextually relevant and responsive; clinical care changes that are contextually relevant and responsive; a clinical focus that allows for 'next practice' and not just 'best practice'; and a language policy that acknowledges that many people speak several languages and so teaching and learning (and clinical service provision) in only English or Afrikaans creates challenges which need to be addressed. Khoza-Shangase and Mophosho (2018) note that it is important that issues of diversity are addressed if effective clinical care is to be provided in line with the goals of the government's universal health care strategy, through implementation of National Health Insurance.

Information provided to caregivers

Five studies reviewed, all conducted in the United States, investigated information provided to caregivers following a failed hearing screening or confirmation of the hearing impairment. In Elpers, Lester, Shinn, and Bush's (2016) study, caregivers reported poor communication of the hearing screening results. These results were reportedly communicated to caregivers a few days or weeks after discharge from the hospital via telephone or posted mail. In Larsen, Munoz, DesGeorges, Nelson, and Kennedy's (2012) study, only 48 percent of the caregivers reportedly received resources pertaining to childhood hearing impairment and only 33 percent were informed about available caregiver support organisations.

Only one study's findings revealed that caregivers were provided with adequate information aligned with the principles of FCEI. Results in Decker and Valloton's (2016) study revealed that caregivers were reportedly informed about the importance of talking frequently throughout the day in everyday routines and activities; promoting listening skills and language by focusing on sound; incorporating other communication channels; and the essential role of caregivers in early intervention.

In studies by Jackson (2011), as well as Findlen, Malhotra, and Adunka (2019), caregivers across the United States reported that they found the following resources most useful during information sharing: written material; verbal/visual demonstrations; hearing aid resources; discussion with other caregivers of children with hearing impairment; internet sources; explanations provided by professionals; parent-friendly books; discussion with adults with hearing impairment; videos and DVDs; brochures and pamphlets; and detailed professional books.

The information provided to caregivers is essential to ensure their involvement in the intervention process. Information sharing dispels any misconceptions and alleviates the emotional turmoil associated with a confirmed hearing impairment. This information enables caregivers to make informed decisions jointly with professionals. Therefore, audiologists need to decide what information is essential to include in feedback sessions, as both the type and amount of information presented may impact caregiver recall. The degree of accurate recall and understanding of information has significant implications for follow-up of treatment options, as well as commitment and adherence to treatment recommendations. Thus, studies investigating caregivers' preferred mode of information sharing are vital, especially in low literacy populations such as South Africa where only 28 percent of 20 to 24 year olds have a grade 12 qualification.

Caregivers' information needs

In studies by Alyami, Soer, and Pottas (2016), Decker and Valloton (2016), Jackson (2011), and Jackson, Wegner, and Turnbull (2010), caregivers reported the following information needs: general information about hearing impairment; information relating to children's development and available community services; available technology; specialised education for children with hearing impairment; and accessing funding for services and support.

The following support needs were also highlighted: support to use signs or sign language; needing professionals to explain the condition to siblings, other children and friends; connecting with other caregivers of children with hearing impairment; caregivers using a specific communication modality; workshops; services provided in natural environments; service coordination; and additional support for family life.

Understanding caregiver information and support needs is essential to ensure that the information provided aligns with their needs as key stakeholders in the intervention process. The method and communicative style in which information is presented also influences caregiver recall and understanding. Consequently, information sharing should be a more reflective practice, characterised by flexibility and adaptability, to ensure that information is presented effectively and appropriately. Furthermore, health care professionals should aim to identify difficulties in comprehension as they raise and tailor information in a given context. Caregivers' reported need for professionals to explain the hearing impairment to siblings, other children and friends (Alyami et al., 2016) has significant implications for clinical practice in LAMI contexts, where the definition of family and caregiver is much wider and more diverse.

Caregiver satisfaction

Five studies reviewed investigated caregiver satisfaction with FCEI programmes. In Ingber and Dromi's (2010) study, caregivers expressed satisfaction with professionals' attitudes and practices towards family participation in the intervention programme. Caregivers reported that professionals were willing to collaborate with them and encouraged them to participate in their child's intervention. Similarly, in Jackson et al.'s (2010) study, caregivers reported improved family interaction, parenting and support following enrolment in an FCEI programme. However, caregivers also reported decreased satisfaction in relation to the expenses associated with their child's hearing impairment, inclusion in their community, support to relieve stress, and having time to pursue their own interests.

Alyami et al. (2016) reported that all participating caregivers expressed satisfaction with the early intervention programme, with 75 percent reporting that the FCEI programme helped them learn auditory training and language activities to use with their child at home. In Findlen et al.'s (2019) study, 86 percent of the caregivers reported overall satisfaction with services provided during annual multidisciplinary assessment and monitoring appointments.

Caregivers' self-reported levels of satisfaction acknowledge their actual experiences with FCEI programmes and make them the most suitable informants to improve accountability of screening, diagnosis and intervention practice. Investigation of caregiver satisfaction with current early intervention initiatives in South Africa is thus warranted to identify gaps and incongruence in knowledge, beliefs and practices. This will ensure that FCEI programmes are grounded in the linguistic, cultural and socio-economic diversity of the South African population and tailored to meet their unique needs.

Constanescu (2012) investigated caregiver satisfaction with remote delivery of early intervention services via computer-based videoconferencing (telehealth) in Brisbane, Australia. All the caregivers expressed satisfaction with the service, with 89 percent reporting that receiving early intervention services via videoconferencing was a better alternative to travelling for regular face-to-face sessions. However, 61 percent reported experiencing technical difficulties that required troubleshooting during the session. In South Africa, where demand–capacity challenges exist (see chapter 5), the use of tele-audiology might be part of the package of care for FCEI. Chapters 9 and 13 look more closely into telehealth in the form of tele-audiology and EHDI.

Challenges of implementing EHDI

The benefits of FCEI include greater satisfaction of families with the services and care received. However, various challenges have been reported when implementing FCEI programmes in various contexts.

Logistical and access challenges

Five studies reviewed for this chapter focused on logistical challenges associated with the provision of FCEI. In studies by Adedeji, Tobih, Sogebi, and Daniel (2015) in Nigeria, and Merugumala, Pothula, and Cooper (2017) in India, the late identification, diagnosis and initiation of early intervention services for children with congenital and early onset hearing impairment was attributed to a lack of attention to early hearing detection, thus making early intervention difficult. In Merugumala et al.'s (2017) study, delayed initiation of early intervention services was also due to a lack of free public services. Caregivers in the study could not afford the costs at available private health care facilities. Similarly, in a study conducted by Scheepers, Swanepoel, and Le Roux (2014), 72 percent of the caregivers reported that they refused universal newborn hearing screening services because the costs were not covered by their medical scheme or because the cost was not included in the birthing package.

South Africa faces a quadruple burden of disease: HIV/AIDS and tuberculosis, high maternal and child mortality, high levels of violence and injuries, as well as a growing burden of non-communicable diseases. Infant hearing impairment is viewed as less urgent and has consequently received less attention from the Department of Health. The lack of attention to early hearing detection in LAMI contexts such as South Africa, India and Nigeria raises implications for the systematic planning and implementation of EHDI programmes at various levels of service delivery. Comprehensive EHDI programme implementation has three stages: hearing impairments must be identified through hearing screening services; the hearing impairment must be confirmed, described and categorised; and intervention services must be provided. Thus, the urgent implementation of widespread and accessible early intervention services would help to equalise vocational and societal opportunities for children with hearing impairment.

In studies by Elpers et al. (2016), Larsen et al. (2012), and Khoza-Shangase (2019), caregivers reported challenges associated with the many appointments their child had to attend, often in different locations. Additional challenges were long waiting lists for appointments, as well as lack of transport, resulting in difficulties getting to health care facilities and having to travel with extended family members.

Poor access to hearing health care services is not unique to LAMI contexts (Khoza-Shangase, 2019; Merugumala et al., 2017). Penetration of hearing health care services and uptake of intervention remains low even in developed contexts (Elpers et al., 2016; Larsen et al., 2012). Thus, decentralisation of hearing health care services and alternative models of service delivery, such as telehealth, must be explored. Telehealth provides significant promise in improving health care access, quality of service delivery, as well as effectiveness and efficiency. This is especially so in South Africa, where millions of children have to travel more than 30 minutes to reach a health care professional (Hall, Nannan, & Sambu, 2013). However, further research is warranted to ensure that telehealth services are comparable to face-to-face audiological services, and are more affordable and improve the reach of these services to underserved communities, without compromising quality of care or infringing on ethics, human rights and medical law (see chapter 13).

Challenges related to professionals

Three studies reviewed highlighted challenges associated with health care professionals. In Elpers et al.'s (2016) study, caregivers reported that paediatricians or health care providers did not expedite hearing health care and ignored their concerns about their infants' hearing impairment. Furthermore, some paediatricians were unaware of early intervention programmes on offer, which resulted in the child not receiving timely intervention. According to Merugumala et al. (2017), caregivers reported that they had been referred for a hearing evaluation from a general children's clinic, but had challenges with accessing the right hearing health care professionals. In Khoza-Shangase's (2019) study, 48 percent of caregivers reported that the professional they dealt with did not seem to know or understand what was wrong with their child.

For FCEI programmes to be effective and efficient, services must be easily accessible to the clients they aim to serve. Health care professionals' lack of knowledge pertaining to paediatric hearing impairment highlights the need for EHDI programmes to be mandated in South Africa and other LAMI contexts. This will facilitate support for and education of all health care professionals involved in paediatric care. Furthermore, awareness of congenital and early onset hearing impairment by health care professionals involved in paediatric care will provide potential prospects for effective transdisciplinary teamwork between the different health care professionals and possibly prompt earlier identification of the hearing impairment.

Caregiver-related challenges

Fifty percent of caregivers in Elpers et al.'s (2016) study reported a lack of knowledge of treatment options for hearing impairment. Various authors, including Jatto, Ogunkuyede, Adeyemo, Adeagbo, and Saiki (2018) as well as Maluleke, Khoza-Shangase, and Kanji (2019) are of the school of thought that maternal awareness of infant and childhood hearing impairments may prompt earlier intervention in LAMI countries. This is especially so in cases of early and delayed onset hearing impairments that cannot be detected via hearing screening programmes. Maternal awareness can be achieved by broadening the health education given to mothers during antenatal care and at immunisation clinics, especially to include awareness of developmental milestones, infant hearing impairment and its impact on speech and language development (Petrocchi-Bartal & Khoza-Shangase, 2014).

In Merugumala et al.'s (2017) study, 35 percent of caregivers reported that traditional wisdom from elders played a crucial role in health-related decision-making in their families. In South Africa and other sub-Saharan contexts, three factors influence access to health care: economic inequalities, male-partner control and patriarchal and hierarchical social norms. These factors limit many women's ability to acquire health information, make decisions regarding health, and take action to improve health. Decisions regarding women and children's access to health services are often made by the male spouse or by a senior member of the family, such as the father-in-law, mother-in-law or grandmother. These decision-making dynamics have been reported in research around access to maternal health care, power imbalances in sexual relationships and healthy behaviour around HIV/AIDS (Khidir et al., 2020). However, these dynamics apply irrespective of the ailment. Therefore, health care professionals need to be cognisant of the complexity of cultural and contextual decision-making dynamics and explore ways of navigating this in clinical practice.

Is family-centred EHDI viable in South Africa?

According to the HPCSA (2018), early intervention services following diagnosis of hearing impairment must be family-centred and in a community-based model of service delivery that is culturally congruent. Establishing FCEI programmes for children with hearing impairment can mitigate the inequities associated with access to health care. This is particularly relevant to the South African context where access to health care services is significantly affected by an overburdened health care system, inequalities and maldistribution of health care professionals, linguistic barriers between health care professionals and patients, as well as cultural diversity. Typically, these challenges mostly affect already vulnerable members of the population in rural and poverty-stricken black communities.

Despite 8.5 percent of South Africa's gross domestic product being spent on health care, the country has poor health outcomes compared to other middle-income countries (Rispel, 2016). In addition to the quadruple burden of disease, South Africa has a crisis of inequalities and maldistribution of health care professionals between urban and rural areas and between the public and private health sectors. This compromises access and coverage, especially for vulnerable populations. Half of the R332 billion allocated annually to health care is spent in the private sector, catering to the socio-economic elite in urban areas, while more than 80 percent of the population depends on the under-resourced, overburdened public sector (Rispel, 2016).

Furthermore, despite South Africa having 12 official languages, which the Constitution states must all enjoy equal esteem and treatment, English is the prominent language in political, educational and social settings. English is viewed as a language of power and prestige, despite being spoken by only 10 percent of the population (Pascoe, Klop, Mdlalo, & Ndhambi, 2017). This has resulted in over 11 million black South Africans receiving health care services in a language that is not their home language. South African audiologists are largely female, white, and English or Afrikaans speaking and thus do not represent the linguistic and cultural diversity of the country's population.

In post-apartheid South Africa, these linguistic and cultural differences replicate historical power dynamics, which may result in clients not feeling confident to request clarification or indicate when they have not understood pertinent information (Watermeyer et al., 2012). Most importantly, evidence on global health indicates that groups that do not form part of the dominant culture have worse health outcomes than the dominant populations (Flood & Rohloff, 2018). This creates a cycle of exclusion, with the patient and their family not receiving effective treatment or care (Mophosho, 2018). However, through family-centred EHDI programmes, this cycle of exclusion can be eliminated as the family's roles and responsibilities are strengthened, allowing caregivers their rightful position as advocates, decision makers and partners along with early intervention professionals (Sass-Lehrer et al., 2015). Children spend a significant amount of time with their caregivers and families. The family is thus the most effective and economical system for fostering and sustaining the child's development.

Will orphaned and vulnerable children benefit from family-centred EHDI?

South Africa faces serious challenges around domestic violence, ill-treatment, sexual abuse and neglect of children (Department of Women, Children and People with Disabilities, 2014). Furthermore, it has the highest burden of HIV/AIDS in the world, with 5.7 million people living with the condition

(UNAIDS, 2010). The AIDS pandemic has resulted in 3.7 million orphans who have lost one or both parents, and 95 000 children who are living in child-headed households, where all members in the family are under the age of 18 years (Atmore, Van Niekerk, & Ashley-Cooper, 2012; UNAIDS, 2010). These are the country's orphaned and vulnerable children (OVC).

In Africa, OVC are typically taken in by extended family members based on the family's financial ability and degree of kinship (Langsam, Lehmann, Vaughn, & Kissling, 2014). However, various circumstances result in some children remaining in child-headed households and others being placed in institutional care (children's homes) as a last resort (Epworth Children's Village, 2013; Richter & Norman, 2009). In order to provide care and support to OVC in child-headed households and others in need, the Department of Social Development has established numerous drop-in centres where children are provided with meals before and after school. Caregivers at these centres are available to assist these children with homework and involve them in life-skills programmes. Furthermore, approximately 20 000 public schools throughout the country are recognised as no-fee schools, and these also offer school nutrition programmes to nine million learners (Department of Basic Education, 2019).

There are currently 345 registered children's homes in South Africa, caring for 21 000 children (Foghill, 2016). According to Omidire, AnnaMosia, and Mampane (2015), some children's homes have 12 children to every caregiver, a significantly higher ratio than the required five or six children to one caregiver. Furthermore, the average qualification of caregivers is a grade 12, with most performing their duties on a rotational basis. This results in instability, inconsistencies and compromised quantity and quality of care for these OVC.

There is a need for caregiving skills development and restructuring of the caregiving process for OVC in children's homes and child-headed households to ensure that caregivers are capacitated to deal effectively with the needs and challenges of these children, while taking into consideration their multilingual and multicultural backgrounds. The creation of a family-like environment at children's homes, where caregiving attempts to replicate the traditional role of the family, has been found to be beneficial to children (Omidire et al., 2015). We thus believe that adequate training of caregivers and restructuring the caregiving process to resemble a family set-up will afford OVC the benefits of family-centred EHDI.

Conclusion

The nuclear family is a foreign concept in the African context, where the term 'family' includes a wider circle of paternal and maternal grandparents, uncles, aunts, nephews, nieces, cousins, sons- and daughters-in-law. Family structures and functions are in a constant state of flux due to various factors. However, the roles of different family members are still patriarchal and hierarchical. Men and senior members of the family have the power to make decisions on behalf of the family, but are significantly less involved in day-to-day child-rearing activities than women.

Family-centred EHDI is a viable option for decentralised service delivery in the South African context given the overburdened health care system, South Africa's socio-political history and dynamics, and the reported poor access to health care services, especially by vulnerable populations. However, for these programmes to be effective, the following factors need to be considered:

- the linguistic and cultural diversity of the South African population and its influence on access to health care, health care seeking behaviour and decision-making dynamics
- aspects of family-centred EHDI programmes such as caregiver involvement, information and support needs, and caregiver satisfaction with current early intervention services
- tailoring of current caregiving programmes for OVC with regard to caregiver training and the caregiving process in order to ensure that these children also benefit from family-centred EHDI
- alternative and feasible service provision avenues, such as tele-audiology, that mitigate the reported barriers associated with access to health care, in order to ensure contextually relevant and responsive care of children with hearing impairment.

References

Adedeji, T. O., Tobih, J. E., Sogebi, O. A., & Daniel, A. D. (2015). Management challenges of congenital and early onset childhood hearing loss in a sub-Saharan country. *International Journal of Pediatric Otorhinolaryngology, 79*, 1625–1629. doi: 10.1016/j.ijporl.2015.06.003.

Aldersey, H. M. (2012). Family perception of intellectual disability: Understanding and support in Dar es Salaam. *African Journal of Disability, 1*(1), Art.#32, 12 pages. doi: 10.4102/ajod.v1.i1.32.

Alyami, H., Soer, M., & Pottas, L. (2016). Deaf or hard of hearing children in Saudi Arabia: Study of early intervention services. *International Journal of Pediatric Otorhinolaryngology, 86*, 142–149. doi: 10.1016/j.ijporl.2016.04.010.

American Psychological Association. (2009). Parents are essential to children's healthy development. Retrieved from https://www.apa.org/pi/families/resources/parents-caregivers.

Atmore, E., Van Niekerk, L., & Ashley-Cooper, M. (2012). Challenges facing the early childhood development sector in South Africa. *South African Journal of Childhood*

Education, 2(1), 120–139. Retrieved from file:///C:/Users/Ntsako/AppData/Local/ Packages/Microsoft.MicrosoftEdge_8wekyb3d8bbwe/TempState/Downloads/ 25-1046-1-PB%20 (1).pdf.

Bruder, M. B. (2000). Family-centered early intervention: Clarifying our values for the new millennium. *Topics in Early Childhood Special Education, 20*(2), 105–116. doi: 10.1177/027112140002000206.

Chataika, T., & McKenzie, J. (2013). Consideration of an African childhood: Disability studies. In T. Curran & K. Runswick-Cole (Eds.), *Disabled children's childhood studies* (pp. 152–163). London, England: Palgrave Macmillan. doi: 10.1057/9781137008220_12.

Constanescu, G. (2012). Satisfaction with telemedicine for teaching listening and spoken language to children with hearing loss. *Journal of Telemedicine and Telecare, 18*, 267–272. doi: 10.1258/jtt.2012.111208.

Dalmau, M., Balcells-Balcells, A., Gine, C., Canadas, M., Casa, D., Salat, Y., … Calaf, N. (2017). How to implement the family-centred model in early intervention. *Annals of Psychology, 33*, 641–651. doi: 10.6018/analesps.33.3.26341.

Decker, K. B., & Valloton, C. D. (2016). Early intervention for children with hearing loss: Information parents receive about supporting children's language. *Journal of Early Intervention, 38*(3), 151–169. doi: 10.1177/1053815116653448.

Department of Basic Education (DBE). (2019). DBE's national school nutrition programme. Retrieved from https://www.gov.za/about-sa/education.

Department of Social Development (DSD). (2013). *White paper on families in South Africa*. Pretoria, South Africa: Department of Social Development. Retrieved from https://www.westwerncape.gov.za.assets/departments/social-development/white-paper-on-families-in-south-africa-2013.pdf.

Department of Women, Children and People with Disabilities. (2014). South Africa's initial country report on the African charter on the rights and welfare of the child. Retrieved from https://www. unicef.org/southafrica/SAF_resources_africanunionreport9.pdf.

Ekberg, K., Scarinci, N., Hickson, L., & Meyer, C. (2018). Parent-directed commentaries during children's hearing habilitation appointments: A practice in family-centred care. *International Journal of Language and Communication Disorders, 53*(5), 929–946. doi: 10.1111/1460-6984.12403.

Elpers, J., Lester, C., Shinn, J. B., & Bush, M. L. (2016). Rural family perspectives and experiences with early infant hearing detection and intervention: A qualitative study. *Journal of Community Health, 41*(2), 226–233. doi: 10.1007/s10900-015-0086-1.

Epley, P., Summers, A. A., & Turnbull, A. (2010). Characteristics and trends in family-centered conceptualizations. *Journal of Family Social Work, 13*, 269–285. doi: 10.1080/10522150903514017.

Epworth Children's Village. (2013). About us. Retrieved from http://www.epworthvillage.org.za/about-us/history/.

Erbasi, E., Scarinci, N., Hickson, L., & Ching, Y. C. (2018). Parental involvement in the care and intervention of children with hearing loss. *International Journal of Audiology, 57*(Suppl. 2), S15–S26. doi: 10.1080/14992027.1220679.

Findlen, U. M., Malhotra, P. S., & Adunka, O. F. (2019). Parent perspectives on multidisciplinary pediatric hearing healthcare. *International Journal of Pediatric Otorhinolaryngology, 116*, 141–146. doi: 10.1016/j.ijporl.2018.10.044.

Flood, D., & Rohloff, P. (2018). Indigenous languages and global health: Comment. *The Lancet, 6*, e134–e135.

Foghill, L. (2016). Where have the children gone? Retrieved from https://www.hope-andhomes.org/blog-article/where-have-the-children-gone/.

Hall, K., Nannan, N., & Sambu, W. (2013). *Child health and nutrition: South African child gauge.* Cape Town, South Africa: Children's Institute.

Health Professions Council of South Africa (HPCSA). (2018). *Early hearing detection and intervention (EHDI): Guidelines.* Pretoria, South Africa: HPCSA. Retrieved from https://www.hpcsa.co.za/Uploads/editor/UserFiles/downloads/speech/Guidelines_for_EHDI_2018.pdf.

Henderson, R. J., Johnson, A., & Moodie, S. (2014). Parent-to-parent support for parents with children who are deaf or hard of hearing: A conceptual framework. *American Journal of Audiology, 23*(4), 437–488. doi: 10.1044/2014_AJA-14-0029.

Ingber, S., Al-Yagon, M., & Dromi, E. (2010). Mothers' involvement in early intervention for children with hearing loss: The role of maternal characteristics and context-based perceptions. *Journal of Early Intervention, 32*(5), 351–369. doi: 10.1177/1053815110387066.

Ingber, S., & Dromi, E. (2010). Actual versus desired family-centred practice in early intervention for children with hearing loss. *Journal of Deaf Studies and Deaf Education, 15*(1), 59–71.

Iversen, M. D., Shimmel, J. P., Ciacera, S. L., & Prabhakar, M. (2003). Creating a family-centered approach to early intervention services: Perceptions of parents and professionals. *Pediatric Physical Therapy, 15*(1), 23–31. doi: 10.1097/01.PEP.0000051694.10495.79.

Jackson, C. W. (2011). Family supports and resources for parents of children who are deaf or hard of hearing. *American Annals of the Deaf, 156*(4), 343–362.

Jackson, C. W., Wegner, J. R., & Turnbull, A. P. (2010). Family quality of life following early identification of deafness. *Language, Speech, and Hearing Services in Schools, 41*, 194–205.

Jatto M. E., Ogunkuyede, S. A., Adeyemo, A. A., Adeagbo, K., & Saiki, O. (2018). Mothers' perspectives of newborn hearing screening programmes. *Ghana Medical Journal, 52*(3), 158–162. doi: 10.4314/gmj.v52i3.9.

Kanji, A., & Khoza-Shangase, K. (2016). Feasibility of newborn hearing screening in a public hospital setting in South Africa: A pilot study. *South African Journal of Communication Disorders, 63*(1), a142. http://dx.doi.org/10.4102/sajcd.v63i1.150.

Khidir, H., Mosery, N., Greener, R., Milford, C., Bennet, K., Kaida, A., ... Matthews, L. T. (2020). Sexual relationship power and periconception HIV-risk behaviour among HIV-infected men in serodifferent relationships. *AIDS and Behaviour, 24*, 881–890. doi: 10.1007/s10461-019-02536-2.

Khoza-Shangase, K. (2019). Early hearing detection and intervention in South Africa: Exploring factors compromising service delivery as expressed by caregivers. *International Journal of Pediatric Otorhinolaryngology, 118,* 73–78. doi: 10.1016/j. ijporl.2018.12.021.

Khoza-Shangase, K., Kanji, A., Petrocchi-Bartal, L., & Farr, K. (2017). Infant hearing screening from a developing country context: Status from two South African provinces. *South African Journal of Child Health, 11*(4), 159–163. doi: 10.7196/SAJCH. 2017.v11i4.1267.

Khoza-Shangase, K., & Mophosho, M. (2018). Language and culture in speech-language and hearing professions in South Africa: The dangers of a single study. *South African Journal of Communication Disorders, 65*(1), a594. doi: 10.4102/sajcd.v65i1.594.

Kuo, D. Z., Houtrow, A. J., Arango, P., Kuhlthau, K. A., Simmons, J. M., & Neff, J. M. (2012). Family-centered care: Current applications and future directions in pediatric health care. *Maternal and Child Health Journal, 16*(2), 297–305. doi: 10.1007/ s10995-011-0751-7.

Langsam, S., Lehmann, C., Vaughn, L. M., & Kissling, A. (2014). Sociocultural issues as barriers to HIV-infected orphan care in Southern Africa. *Clinical Research in HIV/ AIDS Prevention, 2*(1), 27–34. doi: 10.14302/issn.2324-7339.jcrhap-13-239.

Larsen, R., Munoz, K., DesGeorges, J., Nelson, L., & Kennedy, S. (2012). Early hearing detection and intervention: Parent experiences with the diagnostic hearing assessment. *American Journal of Audiology, 21,* 91–99. doi: 10.1044/1059-0889 (2012/11-0016).

MacKean, G. L., Thurston, W. E., & Scott, C. M. (2005). Bridging the divide between families and health professionals' perspectives on family-centred care. *Health Expectations, 8*(1), 74–85.

Magnuson, K., & Schindler, H. (2019). Supporting children's early development by building caregivers' capacities and skills: A theoretical approach informed by new neuroscience research. *Journal of Family Theory or Review, 11*(1), 59–78. doi: 10.1111/ jftr.12319.

Maluleke, N. P., Khoza-Shangase, K., & Kanji, A. (2019). Communication and school readiness abilities of children with hearing impairment in South Africa: A retrospective review of early intervention preschool records. *South African Journal of Communication Disorders, 66*(1), a604. doi:10.4102/sajcd.v66i1.604.

Masuku, K. P., & Khoza-Shangase, K. (2018). Spirituality as a coping mechanism for family caregivers of persons with aphasia. *Journal of Psychology in Africa, 28*(3), 245–248. https://doi.org/10.1080/14330237.2018.1475518.

Merugumala, S. V., Pothula, V., & Cooper, M. (2017). Barriers to timely diagnosis and treatment for children with hearing impairment in a southern Indian city: A qualitative study of parents and clinic staff. *International Journal of Audiology, 56*(10), 733–739. doi: 10.1080/14992027.1340678.

Moeller, M. P., Carr, G., Seaver, L., Stredler-Brown, A., & Holzinger, D. (2013). Best practice in family-centered intervention for children who are deaf or hard of hearing: An international consensus statement. *Journal of Deaf Studies and Deaf Education, 18,* 429–445. doi: 10.1093/deafed/ent034.

Moodie, S. (2018). Family-centred early intervention: Supporting a call to action. *ENT & Audiology News, 27*(5). Retrieved from https://www.entandaudiology news.com/features/audiology-features/post/family-centred-early-intervention-supporting-a-call-to-action.

Mophosho, M. (2018). Speech-language therapy consultation practices in multilingual and multicultural healthcare contexts: Current training in South Africa. *African Journal of Health Professions Education, 10*(3), 145–147.

Morelli, G., Quinn, N., Chaudhary, N., Vicedo, M., Rosabal-Coto, M., Keller, H., … Takada, A. (2018). Ethical challenges of parenting interventions in low- to middle-income countries. *Journal of Cross-Cultural Psychology, 49*(1), 5–24.

Niklas, F., Cohressen C., & Teyler, C. (2018). Making a difference to children's reasoning skills before school-entry: The contribution of the home learning environment. *Contemporary Educational Psychology, 54,* 79–88. doi: 10.1016/j.cedpsych.2018.06.001.

Olusanya, B. O. (2008). Priorities for early hearing detection and intervention in sub-Saharan Africa. *International Journal of Audiology, 47*(1), S3–S13.

Omidire, M. F., AnnaMosia, D., & Mampane, M. R. (2015). Perceptions of the roles and responsibilities of caregivers in children's homes in South Africa. *Revista de Asistenta Sociala, 2,* 113–126. Retrieved from https://www.researchgate.net/publi cation/281584882_Perceptions_of_the_Roles_and_Responsibilities_of_Caregivers_ in_Children's_Homes_in_South_Africa/link/55eead9b08aedecb68fcab38/download.

Pascoe, M., Klop, D., Mdlalo, T., & Ndhambi, M. (2017). Beyond lip service: Towards human rights-driven guidelines for South African speech-language pathologists. *International Journal of Speech-Language Pathology, 20*(1), 1–8. doi: 10.1080/17549507.2018.1397745.

Petrocchi-Bartal, L., & Khoza-Shangase, K. (2014). Hearing screening procedures and protocols in use at immunisation clinics in South Africa. *South African Journal of Communication Disorders, 61*(1), a66. http://dx.doi.org/10.4102/sajcd.v61i1.66.

Petrocchi-Bartal, L., & Khoza-Shangase, K. (2016). Infant hearing screening at primary health care immunization clinics in South Africa: The current status. *South African Journal of Child Health, 10*(2), 139–143.

Richter, L. M., & Norman, A. (2009). AIDS orphan tourism: A threat to young children in residential care. *Vulnerable Children and Youth Studies, 5*(3), 217–229. doi: 10.1080/17450128.2010.487124.

Rispel, L. (2016). Analysing the progress and fault lines of health sector transformation in South Africa. In *South African Health Review* (pp. 17–23). Midrand, South Africa: Health Systems Trust. Retrieved from https://www.hst.org.za/publica tions/South%20African%20Health%20Reviews/2%20Analysing%20the%20prog ress%20and%20fault%20lines%20health%20sector%20transformation%20in%20 South%20Africa%20.pdf.

Sacks, S., Shay, S., Repplinger, L., Leffl, K. R., Sapolich, S. G., Suskind, E., … Suskind, D. (2014). Pilot testing of a parent-directed intervention (Project ASPIRE) for underserved children who are deaf or hard of hearing. *Child Language Teaching and Therapy, 30*(1), 91–102. doi: 10.1177/0265659013494873.

Sass-Lehrer, M., Porter, A., & Wu, C. L. (2015). Families: Partnerships in practice. In M. Sass-Lehrer (Ed.), *Early intervention for deaf and hard of hearing infants, toddlers and their families* (pp. 65–102). Oxford, England: Oxford University Press.

Scheepers, L. J., Swanepoel, D., & Le Roux, T. (2014). Why parents refuse newborn hearing screening and default on follow-up rescreening: A South African perspective. *International Journal of Pediatric Otorhinolaryngology, 78,* 652–658.

Swanepoel, D., Ebrahim, S., Joseph, A., & Friedland, P. (2007). Newborn screening in a South African private health care hospital. *International Journal of Pediatric Otorhinolaryngology, 71,* 881–887.

Swanepoel, D., Störbeck, C., & Friedland, P. (2009). Early hearing detection and intervention in South Africa. *International Journal of Pediatric Otorhinolaryngology, 73,* 783–786.

Theunissen, M., & Swanepoel, D. W. (2008). Early hearing detection and intervention services in the public health sector in South Africa. *International Journal of Audiology, 47*(1), S23–S29.

Turan, Z. (2012). Early intervention with children who have a hearing impairment: Role of the professional and parent participation. In S. Naz (Ed.), *Hearing loss* (pp. 117–132). Rijeka: InTech. Retrieved from http://cdn.intechopen.com/ pdfs/33866/InTechEarly_intervention_with_children_who_have_a_hearing_ impairment_role_of_the_professional_and_parent_participation.pdf.

UNAIDS. (2010). South Africa launches massive HIV prevention and treatment campaign. Retrieved from https://www.unaids.org/en/resources/presscentre/press releaseandstatementarchive/2010/april/20100423sacampaign.

Watermeyer, J., Kanji, A., & Cohen, A. (2012). Caregiver recall and understanding of pediatric diagnostic information and assessment feedback. *International Journal of Audiology, 51*(12), 864–869. doi: 10.3109/14992027.2012.721014.

Watermeyer, J., Kanji, A., & Sarvan, S. (2017). The first step to early intervention following diagnosis: Communication in pediatric hearing aid orientation sessions. *American Journal of Audiology, 26,* 576–582. doi: 10.1044/2017_AJA-17-0027.

Woods, J. J., Wilcox, M. J., Friedman, M., & Murch, T. (2011). Collaborative consultations in natural environments: Strategies to enhance family-centered support services. *Language, Speech, and Hearing Services in Schools, 42,* 379–392. doi: 10.1044/0161-1461 (2011/10-0016).

World Health Organization (WHO). (2018). Deafness and hearing loss: Fact sheet. Retrieved from http://www.who.int/mediacentre/factsheets/fs300/en/.

World Health Organization (WHO). (2019). Hearing loss and rising prevalence and impact. *Bulletin of the World Health Organisation, 97,* 646–646A. doi: 10.2471/ BLT.19.224683.

Yoshinaga-Itano, C. (2014). Principles and guidelines for early intervention after confirmation that a child is deaf or hard of hearing. *Journal of Deaf Studies and Deaf Education, 19*(2), 143–175. doi: 10.1093/deafed/ent043.

12 HIV/AIDS and the Burden of Disease in Early Hearing Detection and Intervention

Katijah Khoza-Shangase

Early hearing detection and intervention (EHDI) is a significant challenge in South Africa. Various reasons have been given for the failure to successfully implement EHDI, including a lack of government mandate for universal newborn hearing screening (UNHS), resource constraints and the burden of disease. This chapter explores EHDI in South Africa in the context of the HIV/AIDS pandemic. It presents evidence on HIV and general child development in the paediatric population, followed by a review of literature on HIV and auditory and otological manifestations. Thereafter, available evidence on HIV perinatal exposure and auditory manifestations is presented. The chapter then puts forward solutions and recommendations, with implications for EHDI as well as research in this population.

A number of studies have established a link between HIV/AIDS and hearing loss in both paediatric and adult populations (Araújo et al., 2012; Assuiti, Lanzoni, Santos, Erdmann, & Meirelles, 2013; Buriti, Oliveira, & Muniz, 2013; Chao et al., 2012; Fasunla et al., 2014; Hrapcak et al., 2016; Khoza-Shangase, 2011; Khoza-Shangase & Anastasiou, 2020; Khoza-Shangase & Turnbull, 2009; Maro et al., 2016; Matas, Santos Filha, Juan, Pinto, & Gonçalves, 2010; Taipele et al., 2011; Torre, 2015). This evidence highlights the need for the audiology community to consider HIV/AIDS in planning clinical and research services. This need is particularly important in contexts such as South Africa, where the prevalence of HIV/AIDS is high (UNAIDS, 2018). The country is home to the largest number of people on antiretroviral (ARV) treatment in the world (UNAIDS, 2018). According to Khoza-Shangase (2020) and Swanepoel (2006), the virus has also created an overwhelming burden and a unique challenge to audiological service delivery in South Africa, with evidence of otological manifestations of HIV/AIDS found in many children (Khoza-Shangase & Anastasiou, 2020).

The most recent UNAIDS (2019) statistics, as detailed in chapter 5, indicate that HIV/AIDS remains a global problem. South Africa, which falls into the category of low and middle-income (LAMI) countries, is the epicentre of the pandemic. Nevertheless, despite the still significantly high numbers of people living with HIV, measurable progress has been made in reducing mother-to-child transmission (UNAIDS, 2019). This is revealed by the decreasing numbers of children with HIV, as well as in the achievement of the UNAIDS 90-90-90 targets. Specific to the paediatric population, globally, 1.7 million children younger than 15 years of age were living with HIV in 2018, a 41 percent decline from 2010. However, only 54 percent of these children were accessing treatment. In the same period, 82 percent of pregnant women living with HIV were reported to have access to ARV medicines to prevent mother-to-child transmission. As far as mortality of people living with HIV is concerned, Johnson and colleagues' (2017) modelling to determine the impact of the antiretroviral therapy (ART) programme on mortality showed that treatment resulted in 1.72 million fewer HIV-related deaths in adults over the period 2000–2014 than would have occurred otherwise. UNAIDS (2019) reported a 33 percent decline in AIDS-related mortality since 2010.

The International Labour Organization (ILO) estimates that the total number of people unable to work fully as a result of HIV complications will decline to about 40 000 in 2020 from a 2005 level of about 350 000, representing an 85 percent decline for men and a 93 percent decline for women (ILO, 2018). A decline from 655 000 to 95 000 over the same period has been estimated for the number who are partially unable to work – an 81 percent decline for men and 91 percent for women. This has significant implications for any country's economy and its citizens' ability to be productive members of society, including managing their health and that of their families. This still raises issues around health priorities and the allocation of resources, including those for EHDI.

Groups that are reportedly most affected by HIV in South Africa include women, sex workers, men who have sex with men, transgender women, people who inject drugs, and children and orphans (Avert, 2018). The Human Sciences Research Council reports that women in South Africa are excessively affected by HIV (HSRC, 2018). According to UNAIDS (2019), 140 000 women became HIV positive in 2018 compared to 86 000 men, and 4.7 million women were living with HIV compared to 2.8 million men. HIV prevalence is reported to be approximately four times higher in young women than in young men (UNAIDS, 2019). The fact that the majority of those affected are women of child-bearing age as well as the economically active has serious economic, psychosocial and health implications for the country. The 2015 national point estimate for HIV prevalence among women who attended antenatal care was 30.8 percent, an estimate that has reportedly remained the same for 10 years, with mother-to-child transmission at 0.9 percent nationally (UNAIDS, 2018).

Access to ART was first rolled out in the South African public health system in 2004 and has allowed approximately three-quarters of HIV-infected adults and children to receive ART (South African National AIDS Council, 2015), compared to an estimated 49 percent of children worldwide (UNAIDS, 2016). Due to the limited availability of trained medical doctors – 0.8 physicians per 1 000 people (Lassiter & Parsons, 2015) and considerably fewer child health specialists – the scaling up of HIV treatment in the public health sector relies on task shifting, with nurses rather than medical doctors prescribing ART and managing HIV-positive children and adults (Knox et al., 2018). However, neurodevelopmental and general audiological assessments in this setting are beyond the scope of practice for many nurse clinicians and non-paediatric medical doctors (Knox et al., 2018). It is in this context that EHDI implementation needs to be deliberated.

HIV infection is a chronic illness (Banks, Zuurmond, Ferrand, & Kuper, 2015), with quality of life issues that require long-term management, such as hearing impairment and communication development. Over the past decade, however, quality HIV care and access to ART has become much more widely available throughout Africa. The expansion in access to ART globally has reduced HIV-related morbidity and mortality and contributed to an increase in life expectancy, including in low-income countries. In many instances, HIV-related morbidity and mortality are now comparable to that of the general population (Mills et al., 2011).

Although South Africa has made significant progress in treatment coverage for HIV/AIDS, including the lauded successes of the prevention of mother-to-child transmission programmes, universal coverage has not yet been achieved. Nonetheless, the 2013 roll-out of the fixed-dose combination ARV medication has had a significant influence on treatment adherence (Davies, 2013). Furthermore, the UNAIDS 90-90-90 targets show a clear and focused strategy for efficient management of this disease in South Africa, with data indicating that 90 percent of those living with HIV know their status, 62 percent are on treatment and 54 percent are virally suppressed (UNAIDS, 2019). Specific to the South African paediatric population living with HIV, 63 percent are on treatment, with a reported 87 percent of HIV-positive pregnant women having accessed antiretroviral treatment to prevent mother-to-child transmission, leading to the prevention of 53 000 new HIV infections among newborns in 2018 (UNAIDS, 2019).

The South African government's HIV/AIDS strategy aims to sustain life and prevent or eliminate the spread of the disease. Khoza-Shangase (2020) argues that it is important that audiologists focus on the quality of life that is sustained by highly active ART (HAART) in the clinical management strategy of this population. She thus stresses that the 2030 target of having 90 percent of infected people diagnosed, 90 percent on treatment, and 90 percent virally suppressed should also include maintenance of at least 90 percent quality of life, including for children infected with HIV.

HIV and general development

Prior to the availability of effective ARTs, neurodevelopmental disabilities were among the earliest recognised features of paediatric HIV infection, affecting as many as 50 percent of children (Columbia University Mailman School of Public Health, 2018). Although early initiation of treatment appears to prevent many of the most severe neurologic impairments, it remains a significant co-morbidity among children living with HIV.

Increased availability of ART in LAMI countries, home to more than 90 percent of HIV-positive children, has resulted in great improvements in survival. As a result, the burden and character of neurodevelopmental disabilities throughout childhood has emerged as an important area for research, clinical care, policy and planning for health, and educational and social services sectors in many high-burden countries (Boivin, Kakooza, Warf, Davidson, & Grigorenko, 2015; Laughton, Cornell, Boivin, & Van Rie, 2013; Le Doare, Bland, & Newell, 2012).

Paediatric HIV is somewhat different from the HIV most commonly identified with adults. In children, HIV symptoms manifest much earlier. Some children, referred to as 'rapid progressors', develop serious signs and symptoms within the first 12 to 24 months of life (Davis-McFarland, 2002). They progress quickly to AIDS-defining conditions and rapidly lose CD4 cells. These cells play an important role in the immune system by helping to orchestrate the body's response to micro-organisms like viruses. Deterioration of CD4 cells leads to the development of various opportunistic infections that are linked to HIV/AIDS sequelae such as hearing loss in children. Because paediatric HIV is neurotropic, manifestations of central nervous system disorders such as developmental disabilities, including language impairment and cognitive deficits, encephalopathy and pyramidal tract signs are expected in a large majority of cases (Davis-McFarland, 2002; Knox et al., 2018). According to Davis-McFarland (2002), a small group of children living with HIV present with minimal or no symptoms of the virus and remain healthy until 9 or 10 years of age.

Researchers at Columbia University's Mailman School of Public Health (2018) note that HIV-positive children in South Africa suffer more developmental disabilities than their HIV-negative counterparts. Their study revealed that HIV-positive children between the ages of four and six years are four times more likely to present with delays in sitting, standing, walking and speaking, and more than twice as likely to present with a hearing disability and cognitive delay when compared to HIV-negative children.

While neurodevelopmental abnormalities are common in children with HIV infection, their detection can be challenging in settings with limited availability of health professionals (Knox et al., 2018). Neurodevelopmental disabilities, including impaired brain growth and motor, cognitive and language development, were among the earliest recognised features of pae-diatric HIV infection, affecting as many as 50 percent of children prior to the availability of effective ARTs (Belman et al., 1996; Epstein et al., 1986; Smith et al., 2006). Though it is difficult to isolate the effect of the virus on the neurological status of infected children, Mwaba, Ngoma, Kusanthan, and Menon (2015) report that 90 percent of HIV-positive children have neurological problems. Early initiation of ART appears to prevent many of the most severe sequelae, but neurologic impairment remains an import-ant co-morbidity among children living with HIV (Chiriboga, Fleishman, Champion, Gaye-Robinson, & Abrams, 2005; Koekkoek et al., 2006; Patel et al., 2009; Van Arnhem et al., 2013). Insults to the brain from HIV and associated illnesses during early childhood development may impede opti-mal social, emotional, physical and educational functioning and outcomes, resulting in impairments, limitations and restrictions that persist through-out childhood and adolescence and beyond (Knox et al., 2018).

Sherr, Croome, Castaneda, Bradshaw, and Romero (2014) reported on developmental and behavioural challenges in children with HIV. They con-ducted a systematic review in 2009, and extended and reanalysed the data in 2014. Their findings revealed an unequal impact on the domains mea-sured, with mixed evidence on language and executive functioning. They reported that 80.1 percent of studies found that HIV had a detrimental cog-nitive effect on children, and that the domains of language and executive functioning are more affected than others. The authors highlighted the need for more definitive control of variables such as environmental factors con-tributing to behavioural and cognitive outcomes. Their review confirmed other reports on the prevalence of cognitive delay in children with HIV. Recommendations offered include the need for internationally agreed mon-itoring tools and studies which control for known contributing factors. I suggest the importance of early detection of and intervention for hearing impairment in this group as a way to positively influence language and exec-utive functioning development.

Sherr and colleagues (2014) stress the importance of research in the cohort of children living with HIV to ensure full understanding of developmental challenges, in order to strategically plan for effective interventions. Sherr et al.'s (2014) findings show that children with HIV may well have special educational needs and face the prospect of cognitive delay in some domains of functioning. The results suggest that centres should be considering rou-tine, regular cognitive monitoring for children from an early age, as well as the provision of interventions to ameliorate or cater for their cognitive needs. Early childhood development and stimulation may be particularly relevant for young children, despite the paucity of data for the youngest age groups. For older children, school provision and adaptations for special needs requirements should be prioritised to accommodate them (see chapter 9).

A review of published evidence on children living with HIV indicates a larger focus on clinical manifestations of the virus than on its sequelae (Miziara, Weber, Filho, & Neto, 2007; Patel et al., 2009; Taipele et al., 2011). However, sufficient evidence exists on the effects of exposure to the virus on language development and communication disorders (Knox et al., 2018; Le Doare et al., 2012; Mwaba et al., 2015; Sherr et al., 2014; Smith et al., 2006; Van Arnhem et al., 2013). According to Davis-McFarland (2002), HIV infection compromises the acquisition and development of communication milestones. If symptoms develop once these milestones have been achieved, regression may occur due to opportunistic conditions such as encephalopathy that often accompany paediatric HIV infection.

HIV and auditory and otological manifestations

There is a dearth of evidence on hearing impairment in the paediatric population infected with HIV/AIDS, both internationally and in South Africa. This has implications for planning and implementing programmes such as EHDI. There is therefore a need for continued efforts to establish an audiological profile in HIV-infected and HIV-exposed but uninfected children. This should include the prevalence of various otological manifestations of HIV in this population, as well as the audiological signs and symptoms of HIV/AIDS in paediatric patients. Such data would aid in planning and executing audiological services like EHDI in this population.

A few, mostly international, studies have investigated hearing loss in HIV-infected children. A limitation of a number of them is the small sample sizes. An overview of findings from these studies is presented in Table 12.1. All the studies presented evidence of a high prevalence of hearing loss in HIV-infected children, ranging from 6.4 to 84.8 percent (Buriti et al., 2013; Chao et al., 2012; Govender, Eley, Walker, Petersen, & Wilmshurst, 2011; Matas, Iorio, & Succi, 2008; Matas et al., 2010; Ndoleriire, Turitwenka, Bakeera-Kitaaka, & Nyabigambo, 2013; Palacios et al., 2008; Taipele et al., 2011; Torre et al., 2012; Torre, Cook, Elliott, Dawood, & Laughton, 2015). This is significantly higher than the prevalence of hearing loss in general population studies in children (Chao et al., 2012; Torre et al., 2012) or in uninfected controls (Torre et al., 2015). There are no South African studies on HIV-exposed but uninfected children.

Auditory system changes are among the many effects of HIV (Khoza-Shangase, 2011). The virus causes various types of hearing loss (conductive, sensori/neural, mixed, central) in affected individuals, with severity ranging from mild to profound, and either unilateral or bilateral. This hearing loss can occur as a result of primary causes (direct action of the virus on the auditory system), secondary causes (opportunistic infections) and iatrogenic

Table 12.1 Overview of otological and audiological manifestations in paediatric HIV/AIDS

Factor	Occurrence in children with HIV/AIDS
Type of hearing loss	Conductive, sensori/neural, mixed, central
Degree of hearing loss	Mild to profound
Laterality	Unilateral or bilateral
Causes of hearing loss	Primary causes: Direct action of the virus itself on the auditory system
	Secondary causes: Opportunistic infections, e.g. otitis media, cytomegalovirus (CMV)
	Iatrogenic causes: Hearing loss due to ototoxic drugs prescribed during the treatment of HIV, including some ARVs
	Perinatal HIV exposure: CMV exposure, mitochondrial mutation
	Perinatal ARV exposure
Signs and symptoms	Otorrhea, tinnitus, vertigo, hearing loss, otalgia, tympanic membrane perforation
Influencing factors	Malnutrition, otorrhea, ear infections, World Health Organization (WHO) stages 3 and 4, type of ARV treatments/exposure

causes (hearing loss due to ototoxic drugs prescribed during the treatment of HIV) (Araújo et al., 2012; Campanini, Marani, Mastroianni, Cancellieri, & Vicini, 2005; Khoza-Shangase, 2020). Furthermore, hearing loss can result from recurrent otitis media, opportunistic infections such as CMV, tuberculosis (TB) or cryptococcus, syphilis, bacterial meningitis, or from side effects of medications such as gentamicin or streptomycin (Assuiti et al., 2013). Some research has suggested that ARV medications, such as certain nucleoside reverse transcriptase inhibitors, may potentially lead to sensorineural hearing loss (Kakuda, 2000), although other research has suggested that ARV medications do not result in hearing loss (Schouten, Lockhart, Rees, Collier, & Marra, 2006). The relationship between HIV and hearing loss is therefore not yet clear, nor have strategies for screening, prevention and treatment been outlined, hence the importance of ensuring comprehensive, systematic and strategic EHDI service planning and implementation in this population.

The audiological and otological complaints most commonly reported in children infected by HIV, with or without hearing loss, are otalgia, otorrhea, vertigo and tinnitus (Campanini et al., 2005; Davis-McFarland, 2002; Hrapcak et al., 2016; Khoza-Shangase & Anastasiou, 2020; Khoza-Shangase & Turnbull, 2009; Miziara et al., 2007; Torre, Cook, Elliott, Dawood & Laughton, 2016; Von Reyn, Palumbo, Moshi, & Buckey, 2016). Modern treatment approaches have changed HIV from a life-threatening terminal condition to a chronic health condition. However, the long-term consequences of the disease and its treatments raise implications for long-term hearing care. All health care professionals working with HIV-positive individuals, including HIV-exposed but uninfected and HIV-infected children, should be made aware of this association between HIV and hearing loss. In the paediatric population, such knowledge will facilitate appropriate EHDI plans.

One of the most common causes of hearing loss in children with HIV infection is otitis media (Davis-McFarland, 2002). Complications of untreated otitis media include conductive hearing loss that has significant implications for the child's communication development and, if left untreated, can progress to a permanent sensorineural hearing loss. The higher incidence of conditions such as nasopharyngeal polyps as well as subcutaneous cysts in patients living with HIV further impacts middle ear functioning, leading to conductive hearing loss. The masses in the nasopharynx block the Eustachian tube, negatively impacting ventilation in the middle ear. This leads to the onset and development of chronic otitis media. Furthermore, a compromised immune system can facilitate the development of mastoiditis, which can lead to conductive or mixed hearing loss. Additional causes of hearing impairment in people living with HIV include opportunistic conditions and infections such as bacterial meningitis, CMV, cryptococcosis, herpes zoster and toxoplasmosis.

Evidence on the otological and audiological manifestations of HIV/ AIDS in the paediatric population is growing. In Brazil, Miziara et al. (2007) explored otitis media in HIV-positive children on ART, aged 0 to 5 years 11 months. Otitis media was present in 33.1 percent of their sample. Children receiving HAART had a higher prevalence of acute otitis media and a lower prevalence of chronic otitis media, highlighting the importance of HAART.

Chronic otitis media has significant implications for poor language development in children (Davis-McFarland, 2002). HIV-positive children can have any of the communication disorders with which other children present. The most common issues are poor language development and loss of language milestones as the child's medical condition worsens. Children with HIV/ AIDS can also have phonological disorders, voice disorders, central auditory processing deficits and learning disorders (Davis-McFarland, 2002). About 25 percent of children with HIV/AIDS will be diagnosed with mental retardation or learning disorders and will require special education services. These can all be exacerbated by otological manifestations that lead to hearing impairment, hence the importance of early detection and intervention.

Torre (2015) notes that there has been an increase in the number of large-scale studies focusing on the association between HIV and hearing loss. He reports that HIV-infected children have poorer hearing than their perinatally exposed but uninfected peers. Furthermore, HIV-infected children also have poorer hearing compared to HIV-unexposed, uninfected children (Torre, 2015). Clear worsening of hearing function in relation to worsening HIV status was found, with measurable differences in auditory brainstem response (ABR) findings in HIV-infected individuals. These differences were not found when distortion product otoacoustic emissions (DPOAEs) were studied in this population. DPOAE findings were similar for HIV-infected and HIV-uninfected individuals. These differences in hearing sensitivity based on HIV status may be a result of auditory neural function. These findings, in terms of the audiology measures used, are important to consider when deciding on test batteries for early hearing detection programmes.

Maro et al. (2016) performed a cross-sectional study on HIV-infected children where they hypothesised that these children would have a higher prevalence of abnormal central and peripheral hearing findings when compared to HIV-negative controls. The authors measured hearing function through a test battery comprising tympanometry, pure-tone audiometry, DPOAEs and ABR. Findings showed that the group of HIV-infected children were significantly more likely to have histories of otorrhea, or vertigo, abnormal tympanograms, reduced DPOAE levels at multiple frequencies, as well as present with a higher proportion of individuals with a hearing loss. ABR latencies did not differ between groups. Furthermore, no relationships were found between treatment regimens or delay in starting treatment and audiological parameters. As far as the reduced DPOAE levels were concerned, Maro and colleagues (2016, p. 443) suggest that a possible cause could 'include effects on efferent pathways connecting to outer hair cells or a direct effect of HIV on the cochlea'.

A study conducted on Peruvian children with HIV also identified risk factors of hearing impairment in these children (Chao et al., 2012). Findings revealed that 38.8 percent of the sample presented with hearing impairment, with identified risk factors including tympanic membrane perforation, abnormal tympanometry, cerebral infection, seizures and a CD4 cell count of less than 500 cells/mm^3. These authors argue that the high prevalence of hearing impairment in their study raises the need for periodic hearing assessment in the routine clinical care of HIV-infected children. I suggest that the risk factors identified in this study raise implications for the risk factors used in hearing screening programmes, as well as for the types of measures used during early hearing detection implementation. For example, inclusion of sensitive middle ear function measures in screening and testing this population seems key given the significant association of abnormal tympanometry to hearing impairment. Hearing screening programmes do not routinely include tympanometry in the screening batteries. The link between hearing loss and low CD4 count may indicate that longer periods of immunocompromise contribute to increased susceptibility to middle ear disease or longer history of recurrent episodes of otitis media in this population. Therefore, any EHDI programme should take this into consideration in its prioritisation, particularly in resource-constrained contexts like South Africa. EHDI programmes should thus include proper identification, prevention and treatment of these risk conditions as part of routine management of HIV-infected children in order to ensure improved quality of life in this population.

Khoza-Shangase and Turnbull (2009) performed hearing screening in a group of paediatric patients attending an HIV/AIDS clinic at a hospital in South Africa. In this study, the estimated prevalence of abnormal hearing screening results was 26 percent. These findings were found at the various stages of the disease, and the symmetry, estimated type and degree of the auditory dysfunction were variable. Furthermore, in this study, otitis media was found to be prevalent in 23 percent of participants and was the most predominant possible cause of hearing loss in the sample evaluated. These findings highlight the need for audiologists and otolaryngologists to be involved in the assessment and management of children living with HIV, with implications for EHDI programmes. Peter (2014) described the audiological profile of school-age children with HIV/AIDS in KwaZulu-Natal, South Africa. Findings from this study revealed abnormal middle ear function in approximately 40 percent of the participants. Conductive hearing loss was the most prevalent type of hearing loss, followed by sensorineural hearing loss and mixed hearing loss. The ABR results in this study, unlike Maro et al.'s (2016) study, revealed auditory dysfunction suggestive of neural dyssynchrony. Torre, Cook et al. (2016), in another South African study, examined middle ear function in HIV-infected children. This study aimed to quantitatively measure middle ear function, using tympanometry, in perinatally HIV-infected (PHIV) and HIV-uninfected children. PHIV children in this study had a higher risk of middle ear problems, although none were statistically significant. Higher parent/caregiver reports of past middle ear infection were found in PHIV children (34.2 percent) than in HIV-uninfected children (25.0 percent). Risk for reported history of middle ear infection was higher in the last stage of the disease when compared to other WHO stages. Outer ear otorrhea was present in two PHIV children and in no HIV-uninfected children. Tympanometry findings were similar in both groups, although PHIV children had a higher rate of outer ear otorrhea. These authors conclude, and I concur, that inclusion of quantitative tympanometry data in assessment of this population is important.

In a recent South African study, qualitative retrospective record reviews of data were collected from 100 medical records at a paediatric HIV/AIDS clinic in a public hospital in Johannesburg (Khoza-Shangase & Anastasiou, 2020).

The study aimed to identify recorded otological manifestations in this population. Findings revealed that almost half (43 percent) of the sample presented with otological manifestations, with otitis media (15 percent) and otorrhea (15 percent) being the most common. Seven percent of the participants with otological manifestations were referred to audiologists and/or ear, nose and throat specialists for assessment and management. These findings raise important implications for the clinical assessment and management of paediatric patients with HIV/AIDS, for the role of all team members, and for the importance of early detection and intervention in this cohort, where speech-language development is still occurring and where successful learning at school is still key (Khoza-Shangase & Anastasiou, 2020). The findings also highlight the need for programmatic approaches to preventive care as far as middle ear pathology in this population is concerned.

In a study in Brazil, Buriti et al. (2013) investigated the occurrence of hearing loss in children with HIV and its association with viral load, opportunistic diseases and ARV treatment. Audiological data revealed that 84.8 percent of the ears assessed presented with hearing loss (mild degree being the most common), and 89.1 percent with abnormal middle ear function, of which 67.4 percent presented with type B tympanograms on immittance testing. In fact, otitis media was found to be the most frequent opportunistic disease, at 61.1 percent of the cases. Statistically significant associations were established between ART use and otitis media. These findings point to the importance of auditory monitoring and intervention as soon as possible in the paediatric population with HIV.

Matas, Leite, Magliaro, and Gonçalves (2006) examined the peripheral auditory system and the auditory brainstem pathway of children with AIDS. Findings from this study revealed that children with AIDS presented with abnormal results more frequently than their matched control, as evidenced by either peripheral or auditory brainstem impairment. These authors assert that AIDS should be considered a risk factor for peripheral and/or auditory brainstem disorders in children.

Hearing function in HIV-infected children was investigated in Malawi by Hrapcak et al. (2016), with the aim of estimating the prevalence and types of hearing loss in this population. These researchers determined factors that predict hearing loss in this group through regression analysis, where age and sex-adjusted odds ratios were calculated. Findings revealed hearing loss in 24 percent of the participants – 82 percent conductive, 14 percent sensorineural and 4 percent mixed. Factors linked to a higher prevalence of hearing loss were history of frequent ear infections and otorrhea, history of WHO stage 3 or 4 of HIV and history of malnutrition. Duration of ART and CD4 count were not found to have any correlation with the prevalence of hearing loss. An additional interesting finding in this study, which has significant implications for EHDI risk factors (particularly parental concern regarding hearing loss), is that only 40 percent of caregivers accurately perceived their child's hearing loss. Another study conducted in Malawi by Devendra, Makawa, Kazembe, Calles, and Kuper (2013) reported on the prevalence of a range of disabilities in children living with HIV (33 percent) compared to their HIV-uninfected siblings (7 percent). Hearing loss accounted for 35 percent of the disabilities found in this study. Of the total number of participants, caregivers reported hearing difficulties in 12 percent of HIV-infected children, compared with only 2 percent of their uninfected siblings.

HIV perinatal exposure and auditory manifestations

HIV is a risk factor for hearing loss in children. However, the potential link between hearing loss and in-utero exposure to maternal HIV infection and HIV medications has not been well studied, and there is a paucity of research on hearing screening results obtained from babies born to mothers infected with HIV. Despite the National Institutes of Health (NIH, 2012) reporting that children exposed to HIV in the womb may be more likely than their unexposed peers to experience hearing loss by age 16, this has not garnered much attention. The NIH estimated that hearing loss affects 9 to 15 percent of HIV-infected children and 5 to 8 percent of children who did not have HIV at birth but whose mothers had HIV infection during pregnancy. Postulations from this study were that, when compared to national averages for other children of the same age, children with HIV infection are about 200 to 300 percent more likely to have a hearing loss. Those whose mothers had HIV during pregnancy but who themselves were born without HIV are 20 percent more likely to have hearing loss. Olusanya, Afe, and Onyia (2009) conducted a study in Nigeria aimed at establishing the characteristics of infants with HIV-infected mothers enrolled under a two-stage UNHS programme. In contrast to the NIH (2012) findings, which indicated a risk of hearing loss in HIV-exposed but uninfected children, findings from this study revealed that maternal HIV status was not significantly associated with the risk of sensorineural hearing loss. However, newborns with HIV-infected mothers had a more than twofold risk of not completing the hearing tests when compared with controls.

Studies have observed about a twofold higher risk of hearing loss for HIV-exposed uninfected (HEU) infants as compared to HIV-unexposed and uninfected infants (Manfredi, Zuanetti, Mishima, & Granzotti, 2011; Olusanya et al., 2009; Torre et al., 2012). Findings from these studies were not, however, statistically significant. Additionally, there is silence around the possible impact of CMV on these findings, although this perinatal infection is well known to be linked to sensorineural hearing loss (Barbi et al., 2003;

Dahle et al., 2000; Fowler & Boppanna, 2006; Yamamoto et al., 2011) and has a higher prevalence in neonates born to mothers with HIV (Doyle, Atkins, & Rivera-Matos, 1996; Mussi-Pinhata, Yamamoto, Figueiredo, Cervi, & Duarte, 1998). The concern about CMV remains relevant even though there is evidence of decreased prevalence of congenital CMV in HEU infants with the advent of HAART (Slyker, 2016). Guibert and colleagues (2009) argue that CMV remains higher in this group than in the general population. It is therefore important to include infants with this risk factor in hearing screening programmes. This is particularly so in contexts where UNHS is still not feasible, and targeted hearing screening is the only viable interim option, as in South Africa.

Torre, Zeldow et al. (2016) argue that because early identification of newborn hearing impairment has important implications for the child's speech, language and educational development, and since congenital CMV infection has been identified as a risk factor for permanent sensorineural hearing loss (Fowler & Boppanna, 2006), screening for CMV co-infection in this group of infants is critical in understanding hearing loss in HEU paediatrics. It is also important for the National Department of Health to ensure that South Africa meets the 90-90-90 targets, particularly in women of child-bearing age, as well as primary prevention of prenatal infections such as CMV.

Torre et al. (2012) report that hearing loss occurred in 20 percent of HIV-infected children in their study and 10.5 percent of HEU children. HIV infection was associated with increased odds of hearing loss in this sample, even when the caregiver educational level was adjusted. Similar to findings in other studies (Hrapcak et al., 2016; Khoza-Shangase & Turnbull, 2009; Torre, Cook et al., 2016), children with a worse stage of HIV diagnosis had over twice the odds of hearing loss. The prevalence of hearing loss was higher in both HIV-infected and HEU children compared with healthy children. The results of this study show that hearing loss is common among children who were perinatally exposed to HIV. HIV-infected children have a higher rate of hearing loss compared to HEU children and both groups of children have a higher rate of hearing loss compared to HIV-unexposed children. This raises important implications for EHDI, such as careful consideration when it comes to possible use of a targeted (risk-based) hearing screening approach. Torre et al. (2012) suggest that future studies should include evaluation of specific risk factors for hearing loss in this population, such as CMV exposure and mitochondrial mutation. They also recommend longitudinal monitoring of these populations to track progression and to establish if there is a risk for greater hearing loss earlier in life that may affect both educational and social development. This highlights the importance of standard screening and assessment protocols for early hearing detection, with appropriate record keeping that will allow for accurate monitoring and test–retest within subject comparisons. It also raises important implications for continuity of care in, and collaborative efforts between, the health and basic education sectors in South Africa.

Fasunla et al. (2014) compared ABR findings in HIV-exposed and -unexposed newborns in sub-Saharan Africa to explore the effects of maternal HIV infection and ART on the hearing of HIV-exposed newborns. Hearing screening of the newborns was done with ABR and compared with maternal HAART, CD4 cell counts, RNA viral loads and newborn CD4 percent. Results revealed sensorineural hearing impairment in 11.1 percent of the HIV-exposed group and in 6.6 percent of unexposed newborns. No significant association was found between the hearing thresholds of HIV-exposed newborns and maternal CD4 cell counts. However, there was an association between hearing thresholds and maternal viral load, with a significant difference between the hearing thresholds of HIV-exposed newborns with CD4 percent of ≤ 25 and those with >25. Furthermore, findings revealed a significant difference in the hearing of HAART-exposed and HAART-unexposed newborns. These findings of a trend towards more hearing loss in HIV-exposed newborns, positively correlated with an increase in the mothers' viral load, suggest the need to consider in-utero exposure to HIV and HAART in newborn hearing, and consequently in EHDI. Fasunla et al. (2014) thus recommend that routine hearing screening be conducted early in all newborns, including HIV-exposed newborns, to identify those with hearing loss.

In another study, Torre, Zeldow et al. (2016) argue that perinatal HIV infection and congenital CMV infection may increase the risk for hearing loss in children living with HIV. They examined infants enrolled in the Surveillance Monitoring of ART Toxicities study of the Pediatric HIV/AIDS Cohort Study network, a prospective study of the safety of in-utero ARV exposures. They determined the proportion of perinatally HEU newborns that were referred for additional hearing testing, and evaluated the association between in-utero ARV exposures and newborn hearing screening results. They also examined congenital CMV infection in infants with and without screening referral. Their findings indicated that 3.1 percent of the infants did not pass the hearing screening and were thus referred for further hearing testing. Additionally, findings indicated that first trimester exposure to Tenofovir was associated with lower odds of a newborn hearing screening referral. However, exposure to Atazanavir was linked to higher odds of newborn screening referral. These findings were, however, not statistically significant. So, over and above CMV exposure and mitochondrial mutation, these findings suggest that maternal ARV use may have varying effects on newborn hearing screenings. They highlight the need for audiologists to be knowledgeable about in-utero ARV exposures in HEU children because of the possibility of higher referrals in these children, hence raising implications for hearing screening programmes. Figure 12.1 provides a global overview of audiological presentation in the general paediatric population in relation to HIV/AIDS.

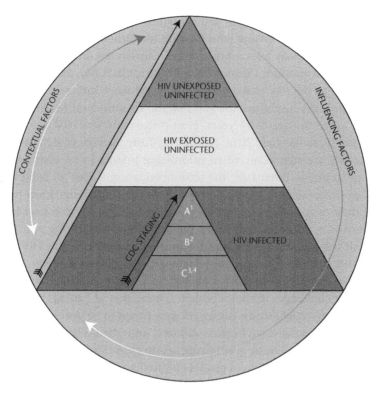

Figure 12.1 Audiological presentation in the general HIV/AIDS paediatric population

Source: M. R. Shangase, 2019

Solutions and recommendations

There is a dearth of substantive, consolidated evidence regarding the impact of HIV/AIDS in the paediatric population. The available evidence, however, is convincing enough to warrant efficient planning for EHDI in this population. There is a clear need for accurate and sensitive measures to identify the auditory manifestations early, and refer them for medical and audiological management.

Evidence suggests that a UNHS programme would be ideal for identifying hearing changes and impairments, regardless of the child's HIV status (Patel & Feldman, 2011; Wroblewska-Seniuk, Dabrowski, Szyfter, & Mazela, 2017), as lower hearing function has been noted even in children who are HIV exposed but uninfected. However, various studies have shown that UNHS is not feasible in the South African context (see chapters 2, 4 and 5), hence the call for targeted newborn hearing screening (TNHS) as an interim measure.

TNHS has both challenges and weaknesses. Besides missing approximately 50 percent of infants with hearing impairment, it relies on agreed upon and contextually relevant risk factors. Current risk factors include HIV/AIDS (Health Professions Council of South Africa [HPCSA], 2018). However, this is listed as the HIV status of the infant. Evidence indicates that maternal HIV and ARV use also raise the risk for sensorineural hearing loss in children up to the age of 16 years, even if the child was HIV exposed but uninfected (Fasunla et al., 2014; NIH, 2012; Torre, Zeldow et al., 2016). The implications are significant when prioritising infants to be included in a TNHS programme. Essentially, the recommendation is that all babies born to HIV-positive mothers should be included in the TNHS programme regardless of their own status. The fact that hearing loss can develop later means that hearing screening programmes should have a monitoring arm for all infants at risk of later development of hearing loss, such as this HIV population. This monitoring cannot be left to parental concern as literature indicates a high prevalence of parents failing to suspect or identify that there are hearing challenges in their children (Hrapcak et al., 2016). In Hrapcak and colleagues' (2016) study, caregivers were found to be unreliable at identifying hearing impairment in their children, and often incorrectly reported children with normal hearing as having hearing loss. Monitoring would also allow for early identification of possible ototoxicity-related hearing loss, and immediate intervention, either medically (change of ototoxic medication if possible and complementary use of oto-protective agents) or audiologically (provision of amplification and enrolment in an aural rehabilitation programme).

The types of auditory and otological manifestations in this population raise implications for the hearing screening and assessment measures that can be used. Commonly, hearing screening measures include otoacoustic emissions as well as automated ABR audiometry. Findings in this population indicate a significantly high prevalence of middle ear disease as well as abnormal ABR audiometry, implying neural dyssynchrony. These conditions thus need to be considered during screening, but there is also a need to include sensitive middle ear measures as part of the screening test battery. This is over and above careful consideration of audiological measures for diagnostic audiology that would allow for monitoring of thresholds across frequencies, including high frequencies such as auditory steady state response. Clear strategies for prevention and treatment are required, considering that most hearing loss in this population is conductive, likely due to frequent ear infections. Children with frequent ear infections, otorrhea, TB, severe HIV disease or low body mass index should receive more frequent ear assessments and hearing evaluations. Following medical clearance, proper planning for amplification and aural rehabilitation services for children diagnosed with hearing loss is important.

Inclusion of sensitive middle ear measures, such as high frequency tympanometry and/or wideband absorbance tympanometry, in routine assessment will ensure early identification and subsequent early referral for medical management of the leading cause of hearing loss in this population. Such early identification and treatment will prevent consequences of this disease, including conductive and/or mixed hearing loss that will have implications for the child's psychosocial, cognitive, linguistic and academic development.

There are two reasons for including all infants with maternal HIV history, regardless of their own status, in a hearing screening and monitoring programme. Firstly, there is the cumulative benefit of establishing the effects of HIV and its treatments on children longitudinally. Such data will allow for causes of hearing loss in this population to be determined. Establishing causative links can only be done if there is enough evidence, which there currently is not. This evidence has to be collated in a systematic, sensitive and reliable manner that allows for repeated measures data statistical analysis within and across clinical sites as well as within and across patients. Secondly, the direct benefits of early identification and intervention to the patients presenting with audiological or otological symptoms cannot be overemphasised. A goal of any EHDI initiative in this population should be early identification of middle ear disease as well as sensorineural hearing loss due to other causes (opportunistic infections or ototoxic medications) before permanent or more significant consequences occur. This will have a positive impact on this population's general development of cognition and language, which will ultimately have a positive influence on their quality of life.

Sensory modalities are essential quality of life indicators. Cognitive–linguistic skills, psychosocial behaviour, as well as vocational, social and interpersonal skills are all negatively impacted by hearing loss. Hence the importance of implementing systematic hearing monitoring programmes in all clinical sites where HIV/AIDS programmes are run, and of following up and monitoring babies with a maternal history of HIV. This is particularly important in South Africa, where HIV presents a significant burden of disease.

Audiologists need to provide information counselling in HIV prenatal clinics, and form part of the clinical team in paediatric HIV/AIDS clinics. Despite the current dearth of audiological evidence in this population, there is sufficient data, including that from adults, to justify assessing and monitoring ear health and hearing function in this population. Clinical teams have an ethical obligation to inform parents/caregivers of the potential effects of HIV and its treatments on hearing, to allow for early reports and access to intervention. Such raised parental awareness has the benefit of facilitating early identification of hearing changes since the caregiver will be aware, and will also be encouraged to bring the child back for monitoring sessions.

Furthermore, parental education can include information about milestones in communication development as well as communication stimulation strategies to enhance development in this vulnerable population.

Audiologists have the important role of advocacy for early and effective medical management where opportunistic infections lead to hearing impairment. This advocacy role extends to informing attending physicians about possible ototoxic hearing loss in order for alternative treatments to be explored. Because ototoxic treatments are often prescribed for life-serving purposes, primary prevention is not always feasible. Therefore, early detection of hearing loss is of paramount importance as it facilitates provision of management options, which may include adjusting the therapy to a potentially less ototoxic regimen or changing the dosage and frequency (Khoza-Shangase & Masondo, 2020). Audiologically, early detection may also allow for fitting of amplification as early as possible, as a treatment option to enhance access to audition for language development.

Conclusion

HIV/AIDS has become a chronic condition rather than an immediate death sentence, and HIV-infected children are living longer and more successfully. This opens up a whole new world of clinical care and research for the speech-language and hearing professions. Research in this population can take numerous directions, including: the effects of HIV infection on hearing and on auditory processing; the nature, degree, configuration, onset and development, as well as causes of hearing loss; impact of treatments on hearing function; and efficacy studies on intervention approaches for children with communication and cognitive disorders related to HIV infection.

There is a need for research into the heterogeneous auditory manifestations of HIV/AIDS in children, including hearing loss, tinnitus and vertigo, which can occur in varied combinations. Types of hearing loss include conductive, mixed, sensorineural and central. The degree, symmetry and configuration of hearing loss in this population has not been described, and the onset and development of the hearing loss not reported. The various causes of hearing loss include HIV/AIDS as a primary cause, opportunistic infections (secondary) as well as treatments that the patients undergo (iatrogenic). The causes of hearing loss in the HIV-exposed but uninfected paediatric population and HIV-exposed HAART-exposed population require exploration.

As far as assessment and intervention are concerned, it is recommended that early screening of neonates and infants with risk factors for hearing loss and impairment be performed. This should be coupled with audiological monitoring; advocacy for safe administration of drugs, especially ototoxic ones; establishment of audiological units to facilitate hearing screening, including sensitive middle ear measures in the test battery; and information counselling for parents and caregivers on HIV/AIDS and hearing/ otological manifestations. Furthermore, otoscopy and tympanometry should form part of the minimum screening measures implemented during routine check-ups to identify middle ear pathologies in the HIV-infected population. It is also important that ART is started early to preserve healthy CD4 levels, as well as virology control that will reduce the likelihood of middle ear problems. Evidence suggests that children with HIV commonly respond to the same intervention strategies and techniques as HIV-negative children (Davis-McFarland, 2002). However, because of the syndromic nature of HIV/ AIDS, holistic management that considers coexisting medical, psychosocial and clinical issues is important.

References

Araújo, E. S., Zucki, F., Corteletti, L. C., Lopes, A. C., Feniman, M. R., & Alvarenga, K. F. (2012). Hearing loss and acquired immune deficiency syndrome: Systematic review. *Jornal da Sociedade Brasileira de Fonoaudiologia, 24*(2), 188–192.

Assuiti, L. F., Lanzoni G. M., Santos, F. C., Erdmann, A. L., & Meirelles, B. H. (2013). Hearing loss in people with HIV/AIDS and associated factors: An integrative review. *Brazilian Journal of Otorhinolaryngology, 79*(2), 248–255. doi: 10.5935/1808-8694.20130042.

Avert. (2018). HIV and AIDS in South Africa. Retrieved from https://www.avert. org/professionals/hiv-around-world/sub-saharan-africa/south-africa#footnote 15_5f9l2yc.

Banks, L. M., Zuurmond, M., Ferrand, R., & Kuper, H. (2015). The relationship between HIV and prevalence of disabilities in sub-Saharan Africa: Systematic review (FA). *Tropical Medicine & International Health, 20*(4), 411–429. doi: 10.1111/tmi.12449.

Barbi, M., Binda, S., Caroppo, S., Ambrosetti, U., Corbetta, C., & Sergi, P. (2003). A wider role for congenital cytomegalovirus infection in sensorineural hearing loss. *The Pediatric Infectious Disease Journal, 22*(1), 39–42.

Belman, A. L., Muenz, L. R., Marcus, J. C., Goedert, J. J., Landesman, S., Rubinstein, A., ... Willoughby, A. (1996). Neurologic status of human immunodeficiency virus 1-infected infants and their controls: A prospective study from birth to 2 years. *Mothers and infants cohort study. Pediatrics, 98*(6 Pt 1), 1109–1118. pmid: 8951261.

Boivin, M. J., Kakooza, A. M., Warf, B. C., Davidson, L. L., & Grigorenko, E. L. (2015). Reducing neurodevelopmental disorders and disability through research and interventions. *Nature, 527*(7578), S155–S160. doi: 10.1038/nature16029.

Buriti, A. K., Oliveira, S. H., & Muniz, L. F. (2013). Hearing loss in children with HIV/ AIDS. *Codas, 25*(6), 513–520. doi: 10.1590/S2317-17822013.05000013.

Campanini, A., Marani, M., Mastroianni, A., Cancellieri, C., & Vicini, C. (2005). Human immunodeficiency virus infection: Personal experience in changes in head and neck manifestations due to recent antiretroviral therapies. *Acta Otorhinolaryngologica Italica, 25*, 30–35.

Chao, C. K., Czechowicz, J. A., Messner, A. H., Alarcón, J., Kolevic Roca, L., Larragán
  Rodriguez, M. M., ... Zunt, J. R. (2012). High prevalence of hearing impairment
  in HIV-infected Peruvian children. *Otolaryngology—Head and Neck Surgery, 146*(2),
  259–265. doi: 10.1177/0194599811429271.

Chiriboga, C. A., Fleishman, S., Champion, S., Gaye-Robinson, L., & Abrams, E. J.
  (2005). Incidence and prevalence of HIV encephalopathy in children with HIV
  infection receiving highly active anti-retroviral therapy (HAART). *The Journal of
  Pediatrics, 146*(3), 402–407. doi: 10.1016/j.jpeds.2004.10.021.

Columbia University Mailman School of Public Health. (2018). Developmental disabilities reported in HIV-positive children in South Africa. Retrieved from https://
  www.mailman.columbia.edu/public-health-now/news/developmental-disabilities-
  reported-hiv-positive-children-south-africa.

Dahle, A. J., Fowler, K. B., Wright, J. D., Boppana, S. B., Britt, W. J., & Pass, R. F. (2000).
  Longitudinal investigation of hearing disorders in children with congenital cytomegalovirus. *Journal of the American Academy of Audiology, 11*(5), 283–290.

Davies, N. E. C. G. (2013). Fixed-dose combination for adults accessing antiretroviral therapy. *Southern African Journal of HIV Medicine, 14*(1), 41–43. doi: 10.7196/
  SAJHIVMED.913.

Davis-McFarland, E. (2002). Pediatric HIV/AIDS: Issues and strategies for intervention.
  The Asha Leader, 7(4), 10–21. https://doi.org/10.1044/leader.FTR2.07042002.10.

Devendra, A., Makawa, A., Kazembe, P. N., Calles, N. R., & Kuper, H. (2013). HIV and
  childhood disability: A case-controlled study at a paediatric antiretroviral center in
  Lilongwe, Malawi. *PLoS One, 8*(12), e84024. doi: 10.1371/journal.pone.0084024.

Doyle, M., Atkins, J. T., & Rivera-Matos, I. R. (1996). Congenital cytomegalovirus infection in infants infected with human immunodeficiency virus type 1. *The Pediatric
  Infectious Disease Journal, 15*(12), 1102–1106.

Epstein, L. G., Sharer, L. R., Oleske, J. M., Connor, E. M., Goudsmit, J., Bagdon, L.,
  ... Koenigsberger, M. R. (1986). Neurologic manifestations of human immunodeficiency virus infection in children. *Pediatrics, 78*(4), 678–687. pmid: 2429248.

Fasunla, A. J., Ogunbosi, B. O., Odaibo, G. N., Nwaorgu, O. G., Taiwo, B., Olaleye, D.
  O., ... Akinyinka, O. O. (2014). Comparison of auditory brainstem response in
  HIV-1 exposed and unexposed newborns and correlation with the maternal viral
  load and CD4+ cell counts. *AIDS, 28*(15), 2223–2230.

Fowler, K. B., & Boppanna, S. B. (2006). Congenital cytomegalovirus (CMV) infection
  and hearing deficit. *Journal of Clinical Virology, 35*(2), 226–231.

Govender, R., Eley, B., Walker, K., Petersen, R., & Wilmshurst, J. M. (2011).
  Neurologic and neurobehavioral sequelae in children with human immunodeficiency virus (HIV-1) infection. *Journal of Child Neurology, 26*(11), 1355–1364. doi:
  10.1177/0883073811405203.

Guibert, G., Warszawski, J., Le Chenadec, J., Blanche, S., Benmebarek, Y., Mandelbrot,
  L., ... Leruez-Ville, M. (2009). Decreased risk of congenital cytomegalovirus
  infection in children born to HIV-1-infected mothers in the era of highly active
  antiretroviral therapy. *Clinical Infectious Diseases, 48*(11), 1516–1525. doi:
  10.1086/598934.

Health Professions Council of South Africa (HPCSA). (2018). Early hearing detection and intervention (EHDI) guidelines. Retrieved from http://www.hpcsa.co.za/Uploads/editor/UserFiles/downloads/speech/Early_Hearing_Detection_and_Intervention_(EHDI)_2018.pdf.

Hrapcak, S., Kuper, H., Bartlett, P., Devendra, A., Makawa, A., Kim, M., ... Ahmed, S. (2016). Hearing loss in HIV-infected children in Lilongwe, Malawi. *PLoS ONE, 11*(8), e0161421. https://doi.org/10.1371/journal.pone.0161421.

Human Sciences Research Council (HSRC). (2018) The fifth South African national HIV prevalence, incidence, behaviour and communication survey, 2017. Retrieved from https://serve.mg.co.za/content/documents/2018/07/17/7M1RBtUShKFJbN3NL1Wr_HSRC_HIV_Survey_Summary_2018.pdf.

International Labour Organization (ILO). (2018). *The impact of HIV and AIDS on the world of work: Global estimates.* Geneva, Switzerland: International Labour Office.

Johnson, L. F., May, M. T., Dorrington, R. E., Cornell, M., Boulle, A., Egger, M., & Davies, M.-A. (2017). Estimating the impact of antiretroviral treatment on adult mortality trends in South Africa: A mathematical modelling study. *PLoS Medicine, 14*(12), e1002468.

Kakuda, T. N. (2000). Pharmacology of nucleoside and nucleotide reverse transcriptase inhibitor-induced mitochondrial toxicity. *Clinical Therapeutics, 22*(6), 685–708.

Khoza-Shangase, K. (2011). An analysis of auditory manifestations in a group of adults with AIDS prior to antiretroviral therapy. *African Journal of Infectious Diseases, 5*(1), 11–22.

Khoza-Shangase, K. (2020). Pharmaco-audiology vigilance in the treatment of patients with HIV/AIDS: Ototoxicity monitoring protocol recommendation. *Infectious Disorders—Drug Targets, 20*(1), 33–42. doi: 10.2174/1871526518666181016102102.

Khoza-Shangase, K., & Anastasiou, J. (2020). An exploration of recorded otological manifestations in South African children with HIV/AIDS: A pilot study. *International Journal of Pediatric Otorhinolaryngology, 133.* https://doi.org/10.1016/j.ijporl.2020.109960.

Khoza-Shangase, K. & Masondo, N. (2020). What are the current audiological practices for ototoxicity assessment and management in the South African healthcare context? *International Journal of Environmental Research and Public Health, 17,* 2613. doi: 10.3390/ijerph17072613.

Khoza-Shangase, K., & Turnbull, T. (2009). Hearing screening in a group of paediatric patients attending an HIV/AIDS clinic: A pilot study. *African Journal of Infectious Diseases, 3*(2), 57–68.

Knox, J., Arpadi, SM., Kauchali, S., Craib, M., Kvalsvig, J. D., Taylor, M., ... Davidson, L. L. (2018). Screening for developmental disabilities in HIV positive and HIV negative children in South Africa: Results from the Asenze study. *PLoS ONE, 13*(7), e0199860. https://doi.org/10.1371/journal.pone.0199860.

Koekkoek, S., Eggermont, L., De Sonneville, L., Jupimai, T., Wicharuk, S., Apateerapong, W., ... Ananworanich, J. (2006). Effects of highly active antiretroviral therapy (HAART) on psychomotor performance in children with HIV disease. *Journal of Neurology, 253*(12), 1615–1624. doi: 10.1007/s00415-006-0277-x.

Lassiter, J. M., & Parsons, J. T. (2015). Religion and spirituality's influences on HIV syndemics among MSM: A systematic review and conceptual model. *AIDS and Behavior, 20*(2), 461–472. doi: 10.1007/s10461-015-1173-0.

Laughton, B., Cornell, M., Boivin, M., & Van Rie, A. (2013). Neurodevelopment in perinatally HIV-infected children: A concern for adolescence. *Journal of the International AIDS Society, 16,* 18603. doi: 10.7448/IAS.16.1.18603.

Le Doare, K., Bland, R., & Newell, M. L. (2012). Neurodevelopment in children born to HIV-infected mothers by infection and treatment status. *Pediatrics, 130*(5), e1326–e1344. doi: 10.1542/peds.2012-0405.

Manfredi, A. K., Zuanetti, P. A., Mishima, F., & Granzotti, R. B. (2011). Newborn hearing screening in infants born to HIV-seropositive mothers. *Jornal da Sociedade Brasileira de Fonoaudiologia, 23*(4), 376–380.

Maro, I. I., Fellows, A. M., Clavier, O. H., Gui, J., Rieke, C. C., Wilbur, J. C., … Buckey, J. C. (2016). Auditory impairments in HIV-infected children. *Ear and Hearing, 37*(4), 443–451.

Matas, C. G., Iorio, M. C., & Succi, R. C. (2008). Auditory disorders and acquisition of the ability to localize sound in children born to HIV-positive mothers. *The Brazilian Journal of Infectious Diseases, 12*(1), 10–14. doi: 10.1590/s1413-86702008000100004.

Matas, C. G., Leite, R. A., Magliaro, F. C., & Gonçalves, I. C. (2006). Audiological and electrophysiological evaluation of children with acquired immunodeficiency syndrome (AIDS). *The Brazilian Journal of Infectious Diseases, 10*(4), 264–268.

Matas, C. G., Santos Filha, V. A., Juan, K. R., Pinto, F. R., & Gonçalves, I. C. (2010). Audiological manifestations in children and adults with AIDS. *Pro Fono, 22*(3), 269–274. doi: 10.1590/s0104-56872010000300019.

Mills, E. J., Bakanda, C., Birungi, J., Chan, K., Ford, N., Cooper, C. L., … Hogg, R. S. (2011). Life expectancy of persons receiving combination antiretroviral therapy in low-income countries: A cohort analysis from Uganda. *Annals of Internal Medicine, 155*(4), 209–216. doi: 10.7326/0003-4819-155-4-201108160-00358.

Miziara, I., Weber, R., Filho, B., & Neto, C. (2007). Otitis media in Brazilian human immunodeficiency virus infected children undergoing antiretroviral therapy. *The Journal of Laryngology and Otology, 121*(11), 1048–1054. doi: 10.1017/S0022215107006093.

Mussi-Pinhata, M. M., Yamamoto, A. Y., Figueiredo, L. T., Cervi, M. C., & Duarte, G. (1998). Congenital and perinatal cytomegalovirus infection in infants born to mothers infected with human immunodeficiency virus. *The Journal of Pediatrics, 132*(2), 285–290.

Mwaba, S. O. C., Ngoma, M. S., Kusanthan, T., & Menon, J. A. (2015). The effect of HIV on developmental milestones in children. *Journal of AIDS and Clinical Research, 6,* 482. doi: 10.4172/2155-6113.1000482.

National Institutes of Health (NIH). (2012). Children exposed to HIV in the womb at increased risk for hearing loss. Retrieved from https://www.nih.gov/news-events/news-releases/children-exposed-hiv-womb-increased-risk-hearing-loss.

Ndoleriire, C., Turitwenka, E., Bakeera-Kitaaka, S., & Nyabigambo, A. (2013). The prevalence of hearing impairment in the 6 months-5 years HIV/AIDS positive patients attending paediatric infectious disease clinic at Mulago Hospital. *International Journal of Pediatric Otorhinolaryngology, 77*(2), 262–265. doi: 10.1016/j.ijporl.2012.11.013.

Olusanya, B. O., Afe, A. J., & Onyia, N. O. (2009). Infants with HIV-infected mothers in a universal newborn hearing screening programme in Lagos, Nigeria. *Acta Pædiatrica, 98*(8), 1288–1293.

Palacios, G. C., Montalvo, M. S., Fraire, M. I., Leon, E., Alvarez, M. T., & Solorzano, F. (2008). Audiologic and vestibular findings in a sample of human immunodeficiency virus type-1-infected Mexican children under highly active antiretroviral therapy. *International Journal of Pediatric Otorhinolaryngology, 72*(11), 1671–1681. doi: 10.1016/j.ijporl.2008.08.002.

Patel, H., & Feldman, M. (2011). Universal newborn hearing screening. *Paediatrics and Child Health, 16*(5), 301–310. https://doi.org/10.1093/pch/16.5.301.

Patel, K., Ming, X., Williams, P. L., Robertson, K. R., Oleske, J. M., Seage, G. R., 3rd, & International Maternal Pediatric Adolescent AIDS Clinical Trials 219/219C Study Team. (2009). Impact of HAART and CNS-penetrating antiretroviral regimens on HIV encephalopathy among perinatally infected children and adolescents. *AIDS, 23*(14), 1893–1901. doi: 10.1097/QAD.0b013e32832dc041.

Peter, V. Z. (2014). An audiological profile of school aged children with HIV/ AIDS at an antiretroviral clinic in KwaZulu Natal. Master of Communication Pathology (Audiology). Retrieved from https://researchspace.ukzn.ac.za/xmlui/handle/10413/13069.

Schouten, J. T., Lockhart, D. W., Rees, T. S., Collier, A. C., & Marra, C. M. (2006). A prospective study of hearing changes after beginning zidovudine or didanosine in HIV-treatment naïve people. *BMC Infectious Diseases, 6*, 28. doi: 10.1186/1471-2334-6-28.

Sherr, L., Croome, N., Castaneda, K. P., Bradshaw, K., & Romero, R. H. (2014). Developmental challenges in HIV infected children: An updated systematic review. *Children and Youth Services Review, 45*, 74–89.

Slyker, J. A. (2016). Cytomegalovirus and paediatric HIV infection. *Journal of Virus Eradication, 2*(4), 208–214.

Smith, R., Malee, K., Leighty, R., Brouwers, P., Mellins, C., Hittelman, J., … Blasini, I. (2006). Effects of perinatal HIV infection and associated risk factors on cognitive development among young children. *Pediatrics, 117*(3), 851–862. doi: 10.1542/peds.2005-0804.

South African National AIDS Council. (2015). Global AIDS response progress report. Retrieved from https://sanac.org.za//wp-content/uploads/2017/06/MandE-SANAC-Global-AIDSResponse-Progress-Report_2016.pdf.

Swanepoel, D. W. (2006). Audiology in South Africa: Audiología en Sudáfrica. *International Journal of Audiology, 45*(5), 262–266.

Taipele, A., Pelkonen, T., Taipele, M., Roine, I., Bernardino, L., Peltola, H., & Pitkäranta, A. (2011). Otorhinolaryngological findings and hearing in HIV-positive and HIV-negative children in a developing country. *European Archives of Oto-Rhino-Laryngology, 268*, 1527–1532. doi: 10.1007/s00405-011-1579-x.

Torre, P. III. (2015). A review of human immunodeficiency virus on the auditory system. *Perspectives on Hearing and Hearing Disorders: Research and Diagnostics, 19*(2), 55–63.

Torre, P. III, Cook, A., Elliott, H., Dawood, G., & Laughton, B. (2015). Hearing assessment data in HIV-infected and uninfected children of Cape Town, South Africa. *AIDS Care, 27*(8), 1037–1041. doi: 10.1080/09540121.2015.1021746.

Torre, P. III, Cook, A., Elliott, H., Dawood, G., & Laughton, B. (2016). Middle ear function in human immunodeficiency virus (HIV)-infected South African children. *Journal of Paediatric Care Insight, 1*(1), 13–17. doi: https://doi.org/10.24218/jpci.2016.04.

Torre, P. III, Zeldow, B., Hoffman, H. J., Buchanan, A., Siberry, G. K., Rice, M., … Williams, P. L. (2012). Hearing loss in perinatally HIV-infected and HIV-exposed but uninfected children and adolescents. *The Pediatric Infectious Diseases Journal, 31*(8), 835–841. doi: 10.1097/INF.0b013e31825b9524.

Torre, P. III, Zeldow, B., Yao, T. J., Hoffman, H. J., Siberry, G. K., Purswani, M. U., … Williams, P. L. (2016). Newborn hearing screenings in human immunodeficiency virus-exposed uninfected infants. *Journal of AIDS Immune Research, 1*(1), 102.

UNAIDS. (2016). *Children and HIV: Fact sheet.* Geneva, Switzerland: UNAIDS.

UNAIDS. (2018). *Miles to go: Closing gaps, breaking barriers, righting injustices: Global AIDS update 2018.* Geneva, Switzerland: UNAIDS.

UNAIDS. (2019). *UNAIDS data 2019.* Geneva, Switzerland: UNAIDS. Retrieved from https://www.unaids.org/sites/default/files/media_asset/2019-UNAIDS-data_en.pdf.

Van Arnhem, L. A., Bunders, M. J., Scherpbier, H. J., Majoie, C. B., Reneman, L., Frinking, O., … Pajkrt, D. (2013). Neurologic abnormalities in HIV-1 infected children in the era of combination antiretroviral therapy. *PLoS One, 8*(5), e64398. doi: 10.1371/journal.pone.0064398.

Von Reyn, F., Palumbo, P. E., Moshi, N., & Buckey, J. C. (2016). Auditory impairments in HIV-infected children. *Ear and Hearing, 37*(4), 443–451.

Wroblewska-Seniuk, K., Dabrowski, P., Szyfter, W., & Mazela, J. (2017). Universal newborn hearing screening: Methods and results, obstacles, and benefits. *Pediatric Research. 81*, 415–422. https://doi.org/10.1038/pr.2016.250.

Yamamoto, A. Y., Mussi-Pinhata, M. M., Isaac Mde, L., Amaral, F. R., Carvalheiro, C., Aragon, D. C., … Britt, W. J. (2011). Congenital cytomegalovirus infection as a cause of sensorineural hearing loss in a highly immune population. *The Pediatric Infectious Diseases Journal, 30*(12), 1043–1046. doi: 10.1097/INF.0b013e31822d9640.

13 Ethical Considerations and Tele-Audiology in Early Hearing Detection and Intervention

Alida Naudé and Juan Bornman

Providing early hearing detection and intervention (EHDI) services over a distance challenges audiologists to exploit the potential offered by tele-audiology as a service delivery model, without violating legal constraints or compromising professional ethical responsibilities. The sensible application of current and emerging technology to deliver clinical services can assist in providing specialised expertise not otherwise available, enhance a clinician's productivity and improve access to quality services in a cost-effective manner. This chapter discusses the main ethical challenges related to tele-audiology in EHDI by referring to six concepts: licensure; competence; privacy and confidentiality; informed consent; effectiveness of services and programme validation; as well as reimbursement for services.

Permanent hearing loss is a global health care burden, with congenital hearing loss being the most common neonatal sensory disorder (Chadha & Stevens, 2013). It is crucial to diagnose hearing loss as soon as possible after birth in order to facilitate early intervention, as a hearing loss that is not identified and treated appropriately will result in significant delays in language, cognitive and social development (Doković et al., 2014), with profound later effects on education and employment (Olusanya, Neumann, & Saunders, 2014). Universal standards of infant hearing health care dictate that infant hearing screening should be completed by one month of age and screening tests with results outside the norm should be addressed with definitive follow-up audiological testing by three months of age (Joint Committee on Infant Hearing [JCIH], 2007).

Timely adherence to infant diagnostic testing and hearing loss treatment is a complex process posing significant challenges to parents. This is because it is typically unknown terrain for parents. Risk of non-adherence to the process is even more pronounced in families with greater travel distances, low levels of parental education, low socio-economic status and lack of medical aid (Bust et al., 2015; Cavalcanti & Guerra, 2012; Lester, Dawson, Gantz, & Hansen, 2011). Conducting diagnostic testing can be complicated by limited access to service delivery in rural areas, breakdowns in communication, lack of parental support, financial constraints and poor coordination of service delivery (Merugumala, Pothula, & Cooper, 2017). Access to services is further complicated by the fact that globally, the number of health care workers who have been educated, trained and employed is insufficient for the number of people who need health services. The lack of health care workers has become a widespread crisis requiring immediate action (Global Health Workforce Alliance, 2008). This is true for audiologic services as well.

There are currently no existing evidence-based approaches to decrease non-adherence to infant hearing testing and treatment. The current state of communication and information technology, however, offers a unique opportunity to develop programmes that can bridge distance, improve access to services and facilitate the achievement of critical EHDI programme goals. Therefore, it is unsurprising that the recent advances in technology and the widespread access to the internet by the general public have created the possibility for health care related services to be offered remotely. Neither South Africa nor the audiology field has escaped this trend, leading to a new focus area aptly named tele-audiology.

Tele-audiology can be defined as 'the application of telecommunications technology to deliver professional services at a distance' (American Speech-Language-Hearing Association [ASHA], 2005, p. 1). As such, it is a blanket term for digital audiology solutions and auditory rehabilitation which has partly been driven by commercial developments in remote otoscopy, remote audiometry as well as hearing aids that can be adjusted by a remote professional. In 2009, the Tele-Audiology Network (TAN), an international non-profit organisation, was founded in South Africa to establish clinics that could provide remote diagnostic hearing care services both live and asynchronously. Unfortunately, TAN dissolved and is no longer in operation as a result of a lack of resources at the time. Tele-audiology seeks to change a situation by bringing an array of hearing care services to those who need them for various reasons, including long travel distances, limited access to or lack of available services and financial constraints. Addressing these barriers forms the basis of tele-audiology in South Africa, as established by the National Department of Health, which aims to deliver services at a distance to communities in underserved areas. The goal is to alleviate the human resource crisis noted earlier and improve the links and communication between developed audiology facilities (mostly found in larger metros) and the underdeveloped rural areas (Health Professions Council of South Africa [HPCSA], 2014).

Potential uses of tele-audiology in EHDI include hearing screening with otoacoustic emissions (OAEs) or automated auditory brainstem response (AABR), diagnostic testing (video-otoscopy, immittance testing, evoked potentials) and intervention (hearing aid fitting, verification, counselling as well as cochlear implant programming). Education, training and mentoring of health care practitioners, paraprofessionals and parents can also be accomplished through tele-audiology systems and interactive online modules (Swanepoel, Olusanya, & Mars, 2010).

As technology continues to grow in scope and pace, the potential for remote service delivery will increase, realising the ideal of the JCIH (2007) that all children diagnosed with a hearing loss should have access to the necessary resources to allow them to reach their full potential. This ideal should, however, not only reflect resource availability following the identification of a hearing loss, but also appropriate and equitable assessment resources. All health care practitioners, including audiologists, should therefore be cognisant of holding a balanced approach towards tele-audiology – employing innovative interventions but without losing sight of the client (Fleming, Edison, & Pak, 2009).

This chapter provides an overview of the ethical aspects relating to early hearing detection through screening and intervention in the context of tele-audiology. We review some of the key professional challenges that could emerge, including the topics of competence, standard of care, privacy, informed consent and the use of support personnel, and offer several principles to guide audiologists. We believe that the audiology profession is only as strong as its commitment to ethical obligations and values.

Ethical considerations

The ethical considerations related to tele-audiology are familiar challenges, but situated in a new context. The American Academy of Audiology (AAA), the ASHA and the HPCSA have endorsed advances in tele-audiology for those with hearing loss and related disorders. This was done to expand the availability and accessibility of hearing and related care (AAA, 2008; ASHA, 2005; HPCSA, 2014). All tele-audiology services should involve a health care provider (servicing practitioner) where there is an actual on-site face-to-face consultation and physical examination of the client in a clinical setting. The consulting practitioner will communicate (via teleservices) the information to the servicing audiologist, who will then provide the necessary assistance (HPCSA, 2014). Tele-audiology is relatively new to the scope of audiology services and solid guidelines that monitor and control its implementation are not yet available. Therefore, providing services over a distance challenges audiologists to exploit the potential offered by tele-audiology, without violating legal constraints or compromising professional ethical responsibilities. The sensible application of current and emerging technology to deliver clinical services can assist in providing specialised expertise not otherwise available, enhance a clinician's productivity, and improve access to quality services in a cost-effective manner (ASHA, 2001).

Registration as an audiologist with the HPCSA, under the Health Professions Act (No. 56 of 1974), implies certain responsibilities. For example, audiologists have the duty to meet the ethical standards and guidelines set by the HPCSA and the Board for Speech, Language and Hearing Professions (HPCSA, 2016a). Audiologists who engage in tele-audiology must observe the professional duties imposed in the HPCSA's general ethical guidelines for good practice (HPCSA, 2016a). Tele-audiology is not the preferred approach when the technology does not allow audiologists to meet established clinical standards (Chaet, Clearfield, Sabin, & Skimming, 2017). Duties to clients include, but are not limited to, always acting in the best interest or well-being of the client, respecting clients' privacy and dignity, providing clients with relevant and appropriate information in an accessible and easy to understand format, and maintaining confidentiality at all times as required by the National Health Act (No. 61 of 2003) and the National Patients' Rights Charter.

These duties are in keeping with the principles of the Constitution of the Republic of South Africa (Act No. 108 of 1996) and the obligation imposed on health care practitioners by law. The Bill of Rights, contained in chapter 2 of the Constitution, embodies the basic principles fundamental to the ethics of health care. The Department of Health, in consultation with various other bodies, developed the National Patients' Rights Charter to ensure the realisation of the right of access to health care services (HPCSA, 2016c).

The philosophy of primary health care and its call for 'health for all' was adopted by South Africa in 1994 (Naledi, Barron, & Schneider, 2011). The philosophy forms the basis of South Africa's health policy and is based on the understanding that the solutions to major health problems lie not only in science, but also in the quest for social justice and the improvement of the life of the poor. It also asserts that health and access to health care are fundamental human rights, and supports the promotion of good health, interdisciplinary and intersectoral collaboration in health matters, along with equitable access to health care that is client-centred, acceptable, affordable and sustainable (O'Hare, 2018). It is important that health care services are available and accessible to all communities in South Africa so that they can receive these services when needed, without undue burden. In some cases, audiology services may be available within a community or geographical region, such as in large metros, but remain inaccessible to many people because of inadequate transportation. The internet and other technologies make it easier to provide audiological information and services over long distances, thereby minimising the obstacle of geography. Consequently, tele-audiology has the potential to reduce the burdens associated with the accessibility of services.

However, a lack of financial resources will be a challenge for many clients if they are required to purchase computers, telephones and other devices on which most tele-audiology services depend. The unavailability or inaccessibility of information and communication technology is a serious health care justice concern. An ethical issue related to justice and inequality may arise if certain clients are deprived of tele-audiology due to a lack of knowledge or the required technology, such as the internet or smartphones, alongside limited internet coverage and bandwidth (Langarizadeh, Moghbeli, & Aliabadi, 2017). This is true for many areas of rural South Africa, posing a particular dilemma: the remote areas most in need of tele-audiology are often the areas without the necessary telecommunication coverage.

The main ethical challenges related to tele-audiology in EHDI have bearing on the National Patients' Rights Charter, specifically informed consent, continuity of care, confidentiality and privacy as well as access to health care, including treatment and rehabilitation, provision of special needs to newborn infants, counselling and health information (ASHA, 2010; Denton & Gladstone, 2005; HPCSA, 2008). The core ethical values outlined in the HPCSA guidelines are important and clinically applicable in tele-audiology. Figure 13.1 shows the legal and ethical aspects generally related to tele-audiology. The top row lists the core ethical values and standards for good practice as outlined by the HPCSA (2016a). Specific aspects, marked with a star (☆), are discussed in more detail below: licensure, competence, privacy and confidentiality, informed consent, evaluating effectiveness of services in terms of programme validation, and reimbursement (fees) for services.

Licensure

The primary purpose of professional regulation is consumer protection, which is performed through licensure laws, and countries establish their own licensing statutes, rules and regulations. In South Africa, audiologists are governed by the HPCSA, a statutory body established by the Health Professions Act (Dhai & McQuoid-Mason, 2011). It is audiologists' responsibility to be familiar with the specific laws, regulations and scope of practice documents under which they operate. The HPCSA guidelines are comprehensive and in line with the South African Constitution, placing the client at the centre of health care practice. In South Africa, only audiologists registered with the HPCSA are authorised to perform audiological services (including tele-audiology), irrespective of whether these are in the capacity of consulting or servicing (HPCSA, 2014). In the case of tele-audiology across country borders, audiologists serving South African clients should be registered with the regulating bodies in their original countries as well as with the HPCSA. The reverse is also true for South African audiologists who provide services in other countries.

ETHICS IN TELE-AUDIOLOGY (HPCSA BOOKLET 10)

Non-maleficence Beneficence Human Rights Autonomy Integrity Truthfulness Conflict of interest Access Natural duties Moral obligations Institutional duties Legal duties Compassion Tolerance Competence Self-improvement Community betterment Referrals Professional practice Informed consent Justice Privacy Confidentiality Respect

LEGAL OBLIGATION (HPCSA BOOKLET 3)	SERVICE (HPCSA BOOKLET 5, 9, 11)	RESEARCH AND PUBLICATION (HPCSA BOOKLET 4, 13, 15)	RESOLVING ETHICS ISSUES (HPCSA BOOKLET 2)	PUBLIC STATEMENTS (HPCSA BOOKLET 2, 5)	HUMAN RELATIONS (HPCSA BOOKLET 4, 5)
1. Constitution of the Republic of South Africa, 1996 (Act No. 108 of 1996) – Chapter 2: Bill of Rights 2. Protection of Personal Information Act, 2013 (Act No. 4 of 2013) – National Patients' Right Charter 3. Health Professionals Act, 1974 (Act No. 56 of 1974) – Licensure ☆ 4. National Health Act, 2003 (Act No. 61 of 2003) – Confidentiality ☆ 5. Children's Act, 2005 (Act No. 38 of 2005)	1. Record keeping & fees ☆ – Maintenance of record – Confidentiality – Fees 2. Assessment & treatment – Informed consent ☆ – Evaluating effectiveness ☆ – Avoiding guarantees – Avoiding injury 3. Competence ☆ – Service provision – Referral – Delegation – Maintaining competence	1. Informed consent 2. Avoid injury 3. Accepted standards	1. Prohibit and report ethical violations 2. Cooperation with Ethical Board 3. Non-violation	1. Avoiding misrepresentation 2. Reporting information	1. Privacy/confidentiality ☆ 2. Informed consent ☆ 3. Discrimination 4. Conflict of interest 5. Exploitation 6. Professional relationship 7. Dishonesty/illegal conduct

Source: Adapted from HPCSA, 2016a

Figure 13.1 General and specific ethical guidelines and rules for tele-audiology

Competence

Competence is the ability to provide a level of care according to a set standard and according to the professional's code of ethics (Aiken, 2002). The legal term *imperitia culpae adnumeratur*, referred to in South African law as the Imperitia Rule, is applicable (Dutton, 2015). It states that it is negligent to engage in any assessment or treatment unless one has the skill and knowledge specified by the profession's professional body. Audiologists should continually endeavour to attain the highest level of knowledge and skills required in their area of practice, while acknowledging the limits of their professional knowledge and competence (HPCSA, 2008). The standards of competence are based on the ethical principles of beneficence (actively doing good) and non-maleficence (do no harm) (Knapp & VandeCreek, 2006). These principles imply that competence encompasses more than mere clinical skill. Additional aspects related to competence and tele-audiology include professional responsibility, clinical standards, technical competency and collaborating with colleagues in a professional manner.

Professional responsibility

Audiologists should not only be concerned with how to effectively and ethically deliver services but should also accept responsibility for deciding not to use a particular method or technique. Tele-audiology offers many advantages, including:

- effectively transmitting expertise over a distance to a client
- fostering protocol-defined assessment results that can be used by a range of related professionals, such as a teacher who may be working with the individual
- enhancing the effectiveness of outcomes through promoting the development of standards to meet the need for shared, common information between all the professionals involved in service delivery to the individual and the family.

If tele-audiology can increase the effectiveness of EHDI service delivery and audiologists actively choose not to utilise these services, they are causing harm to the client.

Another responsibility that audiologists bear when offering newborn hearing screening is to provide early intervention services (Olusanya, Luxon, & Wirz, 2006). Ethical issues arise when a diagnosis is made but treatment or management cannot be provided. Knowing that a newborn has a hearing loss without being able to provide treatment and management of the hearing loss is unethical. Therefore, in order to implement a screening programme, some form of intervention or collaboration with other initiatives needs to be available. An example is Worldwide Hearing Care for Developing Countries. This global initiative uses the framework of the World Health Organization's

(WHO) *Guidelines for Hearing Aids and Services for Developing Countries*, which was launched in 2001. One of its main purposes is to provide appropriate and affordable amplification and hearing services.

However, Olusanya et al. (2006, p. 590) ask an important question: 'Should limited intervention services forestall early detection of hearing?' They argue that failure to implement a screening protocol because of current shortages in service delivery may be counterproductive for requisite capacity-building as suggested by the WHO (2001), as a solution to deal with the current resource gap. In addition, they argue that not knowing what is 'wrong' with a child may lead parents to take incorrect actions, thereby causing additional stress to the family (Olusanya et al., 2006).

Rather than taking an all-or-nothing approach, one possible solution could be to share information and knowledge about available resources and support services, thereby providing the best available services at the time, while also explaining these limitations to the parents. Open communication and autonomy are key to providing ethical services.

Clinical standards

Policies and procedures for documentation, maintenance and transmission of records regarding tele-audiology consultations should be maintained at the same standards of care expected in traditional delivery methods. For example, it could be tempting to use online questionnaires to replace taking a documented clinical history, but this does not constitute an acceptable standard of care (HPCSA, 2014). Tele-audiology should focus on providing clients with new avenues to access services and not on capitalising on potential short cuts offered by technology.

Technical competence

The requirement that audiologists be competent regarding tele-audiology technology is embodied in ethical principles. Audiologists should hold the client's welfare paramount, provide services only when reasonable benefit can be expected, ensure that all equipment used in the provision of services is calibrated and working accurately, and not provide services that exceed their level of education, training and experience (ASHA, 2003). The importance of technical competence cannot be overstated. An audiologist may be skilled in providing intervention for a particular disorder yet may not be competent to do so if the provision of those services requires the use of tele-audiology.

Audiologists should be able to judge whether tele-audiology is the best available option for service delivery. At a minimum, this requires the ability to assess whether the anticipated technology and equipment is of sufficiently high quality, meets the recognised technical standards and is operating satisfactorily. Back-up systems should be available. Quality assessment of the technology employed must be an ongoing process, and routine controls and calibration should be available to monitor the accuracy and quality of data collected and transmitted. At all times, well-established procedures should be in place in the event of equipment failure or if a technical problem arises at the client's remote location.

Finally, even if the audiologist is competent to provide services via tele-practice, the client may not be competent to receive services in this manner. Therefore, the audiologist needs to assess what technical competencies the client needs to have given the type of technology to be used. It is also the audiologist's responsibility to ensure that the client is adequately trained in the procedures for tele-practice, is physically and cognitively capable of carrying out these procedures and fully accepts the process. With EHDI services, it is important that these considerations apply to all family members who are involved in assessment and intervention.

Working with colleagues

Other audiologists or assistants need to be considered. It is good clinical practice to document the roles and responsibilities of each party before starting the process. Both consulting and servicing audiologists are responsible for establishing the competency of the other party before agreeing to participate in tele-audiology activities. Both parties are responsible for detailed record taking and record keeping. If an audiologist makes use of support personnel, they should be cognisant of the fact that no matter where the assistant is located, the treating audiologist is solely responsible for the assistant's conduct.

If an audiologist who provides tele-audiology services employs a colleague or a locum with minimal or no experience with the relevant procedures and technology, the practice owner remains fully responsible for all tele-audiology services offered. This will increase their supervisory responsibility towards the new employee. Similarly, when an audiologist takes leave and arranges a locum, it is the audiologist's responsibility to ensure that the locum is competent in terms of tele-audiology technology.

Figure 13.2 provides a checklist to guide the audiologist in factors to consider when reviewing competence in providing tele-audiology services to the paediatric population.

Privacy and confidentiality

The terms 'privacy' and 'confidentiality' are often used interchangeably in everyday language. However, they have distinctly different meanings from a health professions and legal standpoint. The right to privacy is constitutionally and statutorily protected in the National Health Act. Common law also recognises a right to privacy related to medical malpractice, with specific reference to the unlawful publication of private facts about a person (Dutton, 2015).

Category	Statement	√/x
Equipment	I have OAE equipment I have a high-frequency probe tone for tympanometry I have an ABR unit with click, tone burst and bone conduction I have a real ear analyser with RECD capability I have hearing aid software and supplies designed for this population I have a loaner hearing aid programme	
Referrals	I know when to refer following a hearing assessment I know who to refer to following the identification of a hearing loss I can identify the professional team needed I know the reporting requirements I know the recommended timeframe I know what resources are available to the client	
Expertise	I have training and experience in all components of the infant test battery I have training and experience in all aspects of the amplification process for this population I have the requisite knowledge and skills to service this population I have identified my learning gaps in terms of knowledge and skills and identified resources to update my knowledge and skills to competently service this population	
Service provision	I am familiar with the guidelines and position statements applicable to serving this population I am aware of and responsive to a family's needs for support I utilise family-centred practices	

Figure 13.2 Checklist for ethical decision-making in tele-audiology service delivery

Source: Authors

Medical confidentiality relates to the public disclosure of private medical facts. The basis of medical confidentiality is twofold: while it protects the privacy of the patient, it also performs a public interest function.

Audiologists have an ethical as well as legal duty to protect clients' privacy and confidentiality at all times. Tele-audiology poses new challenges in terms of ensuring the confidentiality of clients' information and increasing data security while receiving, storing and transferring the data (Langarizadeh et al., 2017). Confidentiality and privacy are also closely related to veracity and truth telling (Pera & Van Tonder, 2011). A confidential and fiduciary relationship, which is central to trust between the audiologist and the client, arises whenever one person entrusts confidential information to another. Without confidentiality and trust, clients may be reluctant to provide audiologists with the necessary information for efficient assessment, differential diagnosis and effective management. It is the audiologist's task to understand how the fundamental responsibilities of trust, respect and confidentiality play out differently in the context of tele-audiology when compared to the more traditional in-person client–audiologist interaction (Chaet et al., 2017).

Confidentiality comes into play with respect to the personal information shared by clients. The audiologist–client relationship establishes an implied contract of confidentiality, since audiologists need to collect and analyse private information to help clients. Clients have a right to expect that this type of information will be held in confidence. Audiologists are therefore also directly responsible for ensuring that all employees respect confidentiality in the performance of their duties. Anyone receiving personal information in order to provide care is bound by the legal duty of confidentiality, regardless of contractual or professional obligations to protect confidentiality. The additional duties on audiologists to obtain consent and to anonymise data are consistent with the provisions of the National Health Act, which states that all clients have a right to confidentiality, and that information should not be given to others unless the client consents or the audiologist can justify the disclosure. The HPCSA (2016c) guides audiologists in terms of situations that justify divulging information.

Privacy refers to the freedom from intrusion into one's personal matters and information and is constitutionally and statutorily protected (Grace, 2009). As outlined in the Protection of Personal Information Act (No. 4 of 2013), it includes a right to protection against the unlawful collection, retention, dissemination and use of personal information. Although a client voluntarily relinquishes some of their privacy to an audiologist, this does not imply that the client gives up all right to privacy as described in Section 14 of the Constitution (Act No. 108 of 1996), the National Health Act and the Children's Act (No. 38 of 2005).

The Protection of Personal Information Act addresses clients' protected health information and requires that all services (including via tele-audiology) protect the privacy of clients by using secure systems for electronic information. It is audiologists' responsibility to ensure the same level of confidentiality in delivering services, whether via tele-audiology or face-to-face on-site appointments. Three primary aspects of tele-audiology are susceptible to privacy threats.

The first relates to the observation of 'live' tele-audiology sessions. Just as an audiologist would need to obtain consent from clients, or parents in the case of EHDI, for students or other providers to observe a client–audiologist session, informed consent should also be obtained prior to observing a tele-audiology session. The tele-audiology provider should also be located in a private room to prevent unauthorised persons from viewing the session.

Secondly, technology used during tele-audiology makes it easy to record sessions with a client, thereby creating a potential privacy threat. Again, it is the responsibility of the audiologist implementing the tele-audiology session to ensure that the video recordings of sessions are secure from being viewed by unauthorised persons. Security is often raised as a concern with regard to possible hacking or gaining access to the two-way exchange. Hacking, computer viruses and worms are all threats to security (Houston & Behl, 2019). While some technologies may be less susceptible to security breaches, none are immune. The integrity and privacy protection of a client's personal and health information is a high priority in all aspects of health care and no less so in tele-audiology applications. Most EHDI programmes and telehealth networks will already have policies and procedures in place to ensure client confidentiality. Most remote access software includes strong encryption. Moreover, the host computer will typically not contain client data. Although the host site may track the number of tests performed for statistical and billing purposes, it should not record client information. However, caution should be exercised when an existing network or virtual private network is used to connect sites, as the remote laptop or personal computer that is linked directly to the test equipment (such as in the case of AABR and OAE assessment) will contain client data files. This equipment can be lost or stolen. In many jurisdictions, the consequences of such loss are expensive and problematic if the lost or stolen device contains client-identifying information. To prevent inappropriate access to personal information, it may be prudent to assign a unique identifier to each client file that relates to a separate identification/contact information file maintained at a central site (such as the infant's regional EHDI agency). The actual file will contain the client's demographic data while the code in the software will merely be a file identifier. Screen capture software may record the actual test for later training and evaluation purposes, but client information is not visible. The case manager must establish who is responsible for maintaining the client file and for reporting test results.

Thirdly, it is important to abide by privacy regulations when sharing recordings with other providers. Audiologists should obtain signed informed consent from the parents or legal guardians to record sessions to ensure that they are aware that recordings exist. They can also obtain copies of recordings if needed. In fact, one benefit of video recording is that parents can share their child's progress and coaching strategies with others. It is as important to secure access to these recordings as it is to secure written records or verbal communications, for example by using a password protected, encrypted site (Houston, Behl, & Seroka, 2017). It is also important for audiologists to remember that no information about clients can be made available for research or review unless the client has specifically given informed consent (HPCSA, 2016b). Furthermore, appropriate security for storing recordings should be considered. If an audiologist is not familiar with network security, they should take appropriate authoritative professional advice on how to keep information secure before connecting to a network. The HPCSA recommends that such consultations and advice from other professionals be documented (HPCSA, 2016c).

Duty to inform and informed consent

The recognition of clients' rights, specifically autonomy, became more widespread during the twentieth century. This resulted in increased emphasis on the client's right to decide whether or not a particular assessment or intervention should occur. This shift has been described as a move away from the professional standards of disclosure approach to a client-based approach (Dutton, 2015).

Informed consent involves a social relationship between laypeople and health care practitioners built upon complex layers of mutual loyalty, fidelity, respect and support (Dutton, 2015). The sometimes close and overlapping relationships between ethics and the law necessitate that the legal requirements underlying consent be considered. Section 7(3) of the National Health Act defines informed consent as permission for the provision of a specified health service given by a client with the necessary capacity to do so, and who has been informed as detailed in Section 6 of that Act. Applying the information in that Act to audiology implies that the family should be informed of the following:

- the range of diagnostic procedures and treatment options available to the client
- the benefits, risks, costs and consequences associated with each option
- the differences between tele-audiology and services delivered face-to-face on-site
- the client's right to refuse services.

As noted, a successful relationship between an audiologist and a client depends upon mutual trust. Establishing trust can only be achieved if the audiologist respects the client's autonomy. Sufficient information should be provided in a clear and understandable way to enable clients to exercise their right to make informed decisions about their care. This is what informed consent means. The right to informed consent flows from the South African Constitution, the National Health Act, common law and the HPCSA (2016b) guidelines, which address this topic in detail. Here, we touch only on issues implicitly related to tele-audiology.

Booklet 10 of the *Ethical Guidelines for Good Practice* (HPCSA, 2014) specifies that informed consent for the use of telemedicine technologies should be obtained in writing from the client. Figure 13.3 shows an example of the information to be included in informed consent documentation.

Consent can be regarded as a cornerstone of health care, from a legal as well as ethical point of view (Kakar, Gambhir, Singh, Kaur, & Nanda, 2014). The concept goes to the heart of the audiologist–client relationship, as the audiologist does not hold the power to decide what is in the client's best interest. Rather, the audiologist is in the position of serving the client and, in EHDI, the family. The essence of the relationship is respect for the client's autonomy, and protection of individual rights to bodily integrity, privacy and dignity.

Programme validation

An important consideration in any method of providing audiology services, including tele-audiology, is the reliability and validity of the results. That is, will tele-audiology have the same results that on-site testing would provide?

NKOSI & ENSLIN AUDIOLOGY

4567 Main Street, Lyttleton, 0027 Tel: 012 348 0000

CONSENT FOR TELE-AUDIOLOGY SERVICES

Tele-audiology is the use of electronic information and telecommunications technologies to support remote and distance clinical hearing health care

Patient Name: Mr Johannes Maphakela

Patient Address: 189 Logan Street, ...

Consultation Site: ABC clinic

Servicing Audiologist: Ms Sara Nkosi AUxxxxxxxx

I, Mr Johannes Maphakela, consent to the use of tele-audiology for the following services:

O **Appointment scheduling**   O **Interviewing**   O **Audiological assessment**

O **Feedback/result sharing**   O **Therapy/rehabilitation** O **Hearing aid adjustments**

O **Education/informative**   O **Other**_____

I, Mr Johannes Maphakela, agree that the appropriateness of tele-audiology will be determined by Ms Sara Nkosi. I consent to consultations being recorded. Yes ....   No ....

Ms Sara Nkosi commits to the following security measures to be implemented, namely:

O Data encryption   O Password protected screen savers and data files   O Firewall

Confidentiality will be compromised in the following situations:

Information requested by professional organisations and government regulatory bodies.

If your health or life is at risk, as well as in the interest of public health.

I, Mr Johannes Maphakela, give express consent for the transmission of personal medical information to the consulting health care practitioner, Ms Sara Nkosi, as well as the staff employed by this audiology practice.

The cost of these services is detailed below:

Session 1: Procedure A = R87.65   Procedure B = R127.33

Signature Patient   Signature Witness   Signature Audiologist

Figure 13.3 Example of informed consent documentation related to telemedicine practice

Source: Authors

Ensuring that the test and procedures are reliable and valid leads to a successful tele-audiology programme. The AAA (2008) states that all services should be validated by research before implementation in practice.

Validation of practice is a basic tenet of audiology and of EHDI programme protocol. However, the reality of validation is difficult in terms of proving real equivalence. Certain aspects relating to clinical practices are relatively easily validated, such as showing that remote interpretation of infant ABR assessment data is equivalent to an on-site face-to-face assessment (HPCSA, 2014). However, not all facets of service delivery lend themselves readily and equally to validation, an example being the experience of the child's parent during the actual test procedure and the communication of a diagnosis following an infant assessment. While tele-audiology may be ideal for hearing screening or diagnostic testing, some services, like hearing aid fitting and rehabilitation, are more challenging and require a different approach (Nemes, 2010).

Another important consideration when providing audiologic services is determining client satisfaction and the effectiveness of the services provided. The same applies for tele-audiology services. There is increasing support for the use of patient-reported outcome measures (PROMs) and patient-reported experience measures (PREMs) to measure the quality of care, clinical effectiveness, safety and client experience, as well as to guide service improvement (Kingsley & Patel, 2017). PROMs are standardised, validated questionnaires that are completed by the client to ascertain their perceived level of impairment, disability and health-related quality of life. It is a means of measuring clinical effectiveness from the client's perspective. PREMs, on the other hand, gather information on clients' views of their experience while receiving care. They provide an indicator of the quality of care from the client's perspective and can be either relational or functional. Relational PREMs identify clients' experience of their relationship with the health care practitioner, for example if they felt listened to. Consideration of the parental experience during tele-audiology service delivery can provide the audiologist with guidance on how to facilitate a client-centred approach. Functional PREMs focus more on practical issues such as the facilities available. Both PROMs and PREMs can easily be completed via online methods, increasing their value and applicability in tele-audiology.

Tele-audiology is a new area and although the research base is steadily growing, many questions remain unanswered. When establishing tele-audiology services as part of an EHDI programme, administrators and clinicians are advised to carefully review and examine practices to ensure effectiveness and efficiency (Krumm, 2010).

Reimbursement for services

Reimbursement is currently one of the most challenging aspects of implementing a sustainable tele-audiology programme in South Africa, as there are no standards for compensation in private practice. Specific procedural codes to claim from the client's medical aid are not available. As a profession, audiologists need to raise awareness of the value and applicability of tele-audiology service options and advocate these services to medical aid boards. There is a need for evidence to prove that tele-audiology services are reasonable, reliable and cost-effective, especially when the client is unable to physically visit an audiologist. Coding is more complex for the consulting audiologist than for the servicing audiologist, who can use standard available service delivery codes. In the long run, tele-audiology programmes require reliable, adequate revenue and reimbursement for clinical services. All fees should be discussed with the client in advance to ensure transparency and informed consent.

The public health sector does not face the same concerns related to procedural codes, but does face its own unique challenges. Firstly, the public health sector is under pressure to deliver services to over 80 percent of the population (Brand South Africa, 2012). These services have to be delivered despite a misalignment between resources and need (Global Health Workforce Alliance, 2008). The shortage of audiologists and equipment requires a reform plan to revitalise and restructure audiology departments to be able to offer tele-audiology. Secondly, provincial health departments provide and manage health services via a district-based, public health care model. This implies that clients who meet geographical criteria according to a catchment area may register for health care services. Tele-audiology, also focused on minimising the barrier of geography, would in the current structure only be available to clients within the catchment area. Implementation of tele-audiology requires a comprehensive planning assessment, including surveys of the population, workforce, transportation systems, expansion opportunities as well as consultation with key stakeholders in the target community to set priorities for a potential intervention (AlDossary, Martin-Khan, Bradford, Armfield, & Smith, 2017).

Risk management

Tele-audiology is an emerging technology and means of service delivery. The law regarding many of its aspects will only become known as disputes arise and when court judgments are delivered. For this reason, risk management forms an important part of the tele-audiology process. A number of steps can be followed as a strategy to minimise legal risk and create a safe environment for both the audiologist and the client:

- Consult with legal counsel. The South African Association of Audiology (SAAA) has partnered with the brokers Cover for Professionals (CFP) to provide audiologists with affordable malpractice insurance. Other insurance options are also available and more information can be obtained from SAAA or the South African Speech-Language-Hearing Association (SASLHA). Once registered, an attorney will be able to assist the audiologist in identifying and minimising risk. Audiologists should not assume that they are practising good risk management simply by providing the same standard of care when employing tele-audiology as they do when they render on-site services. Legal counsel can analyse all aspects of an audiologist's tele-practice services related to duty of care, standard of care, jurisdiction, as well as the risks associated with the use of the technology.

- Notify insurance carriers if plans exist to initiate tele-practice.
- Ensure proficiency with technology: understand the minimum specifications for the technology and keep up with changes in capabilities and specifications (Dutton, 2015).
- Ensure the appropriacy of tele-audiology to the situation by documenting the benefits considered during decision-making.
- Educate clients on the benefits and limitations of tele-audiology. Recognise when the usefulness of a tele-audiology approach has been exhausted.
- Refer or schedule an on-site face-to-face consultation if tele-audiology does not provide an adequate assessment or if results are ambiguous.
- Set realistic expectations for all parties.
- Clarify contractual issues, including those with equipment vendors and manufacturers.
- Maintain an archive of equipment in use, which includes a system for performing and archiving backups.
- Personalise the tele-audiology encounter as much as possible.
- Document everything, including the equipment used, the resolution, as well as who participated and for what reason (Hall, 2020).

Conclusion

Audiologists have an obligation to provide services to those in need of audiological assessment or intervention. Tele-audiology is a valid and appropriate method of reaching those in need who would otherwise have difficulty in accessing audiologic services. With continuous and fast-paced changes and developments in technology, a variety of options and advances in tele-audiology enhance its appeal. However, tele-audiology is certainly not without its limitations and difficulties.

Despite some inherent challenges, the opportunities for beneficial utilisation of tele-audiology applications in EHDI programmes are numerous. Programmes may adopt EHDI in the context of tele-audiology to deliver many of the standard clinical service components, including screening, initial diagnostic assessments, behavioural assessment, hearing aid and cochlear implant programming, and communication development options. Tele-audiology in the context of EHDI can also make important contributions to many facets of programme infrastructure, including communication, training and quality management.

Audiology as a profession should work towards a sound evidence base for EHDI via tele-audiology, where the client's experience should be similar to services delivered face-to-face. Not only can tele-audiology serve to increase access to services but it can also facilitate a calibrated standard of practice across a programme so that all children and their families receive the best possible service.

References

Aiken, L. H. (2002). Superior outcomes for magnet hospitals: The evidence base. In M. L. McClure & A. S. Hinshaw (Eds.), *Magnet hospitals revisited: Attraction and retention of professional nurses* (pp. 61–81). Washington, DC: American Nurses Publishing.

AlDossary, S., Martin-Khan, M. G., Bradford, N. K., Armfield, N. R., & Smith A. C. (2017). The development of a telemedicine planning framework based on needs assessment. *Journal of Medical Systems, 41*(5), 74.

American Academy of Audiology (AAA). (2008). The use of telehealth/telemedicine to provide audiology services. Retrieved from http://audiology-web.s3.amazonaws.com/migrated/TelehealthResolution200806.pdf_5386d9f33fd359.83214228.pdf.

American Speech-Language-Hearing Association (ASHA). (2001). Telepractices and ASHA: Report of the telepractices team. Retrieved from https://www.asha.org/policy/PS2005-00029.htm.

American Speech-Language-Hearing Association (ASHA). (2003). Code of ethics. Retrieved from https://asha.org/policy.

American Speech-Language-Hearing Association (ASHA). (2005). Audiologists providing clinical services via telepractice: Position statement. Retrieved from https://www.asha.org/policy/PS2005-00029.htm.

American Speech-Language-Hearing Association (ASHA). (2010). Professional issues in telepractice for speech-language pathologists (professional issues statement). Retrieved from http://www.asha.org/policy.

Brand South Africa. (2012). Health care in South Africa. Retrieved from https://www.brandsouthafrica.com/south-africa-fast-facts/health-facts/health-care-in-south-africa.

Bust, M., Hardin, B., Rayle, C., Lester, C., Studts, C., & Shinn, J. (2015). Rural barriers to early diagnosis and treatment of infant hearing loss in Appalachia. *Otology and Neurotology, 36*(1), 93–98.

Cavalcanti, H. G., & Guerra, R. O. (2012). The role of maternal socioeconomic factors in the commitment to universal newborn hearing screening in the northeastern region of Brazil. *International Journal of Pediatric Otorhinolaryngology, 76*(11), 1661–1667.

Chadha, S., & Stevens, G. (2013). Editorial: Promoting ear and hearing care: The WHO perspective. *Hearing Journal, 66*(9), 2.

Chaet, D., Clearfield, R., Sabin, J. E., & Skimming, K. (2017). Ethical practice in telehealth and telemedicine. *Journal of General Internal Medicine, 32*(10), 1136–1140.

Denton, D., & Gladstone, V. (2005). Ethical and legal issues related to telepractice. *Seminars in Hearing, 26*(1), 43–52.

Dhai, A., & McQuoid-Mason, D. (2011). *Bioethics, human rights and health law: Principles and practices (1st ed.)*. Cape Town, South Africa: Juta.

Doković, S., Gligorović, M., Ostojić, S., Dimić, N., Radić-Šestić, M., & Slavnić, S. (2014). Can mild bilateral sensorineural hearing loss affect developmental abilities in younger school-age children? *Journal of Deaf Studies and Deaf Education, 19*(4), 484–495.

Dutton, I. (2015). *The practitioner's guide to medical malpractice in South African law*. Cape Town, South Africa: Siber Ink.

Fleming, D. A., Edison, K. E., & Pak, H. (2009). Telehealth ethics. *Telemed Journal and E-Health, 15*(8), 797–803.

Global Health Workforce Alliance. (2008). Scaling up, saving lives: Task force for scaling up education and training for health workers. Retrieved from https://www.who.int/workforcealliance/documents/Global_Health_FINAL_REPORT.pdf?ua=1.

Grace, P. J. (2009). *Nursing ethics and professional responsibility in advanced practice*. Boston, MA: Jones and Barlett.

Hall, J. W. (2020). Professional liability and teleaudiology services. *The Hearing Journal, 73*(6), 18–19. Retrieved from https://journals.lww.com/thehearingjournal/fulltext/2020/06000/professional_liability_and_teleaudiology_services.6.aspx.

Health Professions Council of South Africa (HPCSA). (2008). Ethical guidelines for good practice in the health care professions: National Patients' Rights Charter (Booklet 3). Retrieved from https://www.hpcsa.co.za/Uploads/Professional_Practice/Ethics_Booklet.pdf.

Health Professions Council of South Africa (HPCSA). (2014). Ethical guidelines for good practice in the health care professions: Guidelines for the practice of telemedicine (Booklet 10). Retrieved from https://www.hpcsa.co.za/Uploads/Professional_Practice/Ethics_Booklet.pdf.

Health Professions Council of South Africa (HPCSA). (2016a). Ethical guidelines for good practice in the health care professions: General ethical guidelines for health care professions (Booklet 1). Retrieved from https://www.hpcsa.co.za/Uploads/Professional_Practice/Ethics_Booklet.pdf.

Health Professions Council of South Africa (HPCSA). (2016b). Ethical guidelines for good practice in the health care professions: Seeking patients' informed consent: The ethical considerations (Booklet 4). Retrieved from https://www.hpcsa.co.za/Uploads/Professional_Practice/Ethics_Booklet.pdf.

Health Professions Council of South Africa (HPCSA). (2016c). Ethical guidelines for good practice in the health care professions: Confidentiality: Protecting and providing information (Booklet 5). Retrieved from https://www.hpcsa.co.za/Uploads/Professional_Practice/Ethics_Booklet.pdf.

Houston, K. T., & Behl, D. (2019). Using telepractice to improve outcomes for children who are deaf or hard of hearing and their families. In *The NCHAM e-book: A resource guide for early hearing detection and intervention*. Retrieved from http://infanthearing.org/ehdi-ebook/2019_ebook/17%20Chapter17UsingTelepractice2019.pdf.

Houston, K. T., Behl, D., & Seroka, K. (2017). Using telepractice to improve outcomes for children who are deaf or hard of hearing and their families. In *The NCHAM e-book: A resource guide for early hearing detection and intervention.* Retrieved from http://www.infanthearing.org/ehdi-ebook/2017_ebook/18%20Chapter18UsingTelepractice2017.pdf.

Joint Committee on Infant Hearing (JCIH). (2007). Year 2007 position statement: Principles and guidelines for early hearing detection and intervention. Retrieved from www.asha.org/policy.

Kakar, H., Gambhir, R. S., Singh, S., Kaur, A., & Nanda, T. (2014). Informed consent: Corner stone in ethical medical and dental practice. *Journal of Family Medicine and Primary Care, 3*(1), 68–71.

Kingsley, C., & Patel, S. (2017). Patient-reported outcome measures and patient-reported experience measures. *British Journal of Anaesthesia, 17*(4), 137–144.

Knapp, S. J., & VandeCreek (Eds.), L. D. (2006). Remedial and positive ethics. In S. J. Knapp & L. D. VandeCreek, *Practical ethics for psychologists: A positive approach* (pp. 3–14). American Psychological Association. https://doi.org/10.1037/11331-001.

Krumm, M. (2010). Emerging applications in teleaudiology. *Starkey Audiology Series, 2*(2), 1–4.

Langarizadeh, M., Moghbeli, F., & Aliabadi, A. (2017). Application of ethics for providing telemedicine services and information technology. *Medical Archives (Sarajevo, Bosnia and Herzegovina), 71*(5), 351–355.

Lester, E. B., Dawson, J. D., Gantz, F. J., & Hansen, M. R. (2011). Barriers to the early cochlear implantation of deaf children. *Otology and Neurotology, 32*(3), 406–412.

Merugumala, S. V., Pothula, V., & Cooper, M. (2017). Barriers to timely diagnosis and treatment for children with hearing impairment in a southern Indian city: A qualitative study of parents and clinic staff. *International Journal of Audiology, 56*(10), 733–739.

Naledi, T., Barron, P., & Schneider, H. (2011). Primary healthcare in SA since 1994 and implications of the new vision for PHC re-engineering. In A. Padarath & R. English (Eds.), *South African Health Review* (pp. 17–28). Durban, South Africa: Health Systems Trust.

Nemes, J. (2010). Tele-audiology, a once-futuristic concept, is growing into a worldwide reality. *Hearing Journal, 63*(2), 19–24.

O'Hare, D. (2018). Primary healthcare revered and revisited. Retrieved from https://www.news.uct.ac.za/article/-2018-08-20-primary-healthcare-revered-and-revisited.

Olusanya, B. O., Luxon, L. M., & Wirz, S. L. (2006). Ethical issues in screening for hearing impairment in newborns in developing countries. *Journal of Medical Ethics, 32*(10), 588–591.

Olusanya, B. O., Neumann, K. J., & Saunders, J. E. (2014). The global burden of disabling hearing impairment: A call to action. *Bulletin of the World Health Organization, 92*(5), 367–373.

Pera, S., & Van Tonder, S. (2011). *Ethics in healthcare (3rd ed.).* Lansdowne, South Africa: Juta.

Swanepoel, W., Olusanya, B. O., & Mars, M. (2010). Hearing health-care delivery in sub-Saharan Africa: A role for tele-audiology. *Journal of Telemedicine and Telecare*, *16*(2), 53–56.

World Health Organization (WHO). (2001). *Guidelines for hearing aids and services for developing countries*. Geneva, Switzerland: WHO.

14 Best Practice in South Africa for Early Hearing Detection and Intervention

Katijah Khoza-Shangase and Amisha Kanji

Sufficient evidence exists to support increased efforts towards early hearing detection and intervention (EHDI) in South Africa. Regardless of the proven benefit of EHDI for the hearing impaired, its implementation remains difficult due to the numerous challenges that have been detailed in various chapters in this book. Confronting these challenges and ensuring successful EHDI programmes that are contextualised to South African realities is important. This chapter provides recommendations, inspired by evidence emanating from earlier chapters, for EHDI implementation. These recommendations take cognisance of the environment to allow for best or next practice. We advance recommendations for EHDI in sub-Saharan Africa, with a special focus on South Africa, bearing in mind the various levels of service delivery in that country's health care setting. We make suggestions around how to confront the realities impacting EHDI implementation in this context, including contextualisation of risk factors for hearing impairment and deliberations on EHDI in the educational context. Furthermore, we offer proposals on how to deal with South African complexities around EHDI, such as EHDI in the context of other sensory impairments, family-centred EHDI, EHDI in the context of HIV/AIDS (burden of disease), as well as how to engage with EHDI in the context of tele-audiology.

A significant number of hearing-impaired children in South Africa will continue to have their rights denied until EHDI is incorporated as part of a cohesive, systematic and comprehensive nationalised health care strategy that is contextually responsive and relevant (Kanji, Khoza-Shangase, Petrocchi-Bartal, & Harbinson, 2018; Khoza-Shangase, Kanji, Petrocchi-Bartal, & Farr, 2017). We strongly believe that ear and hearing health care practitioners bear the ethical responsibility to ensure that the rights of hearing-impaired children are upheld through best practice in EHDI.

EHDI is the gold standard for any practising audiologist and for the families of infants and children with hearing impairment. EHDI programmes aim to identify, diagnose and provide intervention to children with hearing impairment (as well as those at risk for hearing impairment) by six months of age to ensure that they develop and achieve in line with their hearing peers. EHDI remains a significant challenge for low and middle-income

(LAMI) countries, and in South Africa various initiatives are in place to address this gap in transferring theory into practice. The linguistic, cultural and socio-economic diversity of the South African context presents unique challenges to the academic teaching and research endeavours in this field, which prompted this book project. The South African government's heightened focus on increasing access to health care through the re-engineered primary health care (PHC) model and the National Health Insurance (NHI), as well as the early childhood development (ECD) programmes make this an opportune time for establishing and documenting evidence-based research for current undergraduate and postgraduate students. This book provides research-anchored and evidence-based information on EHDI, grounded in an African context. The chapters comprehensively cover both the detection and the intervention aspects of hearing impairment, paying careful attention to contextual relevance and responsiveness. Although the focus of the book is South Africa, contextual realities are similar across the whole of Africa, and parallels can be drawn for most LAMI countries.

EHDI implementation in African countries faces numerous challenges, key of which are resource constraints in terms of health care professionals and significant demand–capacity challenges. In some countries this picture of an overburdened health care system is exacerbated by a shortage of ear and hearing health care professionals in relation to the population that needs to be served. These challenges influence the implementation of early hearing detection services and adherence to the early hearing detection principles which are aimed at facilitating maximum potential in children presenting with hearing impairment. Hence, interim approaches to early hearing detection need to be explored in each context as health service delivery models may differ in each country. This exploration should include primary and middle-level workers in task-shifting models of delivery in newborn hearing screening (NHS), as well as the use of PHC settings to ensure universal coverage. Furthermore, innovative service delivery models such as the use of hybrid tele-audiology alongside task shifting may be the solution to increasing access to, and success of, EHDI programmes in Africa. This is particularly important, as the World Health Organization (WHO, 2018) estimates that more than 6.1 percent (approximately 466 million people) of the world's population lives with disabling hearing loss, with 7 percent (34 million) of them being children. Mulwafu, Kuper, and Ensink (2016) report that this prevalence is higher in sub-Saharan Africa than in other parts of the world.

Early detection of hearing impairment

Early detection of hearing impairment continues to be a challenge in the wider African context as well as in South Africa specifically. Key to addressing this issue is political will on the part of African governments and their departments of health in mandating universal newborn hearing screening (UNHS) and providing the resources required for the early detection of hearing impairment as part of programmatic planning, such as within the respective countries' ECD priorities. In chapter 2, Kanji argues that framing early hearing detection services under sustainable development goals (SDGs) that include indicators related to maternal, newborn and child health, and universal coverage may facilitate support from governments. This programmatic approach is also required for comprehensive implementation and sustainability of EHDI initiatives. Kanji posits that the use of foreign aid during the SDG period may be effective in supporting the implementation of UNHS services if mandated by governments.

Over and above procurement of appropriate screening equipment, serious planning is needed around the personnel required for the provision of ear and hearing health services in these contexts. Equipment that is sensitive and easy to use opens up opportunities for using non-professionals, as in task shifting, to increase the reach in contexts where professionals are not available. Increased training of audiologists and otorhinolaryngologists is recommended, as well as of mid-level workers such as audiology assistants and non-professionals (volunteers who can serve as screeners) in screening programmes managed by audiologists. Due to the documented shortage of audiologists in the African context, access to global human resources for supervision through tele-audiology should be seriously explored.

The training of non-professionals should adhere to minimum standards set out by regulating bodies such as the Health Professions Council of South Africa (HPCSA) and the Botswana Health Professions Council. In countries where such regulatory bodies and training institutions do not exist, South Africa could serve an advisory role and also share best practice. For example, audiologists need to engage with EHDI guidelines in their respective countries, and contextualise them to their contexts. In South Africa, one contextually responsive solution may be to begin with an approach to NHS that is not only feasible within the broader context, but per level of health care service delivery. Screening at both PHC and hospital level may increase coverage rates and facilitate the screening of both well babies and high-risk neonates. Each African country would need to engage with such factors to determine what is best for their context to ensure increased access and success of NHS programmes. In countries where audiologists or hearing health care services are limited or non-existent, South Africa needs to lead the way with possible solutions. These could include international collaborations in terms of training, as well as tele-supervision and tele-mentoring where the use of tele-practice could be explored within PHC levels of service delivery.

PHC re-engineering in contexts such as South Africa needs to be considered as a platform for early detection services, particularly as this strategy forms the cornerstone to addressing the social determinants of health (Scott, Schaay, Schneider, & Sanders, 2017). PHC also provides a commitment to universal health coverage and primary care, which are important when considering early detection of hearing impairment. In addition, a key emphasis on health reforms in resource-constrained contexts such as South Africa is ensuring the inclusion of not only curative but also preventative and promotive primary health services (Ataguba, Day, & McIntyre, 2015). Early detection of hearing impairment is thus important, particularly as it is a secondary prevention strategy within PHC service delivery.

In the resource-constrained African context, careful deliberations around approaches to early detection are imperative. They should take into consideration context and adopt a realist approach that aims for scaled, systematic implementation of screening programmes. Early detection of hearing impairment through NHS is the initial step to any EHDI programme. Although considered the gold standard worldwide, UNHS may not be feasible for some LAMI contexts, where contextual challenges to implementation exist. While UNHS is the goal that LAMI countries such as South Africa need to strive toward, attention needs to be paid to specific and local needs of the context. This will ensure that the approach to early detection is contextually relevant, realistic, appropriate and sustainable. 'As health care professionals we need to acknowledge the limitations but not allow it to preclude us from providing quality services within our means' (Kanji, 2018, p. 3). Targeted newborn hearing screening (TNHS) is a possible interim approach that may be implemented in such contexts.

Audiologists need to evaluate the contexts in which they work, and decide on the most suitable approach to early detection of hearing impairment. Once the chosen approach has been established, there needs to be consideration of how to develop the programme, including data capturing that allows for proper and accurate assessment and monitoring of the programme's efficacy, success and sustainability. Audiologists need to record data accurately in order to monitor the efficiency of programmes, document prevalence and incidence rates for hearing impairment and use the data to motivate for funding of the programme. This can only be done if the programme is evaluated regularly against key benchmarks specified in the regulating body's guidelines, such as the HPCSA (2018) EHDI guidelines. Audiologists should also share key challenges and successes of the programmes at appropriate forums in order to develop such programmes at provincial and national levels. Differences between levels of service delivery also need to be explored and tiered approaches may be necessary to ensure the highest possible coverage rate, while ensuring continuity of care within a migration-aware health care system. A migration-aware health system calls for a response to migration and health that acknowledges that people move internally within South Africa, and in the case of EHDI, that children move from sector to sector, which has implications for EHDI nationally. Continuity of care for the hearing-impaired child should be ensured for maximal benefit from EHDI initiatives.

The feasibility of implementing early detection of hearing impairment, in the form of infant hearing screening, at the various levels of health care service delivery in the South African context requires exploration. There are inherent inequities in the various health care contexts and levels of service delivery – the public health care sector's primary, secondary and tertiary contexts, as well as the private health care sector. Practicability and efficiency at each level of service delivery should be interrogated to ascertain feasibility in each context. Evidence indicates that:

- Midwife obstetric unit (MOU) three-day assessment clinics appear to be the most viable (Kanji et al., 2018; Khoza-Shangase & Harbinson, 2015).
- Screening at PHC immunisation clinics appears to be an appropriate platform, provided assets are fine-tuned and barriers are formally addressed, especially regarding staffing (Khoza-Shangase et al., 2017; Petrocchi-Bartal & Khoza-Shangase, 2016).
- Screening in the private hospital sector requires formal inclusion as part of the birthing package, with full medical aid cost reimbursement (Störbeck & Moodley, 2011; Swanepoel, Ebrahim, Joseph, & Friedland, 2007; Swanepoel, Störbeck, & Friedland, 2009).
- Aspects such as availability of hearing screening space, measurement and monitoring of ambient noise levels and discharge timing influence the practicability and efficiency of screening in various health care contexts (Bezuidenhout, Khoza-Shangase, De Maayer, & Strehlau, 2018).

In chapter 4, Petrocchi-Bartal, Khoza-Shangase and Kanji note that factors that may facilitate or impede the practicability and efficiency of early hearing screening may vary depending on the level and setting of the health care context. They make suggestions about how to maximise efficiency in each South African service delivery level.

Due consideration of NHS practicability and efficiency is necessary and should recognise, acknowledge and take into account the complexities of conducting NHS. These complexities are unique to the various levels of service delivery in the public and private sectors, as different levels introduce various influencing factors. As Kanji et al. (2018) state, the level of health care influences the practicability and efficiency factors and may act as an NHS facilitator or inhibitor.

In South Africa, current published evidence tends to support the MOU three-day assessment clinic as the most accessible and efficient context for hearing screening programme implementation (Kanji et al., 2018; Khoza-Shangase & Harbinson, 2015). Incorporating these context-specific findings into the NHI planning process would be strategic and would ensure that

NHS implementation becomes part of the government's re-engineered PHC strategies for successful mandating of hearing screening. This would ensure that barriers around human resources and equipment are addressed prior to national implementation. Training of staff deployed to PHC clinics, as part of task shifting, could also be proactively done to include hearing screening. The recommendation by Kanji (2016) of a two-tiered approach to NHS involving early hearing screening of high-risk babies in the hospital setting, with screening of well babies at clinic level, should also be explored to ensure high coverage.

Because of the constantly changing health care landscape in a LAMI country like South Africa, continued reassessment of the best service delivery level for hearing screening and the associated assets and barriers regarding practicability and efficiency must remain a priority for the audiology community. This unflagging attention will facilitate implementation of the HPCSA (2018) EHDI guidelines in a dynamic process that responds to context and confronts the realities with which early detection of hearing impairment has to contend. In South Africa, these realities include lack of a government mandate for UNHS, significant resource constraints, a high burden of disease and poor social determinants of health.

In chapter 5, Khoza-Shangase presents possible solutions and recommendations for confronting these barriers to early detection. Firstly, the South African audiology community needs to plan strategically to implement successful EHDI programmes. Each of the country's nine provinces needs to establish an EHDI programme responsible for creating, maintaining and improving the system of services needed to serve children with hearing impairment and their families. This would apply to all levels of health care for increased access, as well as within the proposed NHI system. We suggest that the provinces host national strategic planning activities to identify EHDI programme coordinators. They will in turn identify ways to implement the HPCSA (2018) EHDI guidelines using a strengths, weaknesses, opportunities and threats (SWOT) analysis and subsequent threats, opportunities, weaknesses and strengths (TOWS) matrix analysis (White & Blaiser, 2011).

Secondly, serious deliberations are needed around the use of tele-audiology, with task shifting as a complementary strategy to deal with the demand–capacity challenges around the availability of audiologists in the country, and should include the documented benefits of telehealth (Krupinski, 2015). Tele-audiology was established for this very reason – to overcome the extreme shortages of audiologists, speech-language pathologists and ear, nose and throat specialists (Fagan & Jacobs, 2009; Mulwafu, Ensink, Kuper, & Fagan, 2017). The health professionals currently located in health centres, usually in big cities and private practices, will be able to increase their reach to communities where people cannot access their services. For UNHS, the barriers to access are exacerbated by the limited working hours of audiologists, who miss babies born outside these hours, and babies born and discharged when audiologists are attending to other work responsibilities. Therefore, tele-audiology can become an alternative model of service delivery, with audiologists serving as programme managers or directors while trained screeners and nurses perform the screening services. This strategy must, however, take into account regulations, scopes of practice and ethics.

Thirdly, if non-audiologists, such as trained screeners and nurses, are involved in NHS, it is important to ensure that they are trained and that there are minimum standards to adhere to. Because nurses are the backbone of PHC, and PHC is the first point of contact in the health system for over 80 percent of the South African population, it is important to ensure that this level of care is well equipped and well resourced to implement NHS. This level of preparedness must include training around hearing screening and referral practices at PHC clinics, with knowledge and skill capacitation of personnel involved (Khan, Joseph, & Adhikari, 2018). The knowledge capacitation would need to be extended to include parents through health education about risk factors and hearing impairment. Studies have supported the need for parental education in order to enhance EHDI implementation in South Africa (Govender & Khan, 2017).

Lastly, it is important to be aware that success in implementation of any programme also relies on a proper data management system. Data management includes the processes of data collection and storage, as well as analysis and interpretation of the data to guide the future planning, implementation and evaluation of EHDI programmes. The data management system must allow for tracking of identified infants as well as coordinated referral pathways within a migration-aware health care system, which South Africa encourages (Vearey, Modisenyane, & Hunter-Adams, 2017). This system should also be intersectoral to facilitate continuity of care for hearing-impaired children, from health services to school services. Evidence suggests that South Africa currently does not have such a data management system (Moodley & Störbeck, 2017).

In summary, considering the realities of the South African health care context, and given that EHDI is key for newborns and infants with hearing impairment, it is important to consider these realities to better implement EHDI in this context. As far as early detection is concerned, Kanji (2018) recommends that South Africa seriously consider TNHS as a starting point or interim approach to early identification, particularly within a hospital setting. Inclusion of the first follow-up visit at MOU clinics as an NHS site is recommended to include those babies without risk factors and those who were born at home. This approach respects both the documented evidence of established risk factors for hearing impairment, and the contextual challenge of resource constraints. It also affirms Kanji's (2018) argument for a 'doing better with less' approach. This approach acknowledges that effective and quality health care is not only dependent on individual professionals but also involves other main stakeholders (Moyakhe, 2014), such as using volunteers and nurses as screeners. It is only when such a strategic approach is adopted that EHDI goals aimed at eradicating the negative impact of hearing impairment can be achieved.

Contextualisation of risk factors for hearing impairment is important, particularly in LAMI countries. In chapter 6, Fitzgibbons, Beswick and Driscoll review the key risk factors used in programmes around the world for their relevance in the South African context. They highlight that the purpose of risk factor registries has changed in developed contexts where UNHS has become the norm. In these contexts, risk factors are used to identify children who may be at risk of developing postnatal hearing loss and require hearing surveillance throughout childhood. The scenario is completely different in LAMI contexts without a universal platform, where risk factor registries are used to identify children requiring assessment for congenital hearing impairment.

Fitzgibbons and colleagues offer important recommendations about risk factors for the South African hearing screening context. They highlight that it is important to clearly define and communicate the purpose of the programme, including the target population and hearing loss condition, as this will ensure appropriate tailoring of risk factors to specific conditions. Examples are birth risk factors to identify permanent congenital and postnatal hearing loss; risk factors if the purpose of the programme is expanded to detection of all hearing losses, including conductive hearing loss, and monitoring children with post-birth causes; and risk factors that require further evidence prior to inclusion in a registry. They also raise the need for increased public and professional awareness around risk factors, with careful cognisance of cultural influences.

Kanji and Khoza-Shangase (2019) note that the quadruple burden of disease in South Africa has a significant influence on the types of risk factors associated with hearing impairment. They argue that the risk for hearing impairment is influenced by four factors: medical advancements, technological advancement, the burden of disease and human advancement (Figure 14.1). According to these authors, any programme purporting to be contextually relevant and responsive should be aware of these influences. In their view, this will allow the South African audiology profession to engage in best practice that is poised for next practice in all its clinical initiatives and endeavours in the paediatric population.

Early intervention for hearing impairment

South Africa needs to consider the various approaches to early intervention, taking careful cognisance of their efficacy in the context, where the goal is

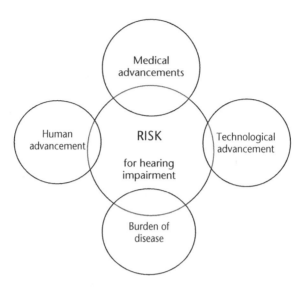

Figure 14.1 Quadruple influence on risk

Source: Kanji and Khoza-Shangase, 2019, p. 53

optimal and timely opportunities to develop linguistic, literary and communicative competence. In chapter 7, Kanji and Casoojee discuss various intervention approaches for children with a hearing impairment to learn to communicate. These range from auditory approaches such as auditory verbal therapy (AVT), incorporating listening and spoken language (LSL) principles, the oral–aural approach and cued speech, to more manual approaches such as total communication or sign language. Considering the global evidence base, it is widely accepted that AVT has its place in the spectrum of therapeutic intervention approaches. There is, however, a need for research-based evidence on adapted therapy methodologies, such as the South African version of LSL, and their benefits and limitations in the context. This is particularly important as linguistic and cultural diversity has an influence on intervention plans, especially in contexts where there is a linguistic and cultural incongruence between clinicians and the majority of the population they serve. Training institutions urgently need to address this issue (Khoza-Shangase & Mophosho, 2018).

There is a lacunae of evidence from countries in sub-Saharan Africa on outcomes of particular early intervention approaches in children with hearing impairment. Many of the intervention approaches and therapy resources used in South Africa have been developed by clinicians and researchers in the developed world due to the absence of South Africa's own contextually relevant resources (Pascoe & Norman, 2011). This has important implications for future studies, which academic and research institutions need to respond to. Contextually relevant efficacy studies would allow for solid arguments for the relevance of EHDI as an approach in these contexts. Contextualised intervention approaches would also facilitate family-centred intervention, with active parental engagement and involvement, in line with the HPCSA (2018) EHDI guidelines. Additionally, Kanji and Casoojee (chapter 7) stress that the mismatch between the language and culture profiles of professionals and patients is particularly relevant when considering oral communication approaches to early intervention such as AVT, as well as in the development, integration and understanding of linguistic profiles such as the Language Assessment, Remediation and Screening Procedure (LARSP) of the different languages in South Africa. This calls for transformation of the student demographic profile as well as curriculum transformation in training institutions, to allow for efficacious intervention at different levels of service models.

The principles of early intervention for hearing impairment should be continuously interrogated, with careful consideration of the appropriateness of individual and group-based approaches in each context. Attention must also be paid to contextual factors which might influence this process. Furthermore, evaluations of the pros and cons of home- and centre-based intervention approaches should be conducted, with reflections on the availability of and access to these options in the African context. This requires government intervention and political will, with early childhood intervention prioritised and mandated. Moreover, health care professionals and teachers in the ECD context in Africa need to collaboratively advocate for access to early intervention services, particularly given the high percentage of childhood disability. In chapter 8, Kanji proposes that all educators or teachers should have some training in childhood disabilities, as this will assist in reducing one of the barriers to inclusive education. This training should be initiated in university curricula.

Implementation of EHDI remains a substantial challenge in the South African educational setting. These challenges are heightened when intervention extends from the health sector to the education sector. These sectors face different realities and do not collaborate seamlessly. Access to education has been a significant focus of the South African government. However, access without a similar emphasis on success is problematic and renders such access unproductive for all stakeholders involved, particularly for learners with barriers to learning, such as the hearing impaired. Efforts to facilitate success should include access to therapeutic services that remediate barriers to learning in order to achieve the goal of inclusive education for the hearing impaired. The use of telehealth in the form of tele-audiology should also be considered.

Translation of policy into practice is heavily influenced by resource constraints. Most children with disabilities in South Africa, including hearing-impaired children, are not taught in classrooms together with their typically developing peers, despite the provisions of Education White Paper 6

(Department of Education, 2001). Notwithstanding various policies and guidelines (see chapter 9), EHDI has also not been successfully implemented in South Africa, for various reasons, and this has a direct impact on inclusive education possibilities. Numerous barriers and challenges to achieving quality and inclusive education for learners with disabilities exist. These include a lack of resources, specifically rehabilitation professionals such as audiologists, and a mismatch between capacity and demand, especially in the basic education sector. We argue strongly for the use of technology in the form of telehealth as one strategy to overcome access barriers in order to enhance the success of early intervention initiatives in the educational setting – a continuity of care imperative. The use of telehealth will allow for transfer and carry-over of early intervention benefits from the health sector to enhance educational outcomes in the educational setting, leading to children with hearing impairment becoming productive and contributing members of society. The application of telehealth to hearing health care in this population is an exciting field with a broad scope of application possibilities, including education and training, screening, diagnosis and intervention. These services are not bound by distance or location and can bridge the gap between patients isolated from the audiological services they require and the facilities that can provide them. Like any new intervention strategy, significant contextually relevant research would need to be conducted in order to ensure a contextually relevant evidence base that will allow for best practice. This evidence gathering should take into consideration contextual issues such as linguistic and cultural diversity, as well as explore task shifting.

Complexities of EHDI

To ensure best practice in EHDI in the African context, four issues need to be considered: EHDI in the context of other sensory impairments, EHDI in the context of family, EHDI in the context of HIV/AIDS, and EHDI in the context of tele-audiology.

All stakeholders, including the families of hearing-impaired children, need to be aware of the impact that other sensory impairments, such as blindness, might have on the assessment and management of children with hearing impairments. This has implications for training, clinical assessment and management, policy formulation and resource allocations, including educational resources for hearing-impaired children with additional sensory impairments. Moroe (chapter 10) highlights the dearth of evidence in this respect from LAMI contexts, particularly from African countries. It is one of the most neglected aspects of early childhood intervention, and is an area requiring increased focus and development as it presents unique challenges for both the attending clinician and the family of the blind and hearing-impaired child.

Family-centred EHDI in South Africa demands that due recognition be given to the unique concept of what constitutes a family in the African context, power and decision-making dynamics within this definition of family, as well as the multilingual and multicultural nature of society. Limited resources, demand–capacity challenges, and the language and culture mismatch between families and clinicians make family-centred interventions not only strategic but ethical as well. In chapter 11, Maluleke, Chiwutsi and Khoza-Shangase argue that family-centred EHDI is a viable option for decentralised service delivery in the South African context given the overburdened health care system, the country's socio-political history and dynamics, and the poor access to health care services, especially by vulnerable populations.

EHDI in the context of the South African HIV/AIDS pandemic needs careful planning. There is sufficient evidence on HIV and general development in the paediatric population, as well as on HIV and auditory and otological manifestations, to warrant attention in planning and executing screening, assessment and intervention plans for this population, with implications for EHDI highlighted and mitigated. This includes evidence of the link between HIV and antiretroviral perinatal exposure and auditory manifestations. However, locally relevant evidence is still required, as most of the published evidence is from developed contexts, where the presentation of the disease and the treatment options and protocols are different to those in LAMI countries. Khoza-Shangase looks more closely into these and related issues in chapter 12.

EHDI in the context of tele-audiology is a reality that cannot be avoided in the South African context because limited resources demand that alternative hearing care service delivery options be adopted to increase access. However, tele-audiology is certainly not without its limitations and challenges, hence the importance of ethical considerations. In chapter 13, Naudé and Bornman argue that despite some inherent challenges, there are numerous opportunities for beneficial utilisation of tele-audiology applications in EHDI programmes, including screening, initial diagnostic assessments, behavioural assessment, hearing aid and cochlear implant programming, and the delivery of communication development options. Tele-audiology in the context of EHDI can also make important contributions to many facets of programme infrastructure, including communications, training and quality management. Ethically, these authors assert that audiology as a profession must work towards a sound evidence base for EHDI via tele-audiology. This is particularly important as telehealth is a rapidly growing field and as such often outpaces the ability of regulatory bodies to develop minimum standards, regulations and guidelines. For tele-audiology to be implemented ethically, adherence to regulations is key.

Conclusion

EHDI, as defined and recommended internationally, may not be feasible and practicable in the African context. However, numerous recommendations and interim solutions are available, as outlined in this book. These recommendations and solutions require increased effort from all stakeholders involved, with sensitivity to the context, while maintaining best practice in a less than ideal context. Doing the best with what Africa has in order to ensure best benefits for the hearing-impaired paediatric population should guide all engagements around EHDI planning, implementation and monitoring. A contextually relevant evidence base should be used to guide interventions, with careful attention to the complexities around EHDI in the African context.

References

Ataguba, J. E., Day, C., & McIntyre, D. (2015). Explaining the role of the social determinants of health on health inequality in South Africa. *Global Health Action*, *8*(1). doi: https://doi.org/10.3402/gha.v8.28865.

Bezuidenhout, K. J., Khoza-Shangase, K., De Maayer, T., & Strehlau, R. (2018). Universal newborn hearing screening in public health care in South Africa: Challenges to implementation. *South African Journal of Child Health*, *12*(4),159–163. doi: 10.7196/SAJCH.2018.v12i4.1522.

Department of Education. (2001). *Education white paper 6. Special needs education: Building an inclusive education and training system*. Pretoria, South Africa: Government Printer.

Fagan, J. J., & Jacobs, M. (2009). Survey of ENT services in Africa: Need for a comprehensive intervention. *Global Health Action*, *2*(1), Art. #1932. doi: 10.3402/gha.v2i0.1932.

Govender, S. M., & Khan, N. B. (2017). Knowledge and cultural beliefs of mothers regarding the risk factors of infant hearing loss and awareness of audiology services. *Journal of Public Health in Africa*, *8*(1), 557. doi: 10.4081/jphia.2017.557.

Health Professions Council of South Africa (HPCSA). (2018). *Early hearing detection and intervention (EHDI): Guidelines*. Pretoria, South Africa: Health Professions Council of South Africa. Retrieved from https://www.hpcsa.co.za/Uploads/editor/UserFiles/downloads/speech/Guidelines_for_EHDI2018.pdf.

Kanji, A. (2016). Early hearing screening in South Africa: Time to get real about context. *South African Journal of Child Health*, *10*(4), 192. doi: 10.7196/SAJCH.2016.v10i4.1298.

Kanji, A. (2018). Early hearing detection and intervention: Reflections from the South African context. *South African Journal of Communication Disorders*, *65*(1), a581.

Kanji, A., & Khoza-Shangase, K. (2019). Early detection of hearing impairment in high risk neonates: Let's talk about the high risk registry in the South African context. *South African Journal of Child Health*, *13*(2), 53–55. doi: 10.7196/SAJCH.2019.v13i2.1675.

Kanji, A., Khoza-Shangase, K., Petrocchi-Bartal, L., & Harbinson, S. (2018). Feasibility of infant hearing screening from a developing country context: The South African experience. *Hearing, Balance and Communication, 16*(4), 263–270. https://doi.org/10.1080/21695717.2018.1519144.

Khan, N., Joseph, L., & Adhikari, M. (2018). The hearing screening experiences and practices of primary health care nurses: Indications for referral based on high-risk factors and community views about hearing loss. *African Journal of Primary Health Care & Family Medicine, 10*(1). https://phcfm.org/index.php/phcfm/article/view/1848/2841.

Khoza-Shangase, K., & Harbinson, S. (2015). Evaluation of universal newborn hearing screening in South African primary care. *African Journal of Primary Health Care and Family Medicine, 7*(1), 1–12.

Khoza-Shangase, K., Kanji, A., Petrocchi-Bartal, L., & Farr, K. (2017). Infant hearing screening from a developing country context: Status from two South African provinces. *South African Journal of Child Health, 11*(4), 159–163. doi: 10.7196/SAJCH.2017.v11i4.1267.

Khoza-Shangase, K., & Mophosho, M. (2018). Language and culture in speech-language and hearing professions in South Africa: The dangers of a single story. *South African Journal of Communication Disorders, 65*(1), a594. https://doi.org/10.4102/sajcd.v65i1.594.

Krupinski, E. (2015). Innovations and possibilities in connected health. *Journal of American Academy of Audiology, 26*, 761–767.

Moodley, S., & Störbeck, C. (2017). Data management for early hearing detection and intervention in South Africa. *South African Journal of Information Management, 19*(1), a779.

Moyakhe, N. P. (2014). Quality healthcare: An attainable goal for all South Africans? *South African Journal of Bioethics and Law, 7*(2), 80–83.

Mulwafu, W., Ensink, R., Kuper, H., & Fagan, J. (2017). Survey of ENT services in sub-Saharan Africa: Little progress between 2009 and 2015. *Global Health Action, 10*(1). doi: 10.1080/16549716.2017.1289736.

Mulwafu, W., Kuper, H., & Ensink, R. J. H. (2016). Prevalence and causes of hearing impairment in Africa. *Tropical Medicine & International Health, 21*, 158–165.

Pascoe, M., & Norman, V. (2011). Contextually relevant resources in speech-language therapy and audiology in South Africa: Are there any? *South African Journal of Communication Disorders, 58*(1), 2–5. doi: https://doi.org/10.4102/sajcd.v58i1.35.

Petrocchi-Bartal, L., & Khoza-Shangase, K. (2016). Infant hearing screening at primary health care immunization clinics in South Africa: The current status. *South African Journal of Child Health, 10*(2), 139–143. doi: 10.7196/SAJCH.2016.v10i2.1114.

Scott, V., Schaay, N., Schneider, H., & Sanders, D. (2017). Addressing social determinants of health in South Africa: The journey continues. *South African Health Review, 2017*(1), 77–87.

Störbeck, C., & Moodley, S. (2011). ECD policies in South Africa: What about children with disabilities? *Journal of African Studies and Development, 3*(1), 1–8.

Swanepoel, D., Ebrahim, S., Joseph, A., & Friedland, P. (2007). Newborn hearing screening in a South African private health care hospital. *International Journal of Pediatric Otorhinolaryngology, 71*(6), 881–887.

Swanepoel, D., Störbeck, C., & Friedland, P. (2009). Early hearing detection and intervention in South Africa. *International Journal of Pediatric Otorhinolaryngology, 73*, 783–786.

Vearey, J., Modisenyane, M., & Hunter-Adams, J. (2017). Towards a migration-aware health system in South Africa: A strategic opportunity to address health inequality. In A. Padarath & P. Barron (Eds.), *South African Health Review 2017* (pp. 89–98). Durban, South Africa: Health Systems Trust. Retrieved from http://www.hst.org.za/publications/south-african-health-review-2017.

White, K. R., & Blaiser, K. M. (2011). Strategic planning to improve EHDI programs. *Volta Review, 111*(2), 83–108.

World Health Organization (WHO). (2018). Prevention of blindness and deafness. Retrieved from https://www.who.int/pbd/publications/en/.

Contributors

Rachael Beswick is the director of Queensland's newborn hearing screening programme, Healthy Hearing. She completed her Bachelor of Speech Pathology, Master's of Audiological Studies and PhD at the University of Queensland, and recently completed her MBA at the Queensland University of Technology. Her primary areas of research lie in screening programmes, risk factors, detection of postnatal hearing loss, and quality assurance processes. She has published several scientific papers, and has presented her research at both national and international conferences.

Juan Bornman is a professor and director of the Centre for Augmentative and Alternative Communication at the University of Pretoria (UP). She has been actively involved in the disability field as a trainer, researcher and activist. Bornman has published more than 60 journal papers and book chapters, written four books and done numerous presentations locally and internationally on the topic of augmentative and alternative communication (AAC). She was awarded a fellowship by the International Society of AAC for exemplary work in the field and in 2018 received the Distinguished Academic Achiever Award from UP. In 2016, together with her team, she won the prestigious Reimagine Education 2016 Regional Awards for Africa.

Aisha Casoojee completed a Bachelor of Communication Pathology at the University of Pretoria in 2002, a Health Professions Council of South Africa (HPCSA) accredited postgraduate course at the University of Stellenbosch (SU) in 2006 and a Master's in Audiology in 2012 at the University of the Witwatersrand (Wits). She qualified as an auditory verbal therapist in 2013 at SU and as a reading therapist in 2014 at Read for Africa. Aisha attended an international course in cochlear implantation at the University of Leiden, The Netherlands, and an international cochlear implantation training workshop in Melbourne, Australia. She worked as a clinician at the Chris Hani Baragwanath Hospital for several years, during which time she was involved in the development and launch of the first fully state-funded cochlear implant programme in South Africa. Aisha currently lectures and provides clinical tutoring to students at the Speech Therapy and Audiology Department in the School of Human and Community Development at Wits.

Rudo Chiwutsi is the current administrator in the Audiology Department at the University of the Witwatersrand. She completed a Bachelor of Arts in 2015, and is currently studying for a postgraduate diploma in disability studies at the University of Cape Town.

Carlie J. Driscoll is an associate professor in the School of Health and Rehabilitation Sciences at the University of Queensland, Australia. She is well known for her research in the fields of paediatric screening and diagnostic audiology. Having overseen many large-scale screening projects in Queensland and in Nanjing, China, and with over 80 papers and three edited books to her name, she is highly experienced in mass community-based testing and test performance analytics. She has taught or coordinated over 70 university courses in audiology, and constructed courses for the interprofessional education of medical and allied health students. She is an editorial consultant for 14 international audiology/medical journals, and sits on the editorial board of the *Journal of the American Academy of Audiology*.

Jane Fitzgibbons is a senior audiologist with the Healthy Hearing Program in Queensland, Australia, and coordinates a diagnostic tele-audiology service for infants referred from newborn hearing screening in regional and remote parts of Queensland. She has worked in infant diagnostic audiology in New Zealand, England and Australia and recently completed a Doctor of Audiology at the AT Still University. Her primary areas of interest include hearing loss risk factors, and innovative use of technology to improve service delivery and clinical training.

Amisha Kanji is an associate professor and former head of Discipline of Audiology at the University of the Witwatersrand. She lectures undergraduate audiology courses, is involved in clinical and research supervision of students, and is the current departmental postgraduate research coordinator and chair of the School of Human and Community Development's Assessment Portfolio. She was awarded the Vice Chancellor's transformation team category award in 2019. Kanji was a member of the Health Professions Council of South Africa's (HPCSA) task team that developed national guidelines for early hearing detection and intervention, and has also served as a member of HPCSA-appointed evaluation panels for speech-language and hearing training programmes. She has a number of peer-reviewed publications to her name and has presented at local and international conferences. Kanji has served as a reviewer for abstract submissions for a number of conferences in the field of audiology, and as a peer reviewer for a number of local and international journals.

Katijah Khoza-Shangase is an associate professor and former head of the Speech Pathology and Audiology Department at the University of the Witwatersrand. She has played an important leadership role in the Health Professions Council of South Africa. Khoza-Shangase has won numerous awards, principally in the area of research and research supervision, and for contributions to the field of audiology. She has a number of publications to her name, including peer-reviewed journal articles, technical and research reports, book chapters and co-edited books. *Black Academic Voices: The South African Experience*, published in 2019, is her most current contribution to the transformation and decolonisation project, and won the 2020 Humanities and Social Sciences Award (Non-fiction category). She also co-edited a Special Issue for the *South African Journal of Communication Disorders* in 2020. Her forthcoming outputs include *Preventive Audiology: An African Perspective*, and *Occupational Noise-Induced Hearing Loss: An African Perspective*, both by AOSIS book publishers.

Ntsako P. Maluleke is an audiologist and lecturer in the Department of Speech-Language Pathology and Audiology at the Sefako Makgatho Health Sciences University in Ga-Rankuwa, Pretoria. She holds an undergraduate degree in speech and hearing therapy and a Master's in Audiology from the University of the Witwatersrand (Wits). She has authored several peer-reviewed articles and presented her research at various conferences. Her research interests include early hearing detection and intervention, childhood and school-age hearing impairment, and family-centred intervention. She is currently a PhD fellow at Wits.

Nomfundo F. Moroe is a senior lecturer and current head of Discipline (Audiology) at the University of the Witwatersrand. She is part of the Department of Higher Education and Training's NGap programme. Moroe is a passionate researcher, with an interest in occupational audiology, complex interventions, deaf culture and deafblindness. She is a Consortium for Advanced Research Training in Africa fellow and is currently conducting postdoctoral research funded by this consortium. She has published several peer-reviewed articles and presented at both national and international conferences.

Alida Naudé is a corporate training audiologist with wide clinical experience of private practice and higher education as a senior lecturer and researcher. She received her PhD in Audiology from the University of Pretoria in 2015, and in 2016 completed her postdoctoral fellowship at the Centre for Augmentative and Alternative Communication. She holds the title of Junior Research Fellow at the University of Pretoria. Special areas of expertise and research include ethics, evoked potentials, vestibular audiology, ototoxicity and infection control. She has co-authored a book, contributed more than 10 articles in accredited journals and served as the editor of a special journal edition about ethics in conjunction with international researchers.

Luisa Petrocchi-Bartal has lectured and supervised students in paediatric audiology for the past 10 years. She completed her Bachelor of Arts in Speech and Hearing Therapy and her Master's in Audiology at the University of the Witwatersrand (Wits). She is a current PhD fellow (Audiology) in early hearing detection and intervention (EHDI) at Wits. She has published several scientific papers in EHDI and has presented her research in this area at national and international conferences. Her other areas of interest include diagnostic audiology and occupational audiology, which were her primary areas of practice for almost 15 years.

Index

Page numbers in *italics* indicate figures or tables.

1:3:6 48–49
90-90-90 targets 72, 220, 221, 231

A

AAA *see* American Academy of
    Audiology
AABR *see* automated auditory brainstem
    response
ABR *see* auditory brainstem response
access
    to ART 220–221
    to education 9, 155, 158–162, 273
    to health care 9, 15–16, 138, 141,
        210, 246–247
    to resources 245
    to services 19, 143, 186, 208–209,
        243–247, 274
Action Plan, Department of Basic
    Education (DBE) 159
adapted therapy methodologies 272
Adeagbo, K. 210
Adedeji, T. O. 208
Adeyemo, A. A. 210
Adhikari, M. 79–80
Adunka, O. F. 206, 207
Advanced Clinical Access 139
advocacy role 77–78, 190, 236, 273
Afe, A. J. 230
African context 5, 143, 205, 212–213,
    265–267, 273, 276
African family, definition of 198–199,
    212–213
Afrikaans language 142
AG Bell Academy for Listening and
    Spoken Language 124–125
age at amplification 117, 120, 123, 131,
    132
age of diagnosis of hearing impairment
    6, 34–35, 48–49, 76, 120–121,
    129, 243, 264
Ahmed, S. 76
aid *see* foreign aid
AIDS *see* HIV/AIDS

Aitken, S. 177
Alport syndrome 98–99
Al-Yagon, M. 202, 203
Alyami, H. 206, 207
American Academy of Audiology (AAA)
    245, 256
American Speech-Language-Hearing
    Association (ASHA) 187, 245
aminoglycoside antibiotics 94–95
amplification devices
    age at amplification 117, 120, 123,
        131, 132
    auditory–verbal therapy (AVT)
        125–126
    cochlear implants 120, 123–125, 127,
        129, 131, 138–139, 158, 164, 244
    communication approaches and 131
    cultural diversity and 121
    hearing aids 120, 123, 124, 131,
        139–141, 148–149, 158, 244
    HIV/AIDS and 236
    JCIH 123
    linguistic diversity and 121
    models of care 138–139, 141,
        144–145, 148–149
ancestral curses *see* beliefs
anger 202–203
Angola 147
AnnaMosia, D. 212
ANSD *see* auditory neuropathy spectrum
    disorder
antibiotics 94–95, 182
antiretroviral therapy (ART) 72, 102,
    219–223, 225, 229, 232, 234, 237
    see also HIV/AIDS
ART *see* antiretroviral therapy
ASD *see* autism spectrum disorder
ASHA *see* American Speech-Language-
    Hearing Association
assisted ventilation 94–95
assistive technologies 201
asynchronous tele-audiology 79, 164, 166
Atazanavir 232

audiologist–client relationship 144,
    252–255, 257
audiologists
    advocacy role of 39, 148–149
    best practice for 266–267, 269–270
    communication approaches 123,
        131–132
    continuity of care 158, 163
    ethical considerations by 245–247,
        249–259
    family-centred early hearing
        detection and intervention 211
    HIV/AIDS and 228–229, 235–236
    newborn hearing screening (NHS) 67,
        73, 76–79
    role of 46, *46–47*
    shortage of 37–38, 53–55, 93,
        141–142
    in sub-Saharan Africa 19–20, 27
auditory brainstem response (ABR) 33,
    227–228, 232, 234
auditory neuropathy spectrum disorder
    (ANSD) 94, 95, 104
Auditory Steady State Response 81, 234
auditory–verbal therapy (AVT) 124–127,
    129, 131–132, 133, 272
Australia 37, 121, 124, 126, 203, 204,
    207–208
autism spectrum disorder (ASD) 178,
    179–181
automated auditory brainstem response
    (AABR) 44, 53, 54, 75, 244, 254
AVT *see* auditory–verbal therapy
awareness programmes 57, 93, 105, 166,
    190, 209–210, 235–236, 259, 270

B
bacterial meningitis 100–101, 225, 226
basal skull fractures 101
Batshaw, M. 182
Bayley Scales of Infant and Toddler
    Development 145
behavioural challenges in children with
    HIV 223
beliefs 80, 91, 121, 143
Belote, M. 180
benchmarks 39, 267

beneficence 249
best practice in South Africa for hearing
        impairment 264–278
    challenges of implementation
        264–265
    complexities of detection and
        intervention 274–275
    early detection 265–271
    early intervention 271–274, *272*
    importance of 264–265, 276
    JCIH 122
bewitchment *see* beliefs
Bezuidenhout, K. J. 53–54, 75
bilateral hearing loss 103
Bill of Rights 45, 66, 159, 246
birthing package, of private hospitals 24,
    37, 42, 58, 268
Blaiser, K. M. 78
blindness 180
'blueberry muffin' rash 96–97
Board for Speech, Language and Hearing
        Professions 22–23, 46, 246
bony labyrinth fracture 101
Bornman, J. 159, 161
Boshoff, L. 182
Botswana 147
Botswana Health Professions Council
        266
Bradshaw, K. 223
Brazil 226, 229
burden of disease
    early hearing detection and 58,
        71–72
    global 117–118
    HIV/AIDS 10, 219, 235
    quadruple 17, 24, 71, 208, 271, *272*
    in sub-Saharan Africa 17
Buriti, A. K. 229
Burke, M. 36
Bush, M. L. 205, 209, 210

C
caesarean sections 104–105
Calles, N. R. 230
Campinha-Bacote, J. 142
capacity vs demand 68–71, *70*, 163, 265
carboplatin 101–102

caregivers *see also* family-centred
early hearing detection and
intervention; parents
  early intervention for hearing
    impairment 118
  HIV/AIDS and 230, 234
  home- vs centre-based early
    intervention 143–146
  information counselling of 237
  JCIH risk factor registry 92–93, 105
  satisfaction of 207–208
  as stakeholders 57
  training of 149
Carel du Toit Centre 146
case managers 121, 203, 254
Casoojee, A. 58
Castaneda, K. P. 223
cCMV *see* congenital CMV infection
CD4 cell count 222, 227–228, 229, 232,
  237
central auditory pathways, damage to
  101
central auditory processing deficits
  226
centre-based early intervention 143–146,
  149, 273
Centre for Deaf Studies 146
cerebral infection 227
CFP *see* Cover for Professionals
Chan, K. Y. 55
Chapman, D. A. 55
Charcot-Marie-Tooth syndrome 99–100
CHARGE syndrome 182
CHC centres/clinics *see* community
  health care (CHC) centres/clinics
chemotherapy 101–102, 105
Chen, G. 55
child-headed households 198, 212
Children's Act 160, 253
Children's Amendment Act 160
Children's Communication Centre 146
children's homes 212
children with disabilities 146–147
China 36
Ching, Y. C. 203–204
Choi, S. 79
cholesteatoma 103

chronic suppurative otitis media (CSOM)
  103
CHWs *see* community health workers
cisplatin 101–102
cleft lip/palate 97, 98
client–audiologist relationship 144,
  252–255, 257
clinics 22–24, 26, 46, 49, *50–51*, 53, *56*,
  57–59, 74, 76, 268–270
CMV *see* cytomegalovirus
coaching 204–205
cochlear concussion 101
cochlear implants 120, 123–125, 127,
  129, 131, 138–139, 158, 164, 244
  see also amplification devices
cognitive delay 222–223
Cohen, A. 204–205
Colgan, S. 36
collaboration 143, 148, 189, 197, 201,
  266
Collins, M. P. 139–141
Columbia University 222
common law 251, 255
communication approaches 145, 186,
  190
communication developmental
  milestones 22, 224
communication disorders 156, 224, 226
communication with clients 96, 250
community health care (CHC) centres/
  clinics *46*, 49, *50*, 53, 69
community health workers (CHWs)
  68–69, 162
community support 45, 48, 53, 128, 131,
  199, 205
compensation *see* reimbursement for
  services
competence 58, 188, 249–251, *252*, 259
computers 253–254 *see also* tele-audiology;
  telehealth
conductive hearing loss 98–99, 102–103,
  105, 226, 228, 271
confidentiality 246, 247, 251–254
conflict in teams 69
congenital abnormalities 118
congenital CMV infection (cCMV)
  95–96, 105

congenital deafblindness 184–185

congenital hearing impairment 35, 91, 177, 243

congenital infections 94, 96, 97

congenital rubella syndrome (CRS) 96–97

congenital toxoplasmosis 97

consanguinity 91, 104, 105

consent 58, 247, 253–255, *256*, 258

Constanescu, G. 207

Constantinescu, G. 125

Constitution of South Africa 45, 66, 159, 162, 198, 211, 246–247, 253, 255

Consultative Group on Early Childhood Care and Development 4

consumer protection 247

contextualisation

    best practices 264–276

    early detection of hearing impairment 39, 44, 48–49, 72–76

    early intervention for hearing impairment 118–119, 133, 149–150

    family-centred early hearing detection and intervention 210

contextualisation, of hearing impairment risk factors 89–114

    history of risk factor registries 89–90

    HPCSA risk factors 102–103

    infant hearing screening 80, 90–91

    JCIH risk factor registry 89, 92–102

    need for contextualisation 8, 20–21, 91–92, 271

    recommendations 105

    risk factors for South African context 103–104

    risk factors from developing nations 104–105

    system change 106

continued professional development 165

continuity of care 155–173

    access to education 155, 158–162

    data management system and 270

    definitions 156–157

    early intervention programmes 155–158, 167

    educational setting 158–162

importance of 9–10

migration and 267–268

referrals and 57

tele-audiology 10, 162–168, 247, 274

Convention on the Rights of Persons with Disabilities (CRPD) 119, 146–147, 160, 186

Convention on the Rights of the Child 119

Cook, A. 228

Cooper, M. 208, 209, 210

coordinators 58, 78, 121, 269

costs of services 35–36, 138–139, 140–141, 145–146, 196–197, 208, 211, 246–247, 257–258

Côte d'Ivoire 23

counselling 123, 235–236, 237, 244, 247

Cover for Professionals (CFP) 258

craniofacial anomalies 97–98, 105

Croome, N. 223

Crouzon/Pfeiffer syndrome 99

CRPD *see* Convention on the Rights of Persons with Disabilities

CRS *see* congenital rubella syndrome

cryptococcosis 226

cryptococcus 225

CSOM *see* chronic suppurative otitis media

cued speech 129–130, 272

cultural awareness 142–143, 150

cultural competence 96, 122, 126–127, 142

cultural diversity

    African context 4–6

    best practice and 265, 271, 272, 274

    early detection of hearing impairment 48–49, 81

    early intervention for hearing impairment 121, 126–128, 132–133, 150

    family-centred early hearing detection and intervention 198, 203, 205, 207, 211, 213

    tele-audiology 166–168

culture-positive postnatal infections associated with sensorineural hearing loss 100–101

Cupples, L. 125–126
curiosity 202–203
curricula 143, 159, 187–188, 203, 205, 273
curses *see* beliefs
cytomegalovirus (CMV) 95–96, 102, 225, 226, 230–232

D

Daniel, A. D. 208
data management systems 22, 28, 39, 57–59, 81, 121, 190, 252–253, 267, 270
Davidson, R. C. 188
Davis-McFarland, E. 222, 224
DBE *see* Department of Basic Education
deafblindness
    causes of 181–183
    definition of 178, 180
    early detection and intervention 185–188, 191
    groups of 181
    impact on children 184–185, 190–191
    prevalence of 177, 183
    in South Africa 183–184
DeafBlind South Africa 184
deaf culture, definition of 128
'deaf', definition of 122–123
decentralisation 68, 209, 213
decision-making 201, 210, 213
Decker, K. B. 206
demand vs capacity and resources 68–71, 70, 163, 265
Democratic Republic of Congo 19
Department of Basic Education (DBE) 156, 159, 166, 203
Department of Health (DoH)
    90-90-90 targets 231
    continuity of care 166
    early detection of hearing impairment 27, 38, 57, 77, 82
    early intervention for hearing impairment 138
    ethical considerations 244, 246

family-centred early hearing detection and intervention 203, 205, 208
Department of Public Service and Administration 156
Department of Social Development (DSD) 77, 198, 203, 212
deprivational index 74
DesGeorges, J. 205, 209
detection of hearing impairment *see* early detection of hearing impairment
developmental delay 3–4, 9, 137, 158, 186, 222–224
developmental disabilities 117–119, 222–224
Devendra, A. 230
diagnosis of hearing impairment, age of 6, 34–35, 76, 120–121, 129, 243, 264
diagnostic testing 74–75, 81–82, 243–244
Discovery 24
discrimination 159, 186
distance senses 184
distortion product otoacoustic emissions (DPOAEs) 227
district hospitals 47, 69, 258
diuretics 94–95, 182
diversity 127, 140, 149–150, 159–160, 205 *see also* cultural diversity; linguistic diversity
documentation 57–58, 250, 251, 255, 256, 259, 267
DoH *see* Department of Health
'doing better with less' approach 75–77, 82–83, 270–271
domestic workers 198
Donohue, D. 159, 161
Dornan, D. 125
Down syndrome 99
DPOAEs *see* distortion product otoacoustic emissions
Dromi, E. 202, 203, 207
DSD *see* Department of Social Development
Durban, study in 80

Durieux-Smith, A. 34–35
duty to inform 254–255

E
EAR *see* Effectiveness of Auditory
    Rehabilitation
ear infections 229, 234
early childhood development (ECD) 4,
    5, 34, 119, 155, 159, 265–266, 273
early childhood intervention (ECI) 4,
    118, 137
early detection of hearing impairment
    7–8, 15–32
  approaches to 33–41, *38*
  best practice for 265–271
  continuity of care 155–156
  deafblindness and 185–189, 191
  health care services 15–16, 18–20, 28
  health priorities 16–18, 28, 266
  HIV/AIDS and 235
  HPCSA guidelines 15
  paradigm shift in 3–11
  prevalence of hearing impairment
    20–21
  preventative care 21
  principles for 22–23
  sensory impairments and 185–189,
    191
  solutions and recommendations
    27–28
  in South Africa 24–27, *25–26*
  in sub-Saharan Africa 23–24
  TNHS 7–8
  UNHS 7–8
early detection of hearing impairment,
    challenges of 66–88
  burden of disease 71–72
  demand vs capacity and resources
    68–71, *70*
  'doing better with less' approach
    75–77, 82–83
  government policy 66–68
  guidelines, lack of 81–82
  newborn hearing screening 72–75
  research on 81–82
  solutions and recommendations
    77–81, 269–270

universal health coverage (UHC)
    67–68
early detection of hearing impairment,
    implementation of 42–65
  contextualisation 48–49
  health care structure of South Africa
    44–46, *46–47*
  levels of health care service 42,
    49–59, *50–52, 56*, 268
  low and middle-income (LAMI)
    countries 42–43
  otoacoustic emissions (OAEs) 44
  UNHS 42–44
early intervention for hearing
    impairment
  best practice for 271–274, *272*
  contextualisation of 48–49
  continuity of care and 155–158, 167
  deafblindness and 185–191
  ethical considerations in 243–245,
    249–250
  HIV/AIDS and 236–237
  paradigm shift in 3–11
  sensory impairments and 185–191
early intervention for hearing impairment,
    approaches to 117–136
  auditory–verbal therapy (AVT)
    124–127, 133
  choice of approach 130–131, 132–133
  contextual risk factors 118–119
  cued speech 129–130
  developmental disabilities 117–119
  guidelines for 119–123
  JCIH 121–123
  research on 120–121, 132–133
  sign language 128–129
  solutions and recommendations
    131–132
  total communication 128
early intervention for hearing
    impairment, models of care in
    137–154
  amplification devices 138–139, 141,
    144–145, 148–149
  definition of 137
  home- vs centre-based 143–146, 150
  importance of 9, 137–138, 150

individual vs group-based 139–143, 150

(re)habilitation 138–139

solutions and recommendations 148–150

special schooling vs mainstream inclusion 146–148, *148*, 150, 273

ear, nose and throat (ENT) specialists 19, 163

Ebrahim, S. 197

ECD *see* early childhood development

ECI *see* early childhood intervention

ECMO *see* extracorporeal membrane oxygenation

Edirippulige, S. 165

education *see also* awareness programmes; continuity of care; schools; training

access to 9, 155, 158–162, 273

barriers to learning 160–161, 167, 273

communication approaches and 123–124

deafblindness and 186

inclusive 147–148, 150, 155, 158–161, 167, 273–274

no-fee schools 158–159, 212

in South Africa 158–162

Education White Paper 6, 160–161, 167, 273

e-education 167

Effectiveness of Auditory Rehabilitation (EAR) 139–140

efficiency 267–268

e-health 167

eighth nerve damage 101

Ekberg, K. 204

elders 210

electronic databases *see* data management systems

Elpers, J. 205, 209, 210

emotional support 201

empowerment 200, 203

encephalopathy 222, 224

encryption 254

English language 142, 211

Ensink, R. J. H. 265

ENT specialists *see* ear, nose and throat (ENT) specialists

environmental risk factors 20

equipment 55, 58, 80, 258, 259, 266

Erbasi, E. 203–204

Eritrea 147

Ethical Guidelines for Good Practice 255

ethics 22–23, 59, 142, 235, 264, 270, 275

ethics, in tele-audiology 243–263

access to services 11, 243–244, 245, 246–247, 275

competence 249–251, *252*

confidentiality 246, 247, 251–254

definitions 244

duty to inform 254–255

HPCSA guidelines 245–247, *248*

importance of 259–260

informed consent 247, 254–255, *256*

licensure 247

privacy 246, 247, 251–254

programme validation 255–257

reimbursement for services 257–258

responsibilities of audiologists 246

risk management 258–259

uses of tele-audiology 244–245, 275

Ethiopia 19, 147

Eustachian tube 226

evaluation of programmes 38–39, 267

Evans, T. 164

exchange transfusion 94–95

extended family 199, 212

extracorporeal membrane oxygenation (ECMO) 94–95

F

facial defects 98

false positive results 55

families

early intervention for hearing impairment 117, 120–133, 143–145, 273

ethical considerations 255

rights of 22

family-centred early hearing detection and intervention 196–218

challenges of implementation 208–210, 213

family-centred early hearing detection
    and intervention (*cont.*)
    contextualisation and 48
    deafblindness 188, 190–191
    definition of African family 198–199,
        212–213
    evidence-based practice 201–208
    importance of 10, 196–197, 274–275
    orphaned and vulnerable children
        (OVC) 211–212, 213
    principles of 199–201
    viability in South Africa 210–211
family health teams 45, 67
family history of hearing loss 93–94, 105
family physicians 19, 69
Fasunla, A. J. 232
feeding schemes 159, 212
fees *see* costs of services
Findlen, U. M. 206, 207
finger spelling 128
foetal alcohol syndrome 98
follow-up rates 55, 76–77
foreign aid 5, 18, 28, 266
fractures 101
Friderichs, N. 58
Friedland, P. 197
funding 46, 58, 143, 267

G

Gauteng, studies in 76, 121, 141
General Household Survey 158–159
genetic conditions 182–183
genetic services 99
gentamicin 225
German measles *see* rubella
Ghana 19
Ghebreyesus, Tedros Adhanom 17–18,
    67
Global AIDS Update (2018) 72
Goh, W. H. 54
Gonçalves, I. C. 229
Govender, S. M. 80
government policies 43–44, 57, 160–161,
    273
government spending on health 18, 28,
    46, 68, 71, 158
Gravel, J. S. 130

group-based vs individual early
    intervention 139–143
group therapy 149, 150
Guibert, G. 231
guidelines for early detection and
    intervention for hearing
    impairment 6, 27, 81–82, 160–161,
    245, 266, 267
Guidelines for Full-Service/Inclusive
    Schools 160
*Guidelines for Hearing Aids and Services for
    Developing Countries,* World Health
    Organization's (WHO) 250
Guidelines for Inclusive Teaching and
    Learning 160
Guidelines for Responding to Learner
    Diversity in the Classroom
    through Curriculum and
    Assessment Policy Statements 160
Guidelines to Ensure Quality Education
    and Support in Special Schools
    and Special School Resource
    Centres 160

H

HAART *see* highly active ART
haemotympanum 101
Hajabubker, M. A. 76
Hall, J. W. 58
'hard of hearing', definition of 122–123
head trauma 101, 105
health care professionals
    advocacy role of 273
    competence of 58, 188, 249–251, 259
    deafblindness and 189, 191
    ethical considerations 245
    family-centred early hearing
        detection and intervention 209
    roles of 251
    shortage of 5, 68–69, 71, 78, 127,
        131–133, 141–143, 149, 158,
        162–163, 201, 211, 221, 258,
        265–266, 269
    in sub-Saharan Africa 18–19
health care services 6, 15–16, 18–20, 28,
    44–46, *46–47*
Health Professions Act 246, 247

Health Professions Council of
    South Africa (HPCSA)
  best practice 266, 267, 269, 273
  continuity of care 160
  deafblindness 186–187
  early detection of hearing
    impairment 15, 22–23, 34, 37–38,
    43, 48–49, 54–55, 57, 72–75, 78,
    81–82
  early intervention for hearing
    impairment 119–120, 123,
    141–142
  ethical considerations 245–247, *248*,
    253, 254, 255
  family-centred early hearing
    detection and intervention 10,
    196, 210
  risk factors for hearing impairment 8,
    90–91, 92, 94, 98, 102–104
  UNHS 7
health technology assessment (HTA) 79,
  165
hearing aids 120, 123, 124, 131,
    139–141, 148–149, 158, 244 *see*
    also amplification devices
hearing screening *see also* early detection
    of hearing impairment; newborn
    hearing screening; targeted
    newborn hearing screening;
    universal newborn hearing
    screening
  best practice 266–268, 270–271
  contextualisation of 72–75, 90–91
  ethical considerations 243, 244
  family-centred early hearing
    detection 197
  HIV/AIDS and 234, 236–237
  multisensory impairments and 189
  principles of 22
  in schools 160
herpes simplex virus (HSV) 96, 105
herpes viruses 100–101
herpes zoster 226
HEU infants *see* HIV-exposed uninfected
    (HEU) infants
Hickson, L. 125, 203–204
hierarchical social norms 210, 213

high frequency tympanometry 235
highly active ART (HAART) 221, 226,
  231, 232, 236
high-risk register (HRR) 33, 35, 37
HI HOPES (Home intervention: Hearing
    and language opportunities
    parent education services) 77–78,
    144–145
Hitchins, A. R. C. 126
HIV/AIDS 219–242
  antiretroviral therapy (ART) 72, 102,
    219–223, 225, 229, 232, 234, 237
  auditory and otological
    manifestations in 224–230, *225*
  best practice for 274–275
  burden of disease 71–72
  families and 198, 211–212
  general development and 222–224
  perinatal exposure and auditory
    manifestations 230–232, *233*, 275
  research on 236
  as risk factor for hearing impairment
    97, 102–103, 105
  solutions and recommendations
    233–237
  in South Africa 10, 219–220
  in sub-Saharan Africa 17–18
HIV-exposed uninfected (HEU) infants
    230–232, 236
Hlayisi, V. 148–149
Hofman, K. 79
Hogan, S. C. 126
home-based care 45, 67, 143–146, 149,
  150, 273
home births 53–54, 76
Home intervention: Hearing and
    language opportunities parent
    education services *see* HI HOPES
hospitals
  birthing package of 24, 37, 42, 58, 268
  early detection of hearing
    impairment in 22, 24, 26–27,
    37, 42, 49, 53, 58, 67, 76, 266,
    268–270
  in South Africa 46, *47*
House, S. S. 188
Houston, T. 125

HPCSA *see* Health Professions Council of
    South Africa
Hrapcak, S. 229, 234
HRR *see* high-risk register
HSV *see* herpes simplex virus
HTA *see* health technology assessment
Huang, L. H. 36
Hughes, M. L. 79
Hui, Y. 54
human resources *see* health care
    professionals
human rights 22, 44–45, 59, 66, 159,
    246, 264
Human Sciences Research Council 220
Hunter syndrome 99–100
hybrid tele-audiology 164
hydrocephalus 97, 98
hyperbilirubinaemia 94–95, 104–105
hypertension, pulmonary 94
hypertensive disorders, maternal 104
hypoxia 94

I

iatrogenic causes of hearing loss
    224–225, 236
ICT (information and communications
    technology) *see* data management
    systems; tele-audiology; telehealth
ILO *see* International Labour
    Organization
IMF *see* International Monetary Fund
immittance testing 229, 244
immunisation 57, 97, 100–101, 182, 189
immunisation clinics 23–24, 53, 56,
    57–58, 268
Imperitia Rule (*imperitia culpae
    adnumeratur*) 249
incidence
    of deafblindness 183
    of hearing impairment 4, 20–21, 197,
        267
    of rubella 181
inclusive education 147–148, 150, 155,
    158–161, 167, 273–274
inclusivity 140
India 76, 208
individual vs group-based early
    intervention 139–143, 150

inequality 17, 45, 201, 210–211
infections 225, 235, 236
information and communications
    technology (ICT) *see* data
    management systems; tele-
    audiology; telehealth
information sharing 200, 203, 204–207,
    235–236, 246–247, 255
information systems *see* data
    management systems
informed choice 22, 201
informed consent 58, 247, 253–255,
    256, 258
Ingber, S. 202, 203, 207
Institute for the Deaf 146
insurance 258–259
Integrated School Health Policy 160
International Labour Organization (ILO)
    220
International Monetary Fund (IMF) 43
internet 79, 163–164, 244 *see also*
    tele-audiology; telehealth
interpreters 205
intersectoral approach 77, 270
intervention for hearing impairment
    see early intervention for hearing
    impairment
in-utero ARV exposure 232
in-utero infections 95–97, 105
invisibilisation 183–184, 186
isiXhosa *see* Xhosa language
isiZulu *see* Zulu language
Israel 202

J

Jackson, C. W. 206, 207
Jatto M. E. 210
jaundice 80, 92
JCIH *see* Joint Committee on Infant
    Hearing
Jervell and Lange-Nielsen syndrome 98–99
Johannesburg, study in 228–229
Johnson, L. F. 220
Joint Committee on Infant Hearing (JCIH)
    continuity of care 157
    deafblindness 186–187
    early detection of hearing impairment
        22, 33–34, 37, 48, 49, 80

early intervention for hearing
impairment 121–123, 131, 138
ethical considerations 245
risk factor registry 89, 91, 92–102,
104
Joint United Nations Programme on
HIV/AIDS (UNAIDS) 71, 72,
219–221
Joseph, A. 197
Joseph, L. 79–80
Joubert, J. 58

K
kangaroo mother care wards 22, 55
Kanji, A.
age at amplification 123
burden of disease 271
caregivers 204–205, 210
follow-up rates 76–77
newborn hearing screening (NHS) 73,
268, 269
risk factors for hearing impairment
37
targeted newborn hearing screening
(TNHS) 59, 75, 82, 91, 270
Kazembe, P. N. 230
Keller, Helen 177
Kennedy, S. 205, 209
Kenya 19, 147
Kerr, G. 138
Khan, M. S. G. 140
Khan, N. 79–80
Khan, N. B. 80
Khoza-Shangase, K.
African context 197, 199, 205
age of diagnosis 123, 157
burden of disease 37, 271
caregivers 57, 209, 210
diversity 49, 132, 142
'doing better with less' approach
75
follow-up rates 77
HIV/AIDS 219, 221, 228
newborn hearing screening (NHS)
74
Kolethekkat, A. A. 76
Krabbenhoft, K. 76–77
Kramer, K. 164

Krupinski, E. 78
Kumar, S. 76
Kuper, H. 230, 265
Kurien, M. 76
Kusanthan, T. 223
KwaZulu-Natal, studies in 69, 80, 228

L
Lam, B. C. 54
LAMI countries *see* low and middle-
income (LAMI) countries
language *see* linguistic diversity
Language Assessment, Remediation and
Screening Procedure (LARSP) 127,
273
language development 186, 201,
222–224, 226
languages, official, in South Africa 127,
142, 198, 211
Larsen, R. 205, 209
LARSP *see* Language Assessment,
Remediation and Screening
Procedure
learning disorders 226
legal aspects 247, *248*, 253, 255, 258–259
Leite, R. A. 229
Le Roux, T. 208
Lesotho 19
Lester, C. 205, 209, 210
Leung, S. S. L. 55
levels of health care service 26–27, 39,
42, *46–47*, 49–59, *50–52, 56*,
267–268
Library Guides Deafblind Resources 184
licensure 247
life-threatening diseases 7, 58, 71, 138,
155
linguistic diversity
African context 4–6
best practice and 265, 272–274
early intervention for hearing
impairment 121, 128, 132–133,
142, 150
family-centred early hearing
detection and intervention 198,
202–203, 205, 207, 211, 213
tele-audiology 166–168
lip reading 128

listening and spoken language (LSL)
  principles 127, 272
Listening and Spoken Language South
  Africa (LSLSA) 132
listening and spoken language specialist
  (LSLS) 127
LOCHI *see* longitudinal outcomes of
  children with hearing impairment
locums 251
logistical challenges 208–209
'long and healthy life' motto 66
longitudinal outcomes of children with
  hearing impairment (LOCHI) 120
loop diuretics 94–95
low and middle-income (LAMI)
    countries
  best practice for 264–265, 267, 271
  continuity of care 156, 157–158, 163,
    165
  deafblindness 181, 190–191
  early detection of hearing
    impairment 7, 33–39, *38*, 42–43,
    49, 68, 73, 75
  early intervention for hearing
    impairment 9, 117, 120, 130, 132,
    138
  family-centred early hearing
    detection and intervention 196
  HIV/AIDS in 222
  prevalence of hearing impairment
    4–5, 20
  risk factors for hearing impairment
    104–105
low body mass index 234
LSL principles *see* listening and spoken
  language (LSL) principles
LSLS *see* listening and spoken language
  specialist
LSLSA *see* Listening and Spoken
  Language South Africa
Luxon, L. M. 55

M
Madagascar 19
Magliaro, F. C. 229
Maguvhe, M. O. 183, 186, 187–188
Maier, J. 180

Mailman School of Public Health 222
mainstream inclusion vs special
  schooling 146–148, *148*
Makawa, A. 230
malaria 103–104, 105
Malawi 23–24, 147, 229, 230
Malhotra, P. S. 206, 207
Malik, M. A. 140
malnutrition 229
malpractice claims 69, 251, 258
Maluleke, N. 123, 210
Mampane, M. R. 212
marginalisation 183–184, 186
Maro, I. I. 227
mastoiditis 103, 226
Matas, C. G. 229
maternal ARV use 234
maternal deaths 16
maternal HIV infection 102, 234
maternal hypertensive disorders 104
MDGs *see* Millennium Development Goals
measles 100, 101
*MEC for Education: KwaZulu-Natal v
  Pillay* 160
medical aid schemes 24, 257–258, 268
meningitis 100–101, 102, 103, 225, 226
Menon, J. A. 223
mentorship 122, 127, 244–245
Merugumala, S. V. 208, 209, 210
Meyer, C. 204
Meyer, M. E. 49
middle ear diseases 228, 234, 235
middle ear disorders 158
middle ear function 226–229
middle ear infection (otitis media) 57,
    80, 102, 118, 225–226, 228–229
  chronic suppurative otitis media
    (CSOM) 103
  otitis media with effusion (OME)
    103, 105
middle ear measures 235, 237
middle ear pathologies 229, 237
middle-level health care workers 28, 73,
  265
midwife obstetric units (MOUs) 26, 37,
    42, *50*, 53–54, 59, 82, 268, 270
migration 5, 81, 267–268, 270

Millennium Development Goals (MDGs) 16, 17, 18, 118, 159
mitochondrial mutation 231, 232
Miziara, I. 226
models of care in early intervention 137–154
    amplification devices 138–139, 141, 144–145, 148–149
    definition of 137
    home- vs centre-based 143–146, 150
    importance of 9, 137–138, 150
    individual vs group-based 139–143, 150
    (re)habilitation 138–139
    solutions and recommendations 148–150
    special schooling vs mainstream inclusion 146–148, *148*, 150, 273
Moeller, M. P. 130
monitoring
    of children 22–23, 122, 201, 234–235
    of programmes 201, 267
Moodley, S. 74, 81
Mophosho, M. 49, 132, 142, 205
mortality rate 17, 220–221
Mosca, R. 187
mother-to-child transmission 220–221
Motshekga, Angie 159
Motsoaledi, Aaron 66
MOUs *see* midwife obstetric units
Muenke syndrome 99
multisensory impairment 178
Mulwafu, W. 19, 265
mumps 100
Munoz, K. 205, 209
Murdoch, B. 125
Mwaba, S. O. C. 223

N
Namibia 147
nasopharyngeal polyps 226
National Development Plan 118, 131, 155, 159
National Education Policy Act 160
National eHealth Strategy 166
National Health Act 79, 165, 246, 251, 253, 255

National Health Insurance Bill (NHI Bill) 44, 45, 66
National Health Insurance (NHI) 5, 44–46, 66–68, 77, 205, 265, 269
National Institute for the Deaf (NID) 128
National Institutes of Health (NIH) 90, 230
National Integrated Early Childhood Development Policy 4, 118, 145
National Patients' Rights Charter 246, 247
National Speech Therapy and Audiology Public Sector Forum (Health) 46
National Treasury 46, 68, 69
Nelson, L. 205, 209
neonatal hyperbilirubinaemia 95
neonatal intensive care units (NICU) *50*, 53, 55, 80, 94–95, 105
neonatal jaundice 92
neonatal wards *50*
neural dyssynchrony 228, 234
neurodegenerative disorders 99–100, 105
neurodevelopmental disabilities 221, 222–223
neurofibromatosis 98–99
newborn hearing screening (NHS) *see also* targeted newborn hearing screening; universal newborn hearing screening
    approaches to 131
    best practice for 265–269
    contextualisation of 7, 72–75
    'doing better with less' approach 76–77
    family-centred early hearing detection and intervention 197
    in LAMI countries 33, 36
    in sub-Saharan Africa 20, 23–24
New Zealand 124
Ngoma, M. S. 223
Ng, P. K. 54
NHI *see* National Health Insurance
NHI Bill *see* National Health Insurance Bill
NHS *see* newborn hearing screening
NICU *see* neonatal intensive care units
NID *see* National Institute for the Deaf

Nigeria 20, 23, 92, 104, 208, 230
NIH *see* National Institutes of Health
90-90-90 targets 72, 220, 221, 231
no-fee schools 158–159, 212
noise exposure 94, 166
non-adherence to programmes 243–244
non-audiologist staff 27, 38–39, 54, 55, 79, 270
non-maleficence 249
non-professional staff 37, 266
nuclear family 198–199, 212–213
nucleoside reverse transcriptase inhibitors 225
nurses 68–69, 79–80, 93, 221, 270, 271

O

OAEs *see* otoacoustic emissions
O'Gara, J. 130
Ogunkuyede, S. A. 210
Olusanya, B. O. 55, 117–118, 177, 230, 250
OME *see* otitis media with effusion
Omidire, M. F. 212
1:3:6 48–49
Onyia, N. O. 230
opportunistic diseases 229, 235, 236
oral–aural approach 123, 124, 272
oral communication approaches 124, 127–128, 129, 273
orphaned and vulnerable children (OVC) 211–212, 213
ossicular chain disruption 101
osteopetrosis 98–99
otalgia 225
otitis media (middle ear infection) 57, 80, 102, 118, 225–226, 228–229
otitis media with effusion (OME) 103, 105
otoacoustic emissions (OAEs) 33, 35, 44, 49, 53–54, 80, 234, 244, 254
otolaryngologists 7, 19, 228
otorhinolaryngologists 266
otorrhea 225, 227, 229, 234
otoscopy 237
ototoxic medications 94–95, 101–102, 103–104, 225, 234–236
outer ear otorrhea 228

OVC *see* orphaned and vulnerable children
oxygen levels 182

P

paediatricians 209
Pan South African Language Board 162
paradigm shift in early hearing detection and intervention 3–14
paraprofessionals 164, 245
parents *see also* caregivers
    auditory–verbal therapy (AVT) 124–127
    challenges faced by 243
    education on hearing impairment for 58, 80, 235–237, 270
    involvement of 120–121, 190, 273
    parent-to-parent support 200
partnerships 143, 189, 201
patient-reported experience measures (PREMs) 257
patient-reported outcome measures (PROMs) 257
patriarchal social norms 199, 210, 213
Pediatric HIV/AIDS Cohort Study network 232
Pendred syndrome 98–99
Percy-Smith, L. 125
perilymph fistula 101
perinatal exposure to HIV 230–232, *233*
perinatally HIV-infected (PHIV) 228
personal information of clients 252–253
Peru 227
pessimism 203
Peter, V. Z. 228
Petrocchi-Bartal, L. 74
Pfeiffer syndrome 99
PHC *see* primary health care
PHIV *see* perinatally HIV-infected
phonological disorders 226
phototherapy, hyperbilirubinaemia requiring 105
Policy Framework on Care and Support for Teaching and Learning 160
political will 266, 273
population growth 15
Pothula, V. 208, 209, 210

Pottas, L. 206, 207
poverty 45, 118
practicability 268
premature births 182
PREMs *see* patient-reported experience
    measures
prenatal viral infections 181–182
prevalence
    of hearing impairment 4, 20–21, 118,
        156, 265, 267
    of risk factors 91
preventative care 17, 19, 21, 45, 67, 166,
    189, 196–197, 267
primary health care (PHC)
    best practice for 265–270
    early detection of hearing
        impairment 26–28, 42, 45–46,
        46–47, 49, *51*, 53, *56*, 57–59,
        67–69, 71, 74, 76, 79–80
    ethical considerations 246
    models of care and 138, 143
    risk factors for hearing impairment
        93
    in South Africa 5, 26–27
    in sub-Saharan Africa 18–19
primary prevention 21
privacy 246, 247, 251–254
private health care sector
    early detection of hearing
        impairment 24, 26, 37, 42–43,
        45–46, 49, *52*, 53, 58–59, 73, 268
    early intervention for hearing
        impairment 127, 142
    ethical considerations 257–258
    family-centred early hearing
        detection and intervention 197,
        211
    in LAMI countries 37
    risk factors for hearing impairment
        90
    in South Africa 24, 26
    in sub-Saharan Africa 21
Professional Board for Speech, Language
    and Hearing Professions 22–23,
    46, 246
PROMs *see* patient-reported outcome
    measures

Protection of Personal Information Act
    253
provincial health departments 46, *47*,
    77, 258, 269
psychosocial skills 120
public health care sector
    best practice for 268
    early detection of hearing
        impairment 26, 37–38, 43, 45–46,
        46–47, 49, *50–51*, 67–71, 73
    early intervention for hearing
        impairment 133, 141–142
    ethical considerations 258
    family-centred early hearing
        detection and intervention 197,
        211
    prevalence of hearing impairment
        21
    in South Africa 6
pulmonary hypertension 94
pyramidal tract signs 222

Q

quadruple burden of disease 17, 24, 71,
    208, 271, *272*
quality of care 257
questionnaires 250, 257

R

Ramaphosa, Cyril 198
Ramma, L. 148–149
'rapid progressors' 222
recommendations *see* solutions and
    recommendations
recordings 253–254
record keeping *see* documentation
referrals 22, 28, 55, 57, 80–81, 185–188,
    229, 270
regional hospitals *47*
regulating bodies 266
Rehabilitation Council of India 180
Rehman, A. 140
reimbursement for services 257–258
reliability of results 255–257
research
    on continuity of care 157, 167
    on deafblindness 184

research (*cont.*)
    on early detection of hearing
        impairment *25–26*, 74, 81–82
    on early intervention for hearing
        impairment 120–121, 129–130,
        132–133, 272–274
    ethical considerations for 254
    on family-centred early hearing
        detection and intervention 197,
        201–208
    on HIV/AIDS 224, 235, 236
    relevance of 4–5
resource constraints 5, 43, 68–71, *70*, 73,
    163, 265, 267, 273–274
respect 252
retinitis pigmentosa 182–183
retinopathy of prematurity (ROP) 182
rights *see* human rights
risk factors for hearing impairment
    89–114
    contextualisation of 91–92, 118–119,
        271
    from developing nations 104–105
    'doing better with less' approach
        75–77
    history of risk factor registries 89–90
    HPCSA risk factors 102–103
    infant hearing screening 80, 90–91
    JCIH risk factor registry 89, 92–102
    need for contextualisation 20–21
    recommendations 105
    registries 8, 89–90, 92–102, 271
    for South African context 103–104
    system change 106
    targeted newborn hearing screening
        (TNHS) 34, 39
risk management for tele-audiology
    258–259
Road to Health booklet 80, 93
role ambiguity and conflict 69, 251
Roman, A. M. 140
Romero, R. H. 223
ROP *see* retinopathy of prematurity
Roux, T. L. 77
rubella 96–97, 105, 181–182, 189
rural areas 78, 79, 163, 164, 210–211, 247
Rwanda 18, 19, 147

S

SAAA *see* South African Association of
    Audiology
Sacks, S. 204
Saiki, O. 210
Sarvan, S. 204–205
SASL *see* South African Sign Language
SASLHA *see* South African Speech-
    Language-Hearing Association
Satti, S. A. 76
Scarinci, N. 203–204
Scheepers, L. J. 77, 208
Schooling 2030 goals 159
schools *see also* continuity of care;
    education
    deafblindness 183, 187–188, 190
    early detection of hearing
        impairment at 79
    feeding schemes at 159, 212
    HIV/AIDS and 223
    no-fee 158–159, 212
    sign language at 129
    special schooling vs mainstream
        inclusion 146–148, *148*, 150, 273
Scott, M. 164
screening *see* hearing screening
Screening, Identification, Assessment
    and Support policy 160
SDGs *see* sustainable development goals
secondary level of health care *47*, 53,
    268
secondary prevention 21, 27, 267
seizures 227
Senegal 19
sensorineural hearing loss 100, 228, 235
sensory impairments in early hearing
    detection and intervention
    177–195
    causes of deafblindness 181–183
    deafblindness in South Africa
        183–184
    definition of deafblindness 178, 180
    early deafblindness detection and
        intervention 185–188, 191
    impact of deafblindness on children
        10, 184–185, 190–191, 274–275
    prevalence of deafblindness 177, 183

sensory impairments vs sensory processing disorders 178–181
solutions and recommendations 189–190
visual impairments 177–178
sensory motor neuropathies 99–100
sensory processing disorders vs sensory impairments 178–181
Sevier, J. D. 79
Shenton, R. C. 36
Sherr, L. 223
Shinn, J. B. 205, 209, 210
sickle cell anaemia 104, 105
Siegfried, N. 79
sign language 128–130, 272
SKI HI Language Development Scale 145
skull fractures 101
SLH professions *see* speech-language and hearing (SLH) professions
social determinants of health 5, 16, 26–27, 46, 67, 75, 155–156, 267
social interaction 140, 200
social support 201, 202–203
socio-economic diversity 207, 265
Soer, M. 206, 207
Sogebi, O. A. 208
solutions and recommendations
deafblindness 189–190
early detection of hearing impairment 27–28, 38–39, 77–81, 105
early intervention for hearing impairment 131–132, 148–150
HIV/AIDS 233–237
South Africa
Convention on the Rights of Persons with Disabilities (CRPD) 147
deafblindness in 183–184
early detection of hearing impairment in 24–27, *25–26*
education in 158–162
family-centred early hearing detection and intervention in 210–211
health care structure of 44–46, *46–47*
HIV/AIDS in 219–220

infant hearing screening in 90–91
tele-audiology in 165–167
South African Association of Audiology (SAAA) 258
South African Health Review 69, 165
South African Schools Act 160, 162
South African Sign Language (SASL) 128–129, 161–162, 198
South African Speech-Language-Hearing Association (SASLHA) 258
South Sudan 147
'special educational needs', definition of 147
special needs, children with 161–162, 223, 226, 247
special schools
continuity of care and 158
for deafblindness 183, 187
mainstream inclusion vs 146–148, *148*, 150, 273
speech-language and hearing (SLH) professions 19, 69–71, *70*, 123, 131–132, 141–142, 162
spinocerebellar ataxia 100
standards 24, 69, 75, 79, 157, 160, 243, 246, 249–250, 266, 270
state *see* government
State of the Nation address (2020) 198
Statistics South Africa 158–159, 161
step-down wards *50*, 53, 55
Steuerward, W. 164
stigma 143
Störbeck, C. 74, 81, 93
strengths, weaknesses, opportunities and threats (SWOT) analysis *see* SWOT analysis
streptomycin 225
studies *see* research
subcutaneous cysts 226
Sudan 76
supervision 251, 266
support systems 122, 201, 206–207
Surveillance Monitoring of ART Toxicities study 232
sustainable development goals (SDGs) 17–18, 27–28, 118, 266
Swanepoel, D. 49, 54–55, 58, 197, 208

Swanepoel, D. W. 77, 79, 163, 219

Swart questionnaire 80

Swaziland 147

SWOT analysis 78, 269

synchronous tele-audiology 79, 164

syndromes associated with hearing loss 98–99, 105

syphilis 96, 105, 225

system change 106

T

tactile communication 128

TAN *see* Tele-Audiology Network

Tanzania 147

targeted newborn hearing screening (TNHS) 7–8, 26–27, 33–37, 43, 75–76, 82–83, 233–234, 267, 270

task sharing 68–69

task shifting 27, 68–69, 149, 162, 164, 221, 265–266, 269, 274

Taylor, M. J. 36

TB *see* tuberculosis

teacher assistants 162, 164

teachers 156, 161–162, 188, 273

teamwork 201

technical competence *see* competence

tele-audiology

    best practice for 265, 266, 269–270, 273–275

    continuity of care 162–168

    early detection of hearing impairment 78–79

    family-centred early hearing detection and intervention 208, 213

tele-audiology, ethics in 243–263

    access to services 11, 243–244, 245, 246–247, 275

    competence 249–251, *252*

    confidentiality 246, 247, 251–254

    definitions 244

    duty to inform 254–255

    HPCSA guidelines 245–247, *248*

    importance of 259–260

    informed consent 247, 254–255, *256*

    licensure 247

    privacy 246, 247, 251–254

    programme validation 255–257

reimbursement for services 257–258

responsibilities of audiologists 246

risk management 258–259

uses of tele-audiology 244–245, 275

Tele-Audiology Network (TAN) 244

telehealth 23, 78, 162, 167–168, 207–209, 269, 273–274

tele-intervention 149

temporal bone fractures 101

Tenofovir 232

tertiary level of health care *47*, 53, 268

tertiary prevention 21

testing *see* diagnostic testing

Theunissen, M. 49, 54–55

threats, opportunities, weaknesses and strengths (TOWS) matrix analysis *see* TOWS matrix analysis

tinnitus 225

TNHS *see* targeted newborn hearing screening

Tobih, J. E. 208

Tooke, L. 182

Torre, P. III 227, 228, 231, 232

total communication 128, 272

TOWS matrix analysis 78, 269

toxoplasmosis 97, 102, 105, 226

tracking of patients 59, 81, 121, 270

traditional healing 93, 203

training

    continued professional development 165

    of health care professionals 19, 127, 131–133, 165, 187, 189, 244–245, 266, 269, 272–273

    of non-professional staff 69, 79, 162, 266, 270

    of teachers 143, 150, 273

travel costs 138, 209

Treacher-Collins syndrome 99

Treasury *see* National Treasury

trust 252, 255

truth telling 252

Tswanya, Y. 183

tuberculosis (TB) 71, 225, 234

Turnbull, A. P. 206, 207

Turnbull, T. 228

tympanic membrane perforation 101, 227

tympanometry 227–229, 235, 237

U

ubuntu 143, 199
Ud Din, N. 140
Uganda 147
UHC *see* universal health coverage
UN *see* United Nations
UNAIDS 71, 72, 219–221
UNHS *see* universal newborn hearing
     screening
United Nations (UN) 27
United States (US) 124, 204–206
universal health coverage (UHC) 67–68,
     267
universal newborn hearing screening
     (UNHS) 3, 7–8, 24–27, 33–37,
     42–44, 73–76, 89–91, 233,
     266–271
universities 165, 273
University of the Witwatersrand (Wits)
     146, 184
upskilling 68, 162
US *see* United States
Usher syndrome 98–99, 182

V

vaccination *see* immunisation
validation of practice 255–257
Valloton, C. D. 206
varicella 100–101
Velocardiofacial syndrome 99
veracity 252
vernix caseosa 53–54
vernix in external auditory canal 44, 54
vertigo 225, 227
very low birth weight (VLBW) 92, 104,
     105
video-otoscopy 244
video recordings 253–254
viral meningitis 100–101
visual communication approaches 123,
     130
Vitamin A supplementation programme
     57
VLBW *see* very low birth weight
voice disorders 226
volunteers 69, 162, 164, 266, 271

W

Waardenburg syndrome 98–99
Watermeyer, J. 204–205
Wegner, J. R. 206, 207
WFDB *see* World Federation of the
     Deafblind
Whispers Speech and Hearing Centre 146
White, K. R. 78
White Paper 6, 160–161, 167, 273
White Paper on National Health
     Insurance 44–45, 66–67
White Paper on the Rights of Persons
     with Disabilities 186, 190
WHO *see* World Health Organization
Wilford, A. 68, 162
Wilkinson, T. 79
Windmill, I. 164
Wirz, S. L. 55
Wits *see* University of the Witwatersrand
women
     as caregivers 199
     HIV/AIDS and 220
World Bank 68
World Federation of the Deafblind
     (WFDB) 183, 185, 190
World Health Organization (WHO)
     17–18, 20, 67–68, 90–91, 119,
     196–197, 229, 250, 265
Worldwide Hearing Care for Developing
     Countries 249–250

X

Xhosa language 142

Y

Yanbay, E. 129
Yang, Y. 144
Yeung, C. Y. 54
Young, A. 93

Z

Zambia 19
Zeldow, B. 231, 232
Zimbabwe 19, 130, 147
Zulu language 142

Printed and bound by CPI Group (UK) Ltd, Croydon, CR0 4YY

27/10/2024

14580398-0005